101
Interesting Cases in
CLINICAL MEDICINE

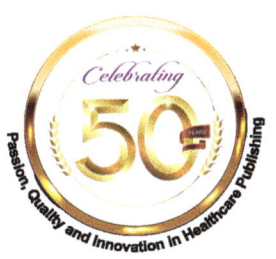

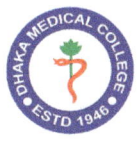

101 Interesting Cases in CLINICAL MEDICINE

Editors

Khan Abul Kalam Azad
MBBS FCPS MD FACP
Professor, Department of Medicine
Principal, Dhaka Medical College, Dhaka
Dean, Faculty of Medicine and
Postgraduate Medical Science and Research
University of Dhaka, Dhaka, Bangladesh

Ahmedul Kabir
MBBS FCPS FACP FRCP
Professor
Department of Medicine
Dhaka Medical College
Dhaka, Bangladesh

Mohammad Robed Amin
MBBS FCPS FACP FRCP
Associate Professor
Department of Medicine
Dhaka Medical College
Dhaka, Bangladesh

Co-Editors

Madhabi Karmaker
MBBS FCPS
Indoor Medical Officer
Department of Medicine
Dhaka Medical College Hospital
Dhaka, Bangladesh

Chowdhury Tamanna Tabassum
MBBS
Postgraduate Trainee
Department of Medicine
Dhaka Medical College Hospital
Dhaka, Bangladesh

Noshin Tabassum
MBBS
Postgraduate Trainee
Department of Medicine
Dhaka Medical College Hospital
Dhaka, Bangladesh

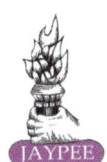

JAYPEE BROTHERS MEDICAL PUBLISHERS
The Health Sciences Publisher
New Delhi | London

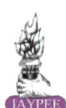 **Jaypee Brothers Medical Publishers (P) Ltd.**

Headquarters
Jaypee Brothers Medical Publishers (P) Ltd
4838/24, Ansari Road, Daryaganj
New Delhi 110 002, India
Phone: +91-11-43574357
Fax: +91-11-43574314
Email: jaypee@jaypeebrothers.com

Overseas Office
J.P. Medical Ltd
83 Victoria Street, London
SW1H 0HW (UK)
Phone: +44 20 3170 8910
Fax: +44 (0)20 3008 6180
Email: info@jpmedpub.com

Website: www.jaypeebrothers.com
Website: www.jaypeedigital.com

© 2020, Jaypee Brothers Medical Publishers

The views and opinions expressed in this book are solely those of the original contributor(s)/author(s) and do not necessarily represent those of editor(s) of the book.

All rights reserved. No part of this publication may be reproduced, stored or transmitted in any form or by any means, electronic, mechanical, photocopying, recording or otherwise, without the prior permission in writing of the publishers.

All brand names and product names used in this book are trade names, service marks, trademarks or registered trademarks of their respective owners. The publisher is not associated with any product or vendor mentioned in this book.

Medical knowledge and practice change constantly. This book is designed to provide accurate, authoritative information about the subject matter in question. However, readers are advised to check the most current information available on procedures included and check information from the manufacturer of each product to be administered, to verify the recommended dose, formula, method and duration of administration, adverse effects and contraindications. It is the responsibility of the practitioner to take all appropriate safety precautions. Neither the publisher nor the author(s)/editor(s) assume any liability for any injury and/or damage to persons or property arising from or related to use of material in this book.

This book is sold on the understanding that the publisher is not engaged in providing professional medical services. If such advice or services are required, the services of a competent medical professional should be sought.

Every effort has been made where necessary to contact holders of copyright to obtain permission to reproduce copyright material. If any have been inadvertently overlooked, the publisher will be pleased to make the necessary arrangements at the first opportunity. The **CD/DVD-ROM** (if any) provided in the sealed envelope with this book is complimentary and free of cost. **Not meant for sale.**

Inquiries for bulk sales may be solicited at: jaypee@jaypeebrothers.com

101 Interesting Cases in Clinical Medicine

First Edition: **2020**

ISBN: 978-93-89129-63-2

Dedicated to

*All the patients of Department of Medicine,
Dhaka Medical College Hospital, for their outstanding
contribution in our clinical preparedness;
who amidst their tremendous sufferings,
showed excellent magnitude of cooperation that paved a great
way to gather more and more clinical knowledge
and to acquire clinical skills.*

Contributors

Sabbiha Nadia Majumder
MBBS MRCP FCPS
Registrar
Department of Medicine
Green Life Medical College and Hospital
Dhaka, Bangladesh

Madhabi Karmaker MBBS FCPS
Indoor Medical Officer
Department of Medicine
Dhaka Medical College Hospital
Dhaka, Bangladesh

Shegufta Mishket Mukerrama MBBS
Postgraduate Trainee
Department of Medicine
Dhaka Medical College Hospital
Dhaka, Bangladesh

Chowdhury Tamanna Tabassum
MBBS
Postgraduate Trainee
Department of Medicine
Dhaka Medical College Hospital
Dhaka, Bangladesh

Mousumi Sanyal MBBS MRCP FCPS
Consultant
Department of Medicine
Better Life Hospital
Dhaka, Bangladesh

Noshin Tabassum MBBS
Postgraduate Trainee
Department of Medicine
Dhaka Medical College Hospital
Dhaka, Bangladesh

Mohammad Sayem
MBBS FCPS MRCP
Consultant
Department of Internal Medicine
AMZ Hospital
Dhaka, Bangladesh

Farnaz Nobi Rima MBBS
Postgraduate Trainee
Department of Medicine
Dhaka Medical College Hospital
Dhaka, Bangladesh

Nawsabah Noor
MBBS ECFMG Certified (USA)
Postgraduate Trainee
Department of Medicine
Dhaka Medical College Hospital
Dhaka, Bangladesh

Proma Halder MBBS
Postgraduate Trainee
Department of Medicine
Dhaka Medical College Hospital
Dhaka, Bangladesh

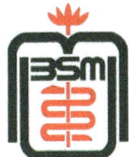

Vice-Chancellor
Bangabandhu Sheikh Mujib Medical University
Shahbag, Dhaka

Foreword

I feel honored and privileged to have the opportunity to write a few words about *'101 Interesting Cases in Clinical Medicine'* by Department of Medicine, Dhaka Medical College of Bangladesh.

Internal medicine is a subject of inquisitiveness and search for the hidden. Sometimes common diseases present in an uncommon way while atypical diseases present in the common way, which requires sound understanding of the whole scenario and critical analysis to finally discover the cases as interesting or rare disease. This book unfolds 101 interesting cases in an amazing way with a sequential exploration of newer dimensions of thinking as one would go through the pages ahead.

This book seems to be very exciting and challenging to readers as they will go through case-by-case exploring the answers of all questions in mind in a fascinating way. I believe these explanations will surely shed light on the important basics of unsolved problems and will lay the foundation of academic case analysis.

At this point I must appreciate the dedication, enormous effort and enthusiasm of the team who worked behind it. I have already seen various publications and reputed works of Department of Medicine of our renowned institution Dhaka Medical College, which is our pride and the editorial board should get a full credential due to their talent, hard work, sincere endeavor, patience, analyzing expertise and their achievements despite all constraints. I believe it is more than a book and surely this amazing work will be beneficial to the medical book lovers and they would feel comfort in going through the pages.

I hope this invaluable work will reach to the widest possible readers, including medical students, postgraduate trainees, and physicians of all stages. I must thank the authors and the team and contributors for producing such a masterwork.

Professor Kanak Kanti Barua
MBBS FCPS (Surgery) MS (Neurosurgery) PhD FICS
Professor and Chairman, Department of Neurosurgery
Vice-Chancellor
Bangabandhu Sheikh Mujib Medical University
Shahbag, Dhaka, Bangladesh

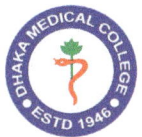

Principal
DHAKA MEDICAL COLLEGE
Dhaka, Bangladesh

Preface

"What the mind does not know, the eyes cannot see". The eyes can only perceive the signs hidden in plain sight when the knowledge is already stored in the mind. For a clinician to see beyond what the ordinary eyes see, both in-depth knowledge and clinical skills are required.

Dhaka Medical College Hospital, Dhaka, Bangladesh, being the country's largest tertiary care hospital is playing its gracious role both in patient care and also in academic activities. While dealing with patients, we came across a significant number of rare diseases as well as common diseases with uncommon presentations. It is worth mentioning that, each of the 101 cases presented here posed much difficulty on their initial presentation-so that in each case, reaching the final diagnosis was not a very straight-forward task. The term 'interesting' focuses on the intriguing presenting features, and the fascinating journey towards diagnosis. Having utmost respect to all our patients, we never had an intention to present any of the debilitating features of patients as interesting. Later the thought of dispersing this hard-acquired knowledge and experience inspired us to take on the endeavor of writing this book.

Many excellent medical textbooks are already available for theoretical knowledge, but this book focuses on improving decision-making capability by guiding the critical thinking process and application of theories.

Problem-based learning is the best way to learn medicine. Every case in the book has some practical problem-related questions for the reader's self-evaluation, followed by correct answers, and discussion on relevant topics and management.

We hope physicians will go through the book and practice the lessons in an enthralling way. We would like to invite suggestions, queries, comments, and constructive criticism from the esteemed readers of this book through email to bsmag.dmch@gmail.com, for further improvement in future editions.

Khan Abul Kalam Azad
Professor of Medicine, Dhaka Medical College
Dean, Faculty of Medicine and
Postgraduate Medical Science and Research
University of Dhaka
Dhaka, Bangladesh

Acknowledgments

We want to express our humble respect and sincere gratitude to all the teachers of the Department of Medicine of Dhaka Medical College, Dhaka, Bangladesh, for their encouragement and valuable suggestions while writing this book. We are also indebted to all the teachers working in Medicine and allied departments of all the government and private medical colleges of Bangladesh for their continuous support and interest for this book.

Our special thanks and gratefulness to all the patients who allowed us to examine them and had given their consent for publishing their photographs, data and other personal information in the book; and to all the doctors who took the responsibility of managing and presenting the cases in weekly grand round.

We are thankful to Professor HAM Nazmul Ahasan and Professor Mohammad Mujibur Rahman for their consent to publish some case reports in the book. We also choose this moment to acknowledge the contribution of Professor Titu Miah, Professor MA Kashem, Associate Professor Mohammad Rafiqul Islam, and Associate Professor Sarmistha Biswas in some specific cases.

Lastly, we are deeply indebted to Shri Jitendar P Vij (Group Chairman), Mr Ankit Vij (Managing Director), Ms Chetna Malhotra Vohra (Associate Director—Content Strategy) and Ms Nedup Denka Bhutia (Development Editor) of M/s Jaypee Brothers Medical Publishers (P) Ltd, New Delhi, India for their endeavor and relentless help which made the book possible to come into the light.

Contents

1. Crippled Young Boy with Recurrent Crying Bouts 1
2. Middle-aged Female with Repeated Bleeding Episodes 5
3. Young Male with Recurrent Jaundice 9
4. Middle-aged Gentleman with Enlargement of Tongue 12
5. Middle-aged Male with Quadriplegia and Speech Disturbance 15
6. Middle-aged Lady with Pulmonary-Renal Syndrome 18
7. Young Male with Quadriparesis 22
8. Middle-aged Man with Vomiting and Weight Loss 25
9. Hyperpigmented Gentleman with Limb Weakness and Hematemesis 29
10. Young Lady with Multiple Blisters and Erosions 34
11. Young Lady with Fever and Polyarthritis 37
12. Young Boy with Recurrent Angioedema 40
13. Young Boy with Bizarre-looking Chest and Abdomen 44
14. Young Man with Recurrent Episodes of Left-sided Weakness 48
15. Young Boy with Arthralgia and Abdominal Pain 51
16. Young Man with Hard Mass in Abdomen 55
17. Middle-aged Male with Progressive Slurring of Speech 58
18. Febrile Middle-aged Man with Hip and Abdominal Pain 62
19. Young Man with Arthralgia, Hyperpigmented Skin Lesions and Fever 66
20. Middle-aged Lady with Progressive Dysphagia 70
21. Delirious Young Man with Fever and Hepatomegaly 73
22. Young Lady with Sudden Unconsciousness 78
23. Young Boy with Chronic Diarrhea and Failure to Thrive 81
24. Middle-aged Man with Fever, Splenomegaly and Arthritis 86
25. Middle-aged Lady with Lumps and Low Back Pain 90
26. Young Boy with Stroke 93

27. Middle-aged Man with Back Pain 96
28. Middle-aged Farmer with Diarrhea and Generalized Itching 100
29. Young Male with Neuropsychiatric Abnormality... 104
30. Middle-aged Lady with Massive Hepatomegaly... 108
31. Young Male with Fever, Rash, Jaundice and Anasarca............................. 113
32. Dizzy Gentleman with Abdominal Pain 117
33. Young Lady with Recurrent Multiple Subcutaneous Nodules.................... 119
34. Adolescent Girl with Unexplained Chronic Liver Disease with
    Short Stature and Primary Amenorrhea 122
35. Middle-aged Male with Ataxia, Dysarthria and Urinary Incontinence........ 127
36. Young Lady Infected with Dual Intracellular Pathogens 130
37. Young Female with Recurrent Painful Reddish
    Skin Nodules with Fever 133
38. Religious Young Boy with Fever During Travel.. 137
39. Middle-aged Male with Recurrent Orogenital Ulcerations......................... 141
40. Young Male with Recurrent Attacks of Fever and Joint Pain 144
41. Middle-aged Woman with Multiple Lumps and Bumps 147
42. Middle-aged Male with Fever, Back Pain and Chest Wall Pain................. 149
43. Young Lady with Multiple Joint Pain and Muscle Weakness..................... 152
44. Middle-aged Male with Hyperpigmentation and Weight Loss.................... 154
45. Young Male with Prolonged Fever and Weight Loss 157
46. Young Boy with Diarrhea and Generalized Swelling 159
47. Unmasking of the Cause of Lymphadenopathy in a Young Girl................ 163
48. Young Boy with a Hidden, Deadly and Rare Complication........................ 166
49. Middle-aged Farmer with a Baggy Abdomen 169
50. Middle-aged Lady with Recurrent Odynophagia and
    Multiple Ulcers 171
51. Middle-aged Man with Weight Gain and Breathlessness.......................... 177
52. Young Lady with Leg Ulcer and Psychosis.. 182
53. Confused Boy with Joint Pain and Fever.. 186

54. Disoriented Young Man with Fever and Acute Abdomen 189
55. Young Male with Passage of Offensive Dark-colored Stool 193
56. Teenage Girl with Progressive Low Back Pain 196
57. Young Man with Dimness of Vision, Facial Numbness and
    Nasal Intonation 199
58. Young Man with Abdominal Pain and Jaundice 203
59. Middle-aged Male with Chronic Sinusitis and Weight Loss 206
60. Meat-loving Young Woman with Abnormal Stool 209
61. Middle-aged Lady with Headache and Facial Nerve Palsy 212
62. Young Housewife with Prolonged Fever and Jaundice 215
63. Febrile Young Girl with Hemiparesis Followed by Neck Swelling 217
64. Young Man with Chronic Diarrhea 221
65. Young Man with Severe Anemia and Generalized Edema 224
66. Young Female with Acute Abdominal Pain and Fever 227
67. Young Boy with Skeletal Deformities 229
68. Gentleman with Bilateral Leg Weakness and
    Generalized Hyperpigmentation 233
69. Middle-aged Man with Acute Confusional State,
    Hematemesis and Melena 236
70. Middle-aged Lady with Recurrent Fractures 241
71. Middle-aged Male with Recurrent Altered Level of Consciousness 245
72. Middle-aged Man with Swelling of Legs and Abdomen 248
73. Young Man with Recurrent Fever and Rashes 251
74. Young Girl with Hemiparesis and Epilepsy 255
75. Young Male with Fluctuating Fever and Myalgia 260
76. Young Boy with Lax Skin 263
77. Young Boy with Recurrent Bleeding Diathesis 267
78. Young Lady having Recurrent Lump in the Abdomen 270
79. Young Female with Cough and Raynaud's Phenomenon 274
80. Multiple Bee Stings with Fatality in a Middle-aged Patient 278

81. Young Lady with Recurrent Hematemesis 281
82. Young Male with Constant Abdominal Pain 284
83. Young Housewife with Severe Abdominal Pain and Distension 288
84. An Unusual Presentation of Chylous Ascites 291
85. Middle-aged Man with Recurrent Limb Weakness 294
86. Young Man with Purpura and Hematuria 297
87. Young Man with Unexplained Jaundice and Fever 301
88. Young Man with Headache and Blurred Vision 304
89. Young Man with Polyarthritis and Renomegaly 306
90. Young Lady with Jaundice and Pruritus 311
91. Little Girl with Relapsed Pott's Disease and Paraplegia 314
92. Young Man with Hepatosplenomegaly and Monoclonal Gammopathy 321
93. Young Female with Recurrent Abdominal Pain 325
94. Middle-aged Lady with Unexplained Anemia 328
95. Young Lady with Palpitation and Hypoplastic Upper Limb 331
96. Young Lady with Disorientation and Blurring of Vision 336
97. Middle-aged Man with Prolonged Fever, Anorexia and Weight Loss 338
98. Young Boy's Long Journey with Unresolved Abdominal Pain 343
99. Young Lady with Abdominal Pain and Respiratory Distress 348
100. Young Man with Prolonged Fever and Rash 351
101. Young Diabetic Male with Persistent Pyuria and Drastic Weight Loss 357

Index 361

CASE 1

CRIPPLED YOUNG BOY WITH RECURRENT CRYING BOUTS

CASE SUMMARY

A 14-year-old young boy, the third child of non-consanguineous parents presented with multiple joint pain, swelling and fixed deformities for 6 years, difficulty of speech for 6 years and progressive generalized wasting of whole body for 5 years. In the beginning, he had intermittent feverish feeling which was not documented, used to come once or twice daily, each time lasted for 3-4 hours, subsided sometimes spontaneously and sometimes after taking antipyretics. Feverish feeling persisted for almost 1 year. He also had asymmetric, progressive polyarthritis of large and small joints. It started initially with the large joints (at first in right elbow, followed by right shoulder joint and subsequently right hip joint). There was no morning stiffness, no involvement of distal interphalangeal (DIP) joints and never complained of back pain. He developed fixed joint deformities in multiple joints for the last 3-4 years. There was progressive wasting of proximal and distal muscles of all four limbs and trunk, leading him to be completely bedridden for the last 1 year. There was no history of circumoral paresthesia, numbness in hands or feet, craniotabes, dental hypoplasia and no ears, nose and throat (ENT) ailment. Additionally, he had difficulty in speech for the last 6 years; it initially started with slurring, and later on, it deteriorated progressively leading to incomprehensible sounds. Moreover, he had emotional lability with frequent crying bouts for the last 1 year. There was no history of temper tantrums, depression, hyperactivity or disinhibition. There was no history of dysphagia, jaundice, convulsion, bowel and bladder dysfunction. There was no consanguinity of marriage, and family history of similar illness was absent. Multiple consultations were made where he was diagnosed as a case of motor neuron disease.

On examination, he was grossly emaciated, body built was below average, undernourished, irritable with frequent cry and vitals were stable. The GALS screening revealed that gait could not be examined. Arm—dystonia present

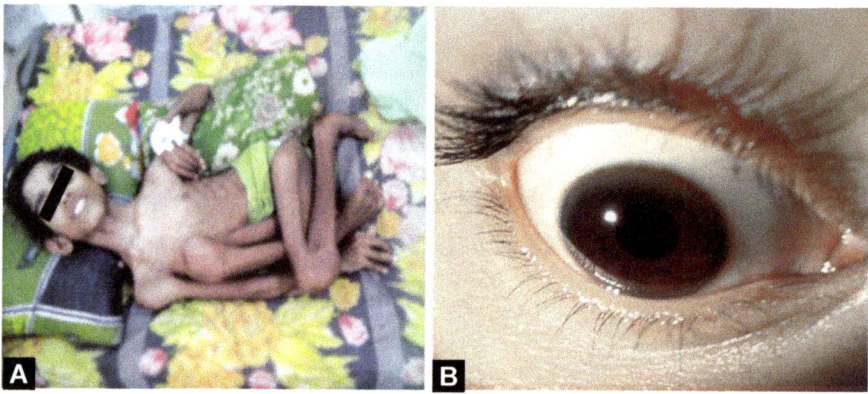

Figs. 1A and B: (A) Torticollis, tortipelvis with swelling and fixed deformity of multiple joints; (B) Gray color ring in the upper part of the limbus.

in both hands, and he had spastic torticollis; legs—on inspection, tortipelvis was present, (Fig. 1A) and multiple joints were swollen, tender and deformed. Fixed deformity was present in both knees and both ankle joints; spine—on inspection from behind scoliosis was present, and spinal movement elicitation was not possible. Examination of the nervous system revealed speech: uttered incomprehensible sounds, intact cranial nerves, muscle bulk were reduced in all four limbs, muscle tone increased, muscle power and reflexes could not be elicited. Plantar responses were flexor bilaterally, sensory function and coordination could not be done appropriately. Examination of the eyes showed the presence of gray colored ring in the upper part of the limbus of both eyes (Fig. 1B). Slit-lamp examination revealed Kayser Fleischer ring in both eyes. Other systemic examination findings were unremarkable.

Investigations showed: Hb level—11.9 g/dL, white blood cells (WBCs)—9,500/cumm (N: 77.8%, L: 18%), platelet (PLT)—393,000/cumm, erythrocyte sedimentation rate (ESR) in first hour—10 mm, urine R/M/E—normal, bedside dipstick test showed trace protein, serum electrolytes—normal, C-reactive protein (CRP)—normal, serum bilirubin—0.93 mg/dL, aspertate aminotransferase (AST)—67 U/L, alanine aminotransferase (ALT)—55 U/L, alkaline phosphatase (ALP)—140 U/L, serum albumin—3.52 g/dL, total protein—7.84 g/dL, corrected calcium—7.5 mg/dL, serum inorganic phosphate—3.17 mg/dL (normal: 4.7 mg/dL), parathormone—41.2 pg/mL (11–67 pg/mL), spot calcium: creatinine—0.60: 1 (normal: <0.14). Ultrasonography (USG) of W/A—normal. X-ray of chest and upper part of the body posteroanterior view revealed: generalized osteopenia, multiple rib fractures with callus formation in the shaft of fourth to seventh ribs in right side, scoliosis toward left, fracture of right humerus and bilateral shoulder dislocation (Fig. 2A). X-ray of lumbosacral spine anteroposterior and lateral view—severe osteopenia and fracture of neck of left femur; X-ray of wrist joint and hand showed coarse trabeculation.

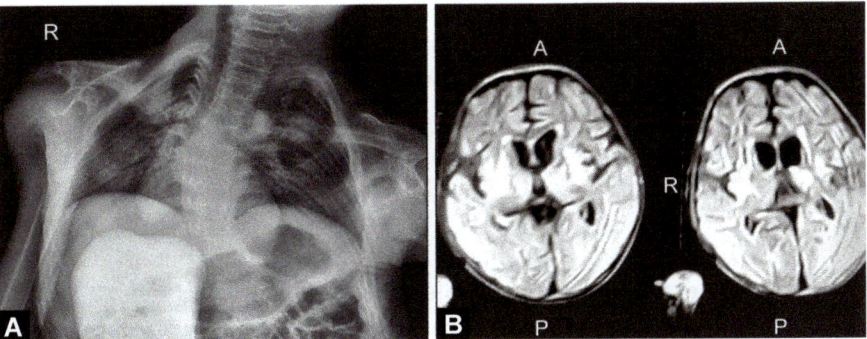

Figs. 2A and B: (A) Chest X-ray posteroanterior view showing generalized osteopenia, multiple rib fractures with callus formation in shaft of 4th to 7th rib in right side. Scoliosis towards left with bilateral shoulder dislocation; (B) Magnetic resonance imaging (MRI) of brain showing hyperintensity in bilateral thalamo-ganglionic capsular area.

QUESTIONS

1. What is the diagnosis?
2. What are the special investigations you need to carry out?

DISCUSSION

For this boy, our differential diagnoses were:
- Juvenile idiopathic arthritis (JIA)
- Rickets
- Wilson's disease.

Some special targeted investigations were carried out to reach the diagnosis: Serum ceruloplasmin—45 mg/dL (normal: 200–600 mg/dL), 24 urinary copper 179 mg/24 hours (>100 mg/24 hours confirms Wilson's disease), magnetic resonance imaging (MRI) of brain showed prominent capsuloganglionic area, ventricles and extraventricular spaces, and hyperintense bilateral thalamo-ganglionic capsular area (Fig. 2B).

Final Diagnosis: Wilson's Disease (Neuropsychiatric and Musculoskeletal Presentation)

The patient's treatment was started with penicillamine and zinc acetate tablets, calcium, vitamin D injection and baclofen tablet. His condition improved remarkably. Within 6 months he was able to walk, and started going to school.

Wilson's disease is a hereditary disorder of the liver and brain. Different types of psychiatric features may be the first presentation of the disease. High index of suspicion is necessary to come up with a straightforward diagnosis.

It rarely presents with *musculoskeletal manifestations also* when there is accumulation of copper.[1] Involvement of large joints, such as knee joint pain, effusion, radiological chondrocalcinosis in young adults and early osteoarthritic changes in imaging should be investigated carefully keeping the diagnosis of Wilson's disease in mind. Psychiatric manifestations may precede neurological symptoms of Wilson's disease in 20% of the cases. This patient initially presented with dysarthria and subsequently emotional lability. Afterwards on the basis of significant biochemical abnormalities and the presence of Kayser-Fleischer ring, he was diagnosed as a case of Wilson's disease.

A patient exhibiting neurologic signs or symptoms associated with Kayser-Fleischer rings and ceruloplasmin levels of less than 20 mg/dL confirms a diagnosis of Wilson's disease. Hepatic copper concentration of more than 250 mg/g of dry weight and a low serum ceruloplasmin level are enough to make a diagnosis of hepatic Wilson's disease.[2]

Chelating agents and medications are used to block copper absorption from the gastrointestinal tract. Zinc and penicillamine are the main treatment options. Trientine, another chelating agent which is more tolerated than penicillamine, can be used. Several other medications are used to combat symptoms, for example, baclofen for dystonia, neuroleptics to treat psychiatric symptoms, levodopa for Parkinsonism and antiepileptics for seizures.

REFERENCES

1. Yu H, Xie JJ, Chen YC, Dong Y, Ni W, ZY. Clinical features and outcome in patients with osseomuscular type of Wilson's disease. BMC Neurol. 2017;17(1):34.
2. Jameson JL, Kasper DL, Longo DL, Fauci AS, Hauser SL, Loscalzo J. Harrison's principles of internal medicine. 20th ed. New York: McGraw Hill Education. 2018. pp. 2982-4.

CASE 2

MIDDLE-AGED FEMALE WITH REPEATED BLEEDING EPISODES

CASE SUMMARY

A 50-year-old housewife presented with recurrent spontaneous bruises and pain in different joints for the last 2 years. Initially her left ankle joint had become swollen spontaneously and was associated with dull aching pain, aggravated on movement and relieved by taking nonsteroidal anti-inflammatory drugs (NSAIDs) without morning stiffness. The overlying skin of the joint was bluish in color. Simultaneously, her right ankle joint and both knee joints became swollen within next 2 days with similar features. She also noticed multiple spontaneous bruises in different parts of her both lower limbs which persisted for few days. Gradually, her pain and swelling of joints disappeared completely with sequential color changes of bruises over about 2 months. But these episodes continued to occur at variable time intervals with occasional gum bleeding while brushing teeth and heavy menstrual blood flow for prolonged duration. With passage of time, she gradually developed pallor and generalized weakness. The previous day before admission, she again developed features of myalgia and painful swelling of right shoulder and elbow joints, 2nd and 3rd proximal interphalangeal (PIP) joints of right hand and enormously swollen face with bluish black discoloration after a minor trauma. She had no history of fever, jaundice, photosensitivity, oral ulcer, features of Raynaud's phenomenon, headache, visual disturbance or convulsion and no hematemesis, melena, or hematuria. She had no bad obstetric history including spontaneous abortion. None of her family members including maternal and paternal uncles had similar complaints. Her parents had no history of consanguinity of marriage.

On examination, she was ill-looking, depressed with average body built. Her whole face was swollen, bluish black in color, tender on palpation with black eye. She also had multiple bruises and ecchymoses of different sizes with varying color changes from bluish to greenish over different parts of her body. She was moderately anemic, vital signs were normal and there were no accessible lymph nodes. Her musculoskeletal system examination revealed swollen right-sided shoulder, elbow, 2nd and 3rd PIP joints with overlying bluish skin; affected joints were tender and warm on palpation and movement of the joints were painful and restricted. Cardiovascular, respiratory and alimentary system examination revealed no abnormality. After disappearance of joint swelling, we reexamined the patient and found no features of synovitis.

Investigations showed complete blood count: severe anemia [Hb—5.8 mg/dL, hematocrit (Hct)—18.1%], which was gradually corrected after 5 units of blood transfusion (Hb—11.7 g/dL and Hct—35.6%). Peripheral blood film showed normocytic anemia with neutrophilic leukocytosis with increased rouleaux formation and normal platelet count. Coagulation profile after admission showed prolonged activated partial thromboplastin time (APTT)—80 sec with normal bleeding time (BT)—3 min 30 sec, clotting time (CT)—2 min 20 sec, thrombin time (TT)—16 sec, and prothrombin time (PT)—17 sec. Other investigations revealed normal alanine aminotransferase (ALT), normal creatinine and urine routine microscopic examination (R/M/E). Antinuclear antibodies (ANA); anti-dsDNA and antiphospholipid antibody were all negative. Further workup on coagulation profile revealed reduced factor VIII activity which was of 2.7% (normal: 50-150%) and reduced factor IX activity 2% (N: 50-150%) and normal von Willebrand factor (VWF) level.

QUESTIONS

1. What is the most likely diagnosis?
2. What further tests can be carried out to find out the cause of prolonged APTT with reduced factor VIII and IX activity?

DISCUSSION

Initially, in this case, we had some differentials considering the history and clinical examination, like—
- Hemorrhagic disorder with possible systemic lupus erythematosus (SLE)
- von Willebrand disease
- Acquired coagulation disorder.

Absence of rash, photosensitivity, oral ulceration, no bad obstetric history, normal urine R/M/E findings and negative ANA and anti-ds DNA virtually excluded the diagnosis of SLE. A normal VWF level and normal bleeding time excluded von Willebrand disease. As factor VIII and IX were found to be deficient, there were two possibilities either inherited deficiency of factor VIII and IX or acquired deficiency due to presence of inhibitors. A female patient with negative family history with bleeding episodes at this age decreased the possibility of inherited hemophilia. We decided to go for mixing study (Table 1).

Table 1: Mixing study.

Test	Initial result	Test result 2 hours after incubation
Activated partial thromboplastin time (APTT) 1:1 dilution	66.8 sec	70.6 sec
Factor VIII 1:1 dilution	33%	2.6%
Factor IX 1:1 dilution	59%	49%

Mixing study is a test which is usually done to differentiate inherited factor deficiency from presence of inhibitors. Inhibitors are antibodies which act against factor VIII and IX and reduce their activity. A prolonged APTT which fails to be corrected in 1:1 mix initially and also after incubation is suggestive of presence of inhibitor.

In our case, as the mixing study failed to correct prolonged APTT in a 1:1 mix immediately and also after 2 hours incubation suggested the presence of inhibitors. At this point, we needed Bethesda test to quantify the inhibitors but unavailability of this facility made us unable to do the test. An ENA (extractable nuclear antigen) panel also failed to detect the presence of specific autoantibody in blood. HBsAg and anti-HCV Ab were also negative. We also didn't find any underlying autoimmune disease or other medical conditions or drugs behind this illness. Thus, we labeled our case as Idiopathic Acquired Hemophilia.

Final Diagnosis: Idiopathic Acquired Hemophilia[1]

Acquired hemophilia (AH) is a rare condition in which autoantibodies, usually of the IgG class are produced against factor VIII or IX and reduce their activity and increase bleeding diathesis.[2] AH is significantly rarer than the inherited form, affecting around 2 per million of the population. It appears in all ethnic groups and has a worldwide prevalence.[3,4] Age distribution is bimodal with a first peak occurring among young women in the postpartum period and a second major peak among elderly patients. The mortality rate is high, ranging from 8% to 22%. This is related to severe hemorrhage that can occur in 85-90% of the patients.[4,5] There is often an underlying medical condition associated with this acquired hemophilia. An association with other autoimmune conditions (SLE, inflammatory bowel disease, rheumatoid arthritis), malignant disease, certain drugs (such as penicillin, sulfonamide, interferon, fludarabine, phenytoin, flupentixol, etc.), pregnancy and infections [hepatitis B virus (HBV), hepatitis C virus (HCV)] have been recognized in various surveys. In approximately half of all cases, there is no obvious underlying cause and the condition is labeled as idiopathic.[6] The patterns of bleeding in AH also differs from that of inherited hemophilia. In AH, bleeding tends to occur in soft tissue, muscle, retroperitoneal space and gastrointestinal or genitourinary tracts. In contrast, hemarthrosis is rare in patients of AH than in patients of hereditary hemophilia. Given the complexity of diagnosis, the condition may be underdiagnosed for many years. The typical laboratory findings of AH are prolonged activated partial thromboplastin time, normal prothrombin time as well as normal platelet count and function. Mixing studies can be used to demonstrate the presence of a time-dependent inhibitor of factor VIII and IX and the antibody titers are measured by Bethesda test.

Treatment of AH is two-pronged. The immediate priority is to control acute bleeding with bypassing agents. Two commonly available bypassing agents are plasma-derived activated prothrombin complex concentrate (aPCC), recombinant activated factor VII (rFVIIa).[5] Immunosuppressants such as cyclophosphamide, and azathioprine should be used to control antibody production. Oral steroids 1 mg/kg for 3-6 weeks can cause remission in one-third to one-half of patients with AH.[4] Human factor VIII is likely to be very rapidly inactivated by a significant titer of inhibitory antibody and therefore of no practical use, even at high doses. It is reported that most deaths in AH occurs in the first few weeks. Thus a prompt recognition of the disorder and an early and aggressive treatment are mandatory.

REFERENCES

1. Karmaker M, Zerin I, Afrose S, Rahman MM, Azad KAK. Acquired hemophilia in female—a case report. J Med. 2017;18(2):119-22.
2. Delgado J, Yimenez-Yuste, Hernandez-Navarro F, Villar A. Acquired hemophilia: review and meta-analysis focused on therapy and prognostic factors. Br J Haematol. 2003;121:21-35.
3. Collins P, Maccartney N, Davies B, Lees S, Giddings J, Maier R. A population-based, unselected, consecutive cohort of patients with acquired hemophilia A. Br J Hematol. 2004;124:86-90.
4. Franchini M, Lippi G. How I treat acquired factor VIII inhibitors. Blood. 2008;112:250-5.
5. Green D, LechnerK. A survey of 125 nonhemophilic patients with inhibitors to factor VIII. Thyrom Haemost. 1981;45:200-3.
6. Hultin MB. Acquired inhibitors in malignant and nonmalignant disease states. Am J Med. 1991;91:9-13.

CASE 3

YOUNG MALE WITH RECURRENT JAUNDICE

CASE SUMMARY

A 20-year-old male presented with recurrent jaundice of variable duration for the last 6 years. Each of these episodes persisted approximately for 3–4 months and was associated with dark urine, pale stool, intense itching, abdominal bloating and significant weight loss. For these complaints, he was admitted in different hospitals for multiple times, got symptomatic treatment and his condition improved. Between these episodes of jaundice, he was completely well. He did not report any fever, arthralgia, hematemesis, melena, confusion, cough or hemoptysis. He had no history of blood transfusion or intravenous drug abuse, intake of herbal medication, unsafe sexual exposure. He was nonsmoker, nonalcoholic, and no similar illness or other familial illness ran in his family.

On examination, he was ill-looking and deeply icteric. Scratch marks were present in different parts of the body, but other stigmata of liver disease were absent. Vitals were within normal limit. Abdominal examination revealed 4 cm firm, non-tender hepatomegaly. Nervous system examination showed, a normal higher psychic function and intact cranial nerves, with normal fundoscopic findings. Slit-lamp examination revealed no Kayser Fleischer ring. The rest of the examination was normal.

On investigation, complete blood count (CBC) was normal except erythrocyte sedimentation rate (ESR)—60 mm in first hour; serum bilirubin—22.8 mg/dL; direct bilirubin—19.4 mg/dL; alanine aminotransferase (ALT)—101 U/L; aspartate aminotransferase (AST)—63 U/L; prothrombin time (PT)—16 sec (control 12 sec); serum alkaline phosphatase—680 U/L; gamma-glutamyl transferase 41 U/L. Urinalysis, serum creatinine, chest X-ray, and upper gastrointestinal (GI) endoscopy- all were normal; ultrasonography (USG) of whole abdomen (W/A) showed mild hepatomegaly with hypoechoic parenchyma and contracted gallbladder, intrahepatic biliary channels were not dilated. Viral markers including HBsAg, anti-hepatitis C virus (HCV) antibody (Ab), anti-hepatitis A virus

(HAV) Ab, anti-hepatitis E virus Ab were negative, anti-herpes simplex virus (HSV)-1 Ab (IgM) and anti-cytomegalovirus (CMV) Ab (IgM)—negative. Hb electrophoresis—normal, serum antinuclear antibodies (ANA), anti-liver-kidney microsome (LKM)—1 Ab, anti-mitochondrial Ab, and anti-Smith (SM) Ab—negative.

QUESTIONS

1. What is the most likely diagnosis?
2. Suggest further investigations to reach the diagnosis.
3. How would you manage the case?

DISCUSSION

This young man had been suffering from recurrent episodes of obstructive jaundice with complete recovery between the episodes for the last 6 years. Initial investigations also showed high alkaline phosphatase (ALP), but intrahepatic biliary channels were not dilated. All usual and possible conditions to produce obstruction were also excluded by doing relevant investigations. So, benign recurrent intrahepatic cholestasis (BRIC) was the most likely diagnosis here. As he is a young patient, Wilson's disease was an important possibility though there was no neuropsychiatric manifestation. Further investigations done in this patient:

- Serum ceruloplasmin—494 mg/L. 24 hrs urinary copper—78.57 mg/24 hrs.
- Magnetic resonance cholangiopancreatography (MRCP): contracted gallbladder (GB), otherwise unremarkable findings.
- Fibroscan of liver: median stiffness: 11.8 kPa
- Liver biopsy: there are scattered mild perivenular and lobular cholestasis, mild-to-moderate cellular swelling, slightly increased lymphoplasmacytic and few eosinophilic infiltrates in sinusoidal spaces and lobules. Pseudo-osette formation is scattered. Portal tracts contain scanty inflammatory cell infiltration. Trichome stain highlighted mild portal fibrosis.

Final Diagnosis: Benign Recurrent Intrahepatic Cholestasis

Benign recurrent intrahepatic cholestasis is a benign hereditary form of cholestasis. Here recurrent attacks of jaundice and pruritus occur with spontaneous resolution without any damage to the liver. Between the attacks, patients are completely asymptomatic.

Both sexes are equally affected. It manifests early in life with the onset in the first decade. Duration of cholestasis varies from 2 to 24 weeks. Associated symptoms include anorexia, steatorrhea and deficiency of fat-soluble vitamins.

The diagnosis is reached by exclusion of other causes of primary and secondary cholestasis. Liver biopsy is needed for confirmation.

Diagnostic criteria of BRIC: Luketic and Shiffman have proposed a diagnostic criteria for BRIC,[1] which include:

- At least two episodes of jaundice separated by a symptom-free interval lasting several months to years
- Laboratory values consistent with intrahepatic cholestasis
- Severe pruritus secondary to cholestasis
- Normal intra- and extrahepatic bile ducts confirmed by cholangiography
- Absence of factors known to be associated with cholestasis.

The goal of treatment is mainly symptomatic to reduce pruritus, improve cholestasis and spontaneous resolution. Treatment options are antihistamines, cholestyramine, ursodeoxycholic acid and rifampicin. Rifampicin has been shown to prevent relapses.[2] Surgical treatment like primary biliary diversion can be tried in refractory cases.[3]

REFERENCES

1. Luketic VA, Schiffman ML. Benign recurrent intrahepatic cholestasis. Clin Liver Dis. 1999;3:509-28.
2. Uegaki S, Tanaka A, Mori Y, Kodama H, Fukusato T, Takikawa H. Successful treatment with colestimide for a bout of cholestasis in a Japanese patient with benign recurrent intrahepatic cholestasis caused by ATP8B1 mutation. Intern Med. 2008;47:599-602.
3. Geethalakshmi S, Mageshkumar S. Benign recurrent intrahepatic cholestasis: a rare case report. Int J Sci Stud. 2014;2(7):222-4.

CASE 4

MIDDLE-AGED GENTLEMAN WITH ENLARGEMENT OF TONGUE

CASE SUMMARY

A 54-year-old male presented with gradual swelling and enlargement of tongue for the last 1 year. He complained of repeated accidental tongue bites and multiple small oral ulcerations all over the tongue, which were painful. The pain was so intense that he developed swallowing and speech difficulty. His dysphagia started with solid food, then it progressed to interfere with intake of liquids too and subsequently he lost approximately 15 kg weight because of this condition. He had long-standing bilateral knee joint pain and walking difficulty. Sometimes, both knees became so painful that he needed to use walking aid. He also developed generalized body ache during this course of illness. On his past medical history, he had vitiligo for the last 24 years. He was a diagnosed case of ischemic heart disease and had a history of stenting with percutaneous coronary intervention to left anterior descending and right coronary arteries about 3 years back before his current symptoms arose but during this 1 year course of illness, he noticed gradual deterioration in his general health with generalized fatigue, bilateral leg swelling and significant exertional dyspnea. On query, he mentioned having occasional passage of loose stool without any blood. Along with all these complaints, he was unable to perform his daily activities. So, he got admitted to our hospital.

On examination, patient was ill-looking and mildly anemic. Bilateral pitting leg edema was present. Vitiligo was present all over his body and around lips. Vital signs were within normal limit. There was generalized enlargement of the tongue with indentation on the lateral border due to pressure from tooth. There was no fasciculation or tongue deviation. The tongue was red on dorsal and ventral surfaces. Dorsal surface was rough; multiple painful small, nodular and plaque-like ulcers were present all over the tongue (Fig. 1). Angular stomatitis was absent. There was no tooth spacing. Shape and

Middle-aged Gentleman with Enlargement of Tongue

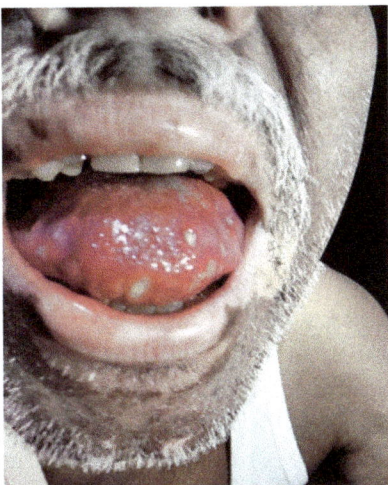

Fig. 1: Dorsal surface of the tongue showing enlargement, redness and multiple small, nodular and plaque-like ulcers.

movement of the chest were normal and symmetric and trachea was central. Breath sound was vesicular with few bilateral basal crackles. Nervous system examination was normal.

Investigations showed Hb—10.3 g/dL; peripheral blood film (PBF)—normocytic normochromic anemia; liver function tests—normal; renal function tests—normal, except urine routine examination revealed 1 + protein; S. electrolytes and S. calcium level—normal; thyroid function test—normal; C-reactive protein, antinuclear antibody, rheumatoid factor test, anti-cyclic citrullinated peptide—negative; X-ray of knee joint—osteoarthritis; X-ray of skull—normal; echocardiography—septal, anterior and lateral wall hypokinesia (OMI); moderate left ventricular systolic dysfunction. Borderline concentric left ventricular hypertrophy; ejection fraction was 38%. Ultrasonography (USG) of W/A—normal. USG of tongue—macroglossia, where echotexture was homogeneous and multiple tiny hypoechoic nodules were seen in the musculature. Urine for Bence Jones protein was positive. Protein electrophoresis was done on two episodes. On first report, there was significant raised alpha-2, and on both reports no monoclonal band was seen; bone marrow study—6–7% of plasma cells.

QUESTIONS

1. What are the causes of gradual swelling of tongue?
2. What are the possibilities in this case?
3. What should be the next plan of investigations?

DISCUSSION

Most common causes of acquired macroglossia are: acromegaly, hypothyroidism and amyloidosis.

Clinical features were not suggestive of acromegaly in our case and we ruled out hypothyroidism by thyroid function tests. Bone marrow study and protein electrophoresis reports were not in favor of multiple myeloma. Our patient's positive history was enlarged tongue with cardiac involvement with occasional diarrhea.

We did a tongue biopsy with Congo red stain and it revealed subepithelial tissue showing focal hyalinization with deposition of eosinophilic structureless substances morphologically resembling amyloid protein. Congo red stain of biopsy material with polarized light was **positive** (Apple-green birefringence in polarized light.) In free light chain assay Kappa–Lambda ratio was increased (8.80).

Final Diagnosis: Primary Systemic Amyloidosis

Amyloidosis is characterized by abnormal deposit of fibril protein within tissues. Usually amyloidosis is systemic, where different organ involvement is present, but rarely amyloidosis can be localized where one organ or one body part is involved. Systemic amyloidosis is sometimes associated with multiple myeloma. Tongue involvement in amyloidosis is not uncommon and typically tongue amyloidosis is secondary to systemic involvement.[1]

Tongue amyloidosis can be localized though unusual. Localized amyloidosis has better prognosis than the systemic disease as surgical treatment is possible in localized disease.[2]

In case of tongue involvement due to systemic disease, local therapy or role of surgery is not clear as recurrence is very common in systemic involvement.[1]

Treatment for systemic amyloidosis: combination chemotherapy with steroid and alkylating agent is effective.

Chemotherapy (Conventional): Melphalan + Prednisolone, Melphalan + Dexamethasone.

Newer agent: Bortezomib, lenalidomide—combination with steroid and alkylating agent.[3]

REFERENCES

1. Thibault I, Vallières I. Macroglossia due to systemic amyloidosis: Is there a role for radiotherapy? Case Rep Oncol. 2011;4(2):392-9.
2. Fahrner KS, Black CC, Gosselin BJ. Localized amyloidosis of the tongue: a review. Am J Otolaryngol. 2004;25(3):186-9.
3. Sher T, Hayman SR, Gertz MA. Treatment of primary systemic amyloidosis (AL): role of intensive and standard. Clin Adv Hematol Oncol. 2012;10(10):644-51.

CASE 5

MIDDLE-AGED MALE WITH QUADRIPLEGIA AND SPEECH DISTURBANCE

CASE SUMMARY

A 60-year-old diabetic, hypertensive man attended the emergency department with sudden onset of asymmetrical weakness of all four limbs with dysphasia and vertigo for 2 weeks. He mentioned to have sudden onset of brief unconsciousness following nausea and vomiting before this weakness. His bowel bladder habit was normal. There was no history of fever, headache, convulsion, trauma to head and neck, heavy weight lifting, vaccination, dysphagia, visual disturbance or hearing difficulties.

On examination patient was conscious and oriented, but speech was influent. There was bilateral 12th nerve (hypoglossal) palsy with normal fundoscopic finding. Signs of meningeal irritation were absent. Motor examination revealed that all reflexes were exaggerated in both upper and lower limbs with bilateral extensor plantar response. All modalities of sensations were intact. Cerebellar sign was absent. Rest of the systemic examination revealed normal findings.

Investigation showed the baseline parameters, including complete blood count within normal limit. Hepatic, renal, and cardiac function tests were unremarkable. Serum lipid profile and plasma glucose was minimally high. Cerebrospinal fluid study was normal.

QUESTIONS

1. What are the differentials?
2. What is the next step of investigation?

DISCUSSION

This middle-aged diabetic patient presented with sudden onset quadriplegia with dysphasia. The differentials were large stroke (most likely involving

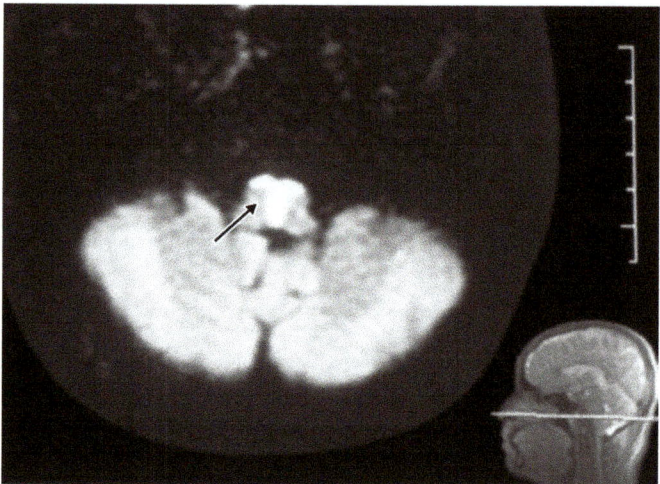

Fig. 1: Diffusion-weight image MRI of brain (characteristic heart sign showing hyperintense signal in both medullas).

the brainstem), brainstem encephalitis, multiple sclerosis, paraneoplastic syndrome.

As CT scan of brain was inconclusive, at first instance, we precisely ruled out large hemorrhagic stroke. Moreover, the patient was well oriented, which disfavors the diagnosis of large hemorrhage. He was afebrile and there was no history of convulsion, and CSF study was normal. All these ruled out brainstem encephalitis.

So another possibility was multiple sclerosis which can involve the brain and spinal cord at the same time. So we decided to do the magnetic resonance imaging (MRI) of brain with spinal cord and studied the cerebrospinal fluid (CSF) pathology. MRI of brain revealed the characteristic "heart sign" infarct involving both the medullas (Fig. 1). Also we screened the MRI of spine in case we missed any demyelination in the spinal cord, and it was normal.

Final Diagnosis: Bilateral Medial Medullary Syndrome

The patient was advised for digital subtraction angiography (DSA). He was given secondary preventive therapy along with physiotherapy.

Medial medullary syndrome is a stroke syndrome which results from anterior spinal artery infarct and/or infarction in vertebral arteries. It is associated with the clinical triad of ipsilateral hypoglossal palsy, contralateral hemiparesis, and contralateral lemniscal sensory loss.

Bilateral infarction of the medial medulla is often rare. The clinical presentation may include quadriparesis or ipsilateral hemiparesis, dysarthria, nystagmus, hypoglossal palsy, signs of brainstem dysfunction, e.g. dysphagia, even sometimes fatal respiratory failure.[1] The most common vascular pathology is vertebral artery atherosclerosis. However, few literature reported vasculitis as a cause of bilateral medial medullary syndrome.[2] MRI brain is the tool of diagnosis and the "heart sign" in the diffusion-weighted MRI is the pathognomic radiological feature. The acute phase MRI of brain may show only linear abnormal signal in midline that is easy to miss.[3] The clinical outcome is poor with mortality rate up to 23.8%.[3] The reported patient did not have the fatal outcome so far as there was early diagnosis, intervention and no respiratory failure.

The beauty of this case lies in the demonstration of varied presentations of brainstem syndrome, which may or may not follow the rules always. Considering the fatal outcome of bilateral medial medullary syndrome, it is crucial for clinicians as well as radiologists to pick up the signs to diagnose it early for possible early intervention by thrombolysis.

REFERENCES

1. Pongmoragot J, Parthasarathy S, Selchen D, Saposnik G. Bilateral medial medullary infarction: a systematic review. J Stroke Cerebrovasc Dis. 2013;22(6):775-80. doi: 10.1016/j.jstrokecerebrovasdis.2012.03.010. Epub 2012 Apr 26.
2. Deshpande A, Chandran V, Pai A, Rao S, Shetty R. Bilateral medial medullary syndrome secondary to Takayasu arteritis. BMJ Case Rep. 2013;2013:bcr0120125600. doi:10.1136/bcr-01-2012-5600.
3. Torabi AM. Bilateral medial medullary stroke: A challenge in early diagnosis. Case Reports in Neurological Medicine. 2013;2013:1.

CASE 6

MIDDLE-AGED LADY WITH PULMONARY-RENAL SYNDROME

CASE SUMMARY

A 55-year-old housewife presented with hemoptysis, respiratory distress and low-grade continued fever for 10 days. On query, she reported having hematuria but denied nasal crusting or any upper respiratory infection or arthralgia. There was no rash, photosensitivity or Raynaud's phenomenon. Eight months prior to this onset of illness, she had similar complaints and was diagnosed as bacteriologically confirmed (bronchoalveolar lavage fluid Xpert MTB positive) pulmonary tuberculosis case. She was treated with antitubercular medication for 6 months, which led to symptom-free period of about 2 months. She was smoker (40 packs/year), nondiabetic, nonalcoholic, and was previously normotensive. No similar illness was found in the family.

On examination, the patient was moderately anemic, temperature: 100°F, pulse: 102 beats/min, blood pressure: 120/80 mm Hg, respiratory rate: 24 breaths/min. Bipedal pitting edema was present with normal jugular venous pressure (JVP), and clubbing was absent. Bedside heat coagulation test revealed heavy proteinuria. Respiratory system examination revealed bilateral coarse crackles without any post-tussive alteration along with pleural rub on the right side. Other system examination findings were normal.

Initial laboratory investigations revealed: hemoglobin (Hb): 7.6 g/dL, eosinophil count: normal, erythrocyte sedimentation rate (ESR): 45 mm in first hour, C-reactive protein (CRP): 24 mg/dL, serum creatinine: 3.12 mg/dL. Urinalysis showed nephrotic-range proteinuria [albumin: +++, 24-hour urine protein test (UTP): 8.81 g] and plenty red blood cell (RBC) with 40% dysmorphism and granular casts. Serum albumin was 2.72 g/dL. Repeated X-ray chest posteroanterior (PA) view (Figs. 1A and B) demonstrated diffuse bilateral inhomogeneous opacities which seemed to change sites; computed tomography (CT) scan of chest (Figs. 2A and B) showed extensive diffuse parenchymal lung disease. Spirometry: suspected restrictive abnormality. X-ray paranasal sinus (PNS) occipitomental (OM) view: normal study.

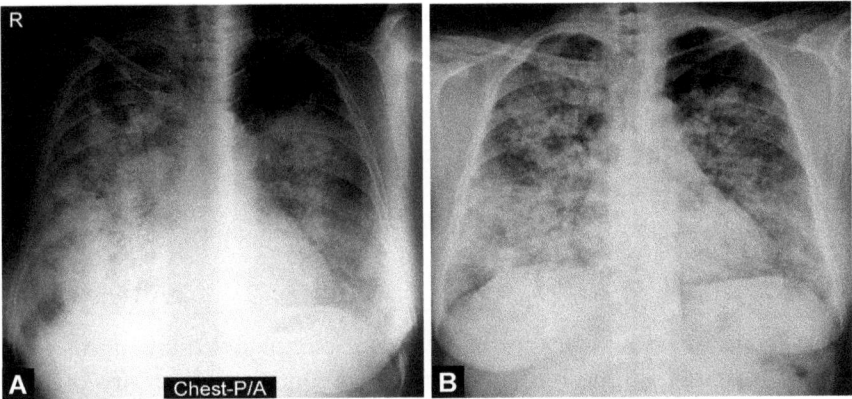

Figs. 1A and B: Chest skiagram posteroanterior (P/A) view. (A) Done on admission showing bilateral inhomogeneous opacities resembling masslike consolidations; (B) Done a week after admission showing bilateral inhomogeneous opacities.

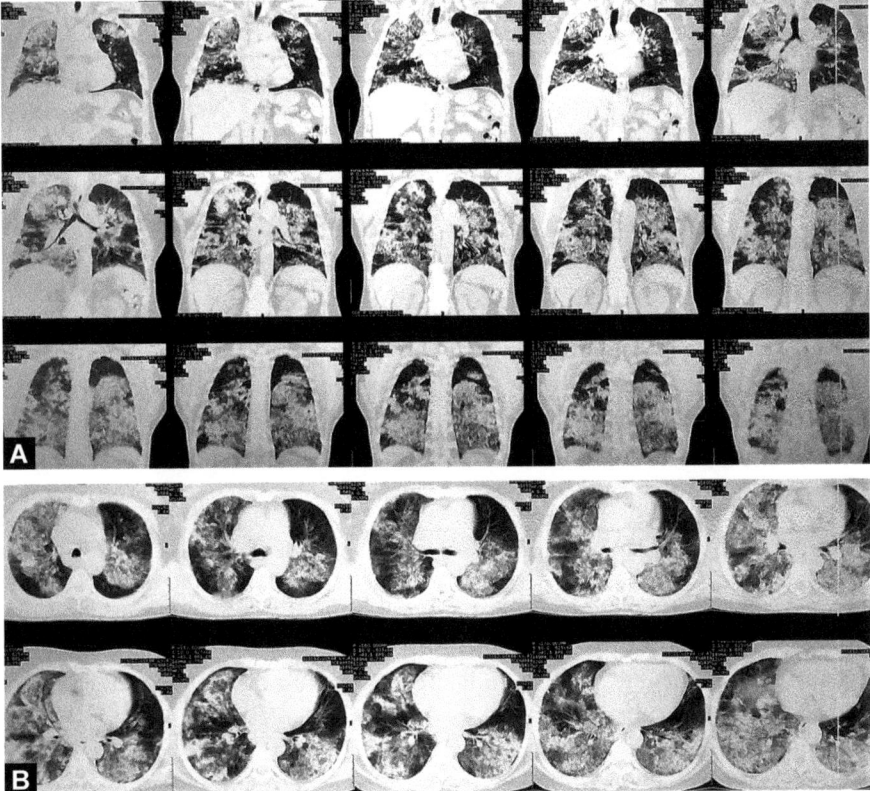

Figs. 2A and B: Computed tomography (CT) scan of chest, multiple coronal, and axial planes showing extensive parenchymal lung disease.

Sputum GeneXpert: negative for MTB. Ultrasonography of whole abdomen showed bilateral renal parenchymal disease.

QUESTIONS

1. What differential would you suggest for this patient with respiratory and renal involvement?
2. What investigations are necessary to reach the diagnosis?

DISCUSSION

Considering the recent history of treatment-completed tuberculosis (TB), positive respiratory findings in physical examination, discovery of renal involvement and thorough investigation findings—we had a strong suspicion of pulmonary-renal syndrome. The differential diagnoses were:

- Goodpasture's syndrome
- Systemic lupus erythematosus (SLE)
- Microscopic polyangiitis (MPA)
- Granulomatosis with polyangiitis.

These differentials warranted further workup, which showed, antinuclear antibody (ANA): negative, MPO-ANCA (P-ANCA): 21.2 U/mL (positive, control: <6 U/mL), PR3-ANCA (C-ANCA): 3.1 U/mL (negative).

SLE was virtually excluded and positive MPO-ANCA was a strong evidence for MPA. To exclude Goodpasture's syndrome (GPS) and other ANCA-positive vasculitides, renal biopsy was done. Histopathology revealed rapidly progressive (crescentic) glomerulonephritis with paucity of immune-complex deposition in direct immunofluorescence study, which went in favor of MPA. The absence of upper respiratory tract involvement and no granulomatous lesions in renal histopathology excluded granulomatosis with polyangiitis (previously called Wegener's granulomatosis). There was neither any neurological involvement and history of atopy nor eosinophilia and any granuloma in renal histopathology, as expected in eosinophilic granulomatosis with polyangiitis (formerly termed Churg-Strauss syndrome). Further evidence could have been obtained from lung biopsy.

Final Diagnosis: Microscopic Polyangiitis

Microscopic polyangiitis is an ANCA-associated necrotizing vasculitis that most commonly affects kidneys, lungs, skin and joints, and is a life-threatening disorder. Patients are usually MPO antibody positive and granulomatous inflammation is usually absent. It is an uncommon disease worldwide and can affect people from all ethnicity and of any age.

Patients who have MPA commonly present with malaise, fever, loss of appetite and weight loss. Other associated symptoms may include rashes, myalgia and/or arthralgia. When MPA affects the lungs, patients may present with breathlessness or hemoptysis. MPA affecting the peripheral nerves may present with paresthesia followed by numbness or loss of strength. Renal involvement by MPA often remains asymptomatic until the kidneys begin to malfunction. Therefore, urinalysis is precisely important. The five most common clinical presentations of MPA are:[1]

- Renal inflammation (~80% of patients)
- Weight loss (>70%)
- Skin lesions (>60%)
- Peripheral nerve damage (60%)
- Fever (55%).

Laboratory investigation findings in MPA include high ESR and CRP. Urinalysis demonstrates variable degree of proteinuria, hematuria with presence of casts, if renal involvement is present. Patients of MPA present with rapidly progressive glomerulonephritis, often in association with alveolar hemorrhage. Repeated X-ray chest shows bilateral inhomogeneous pulmonary infiltrates, which are not fixed. CT scan of chest can aid in better delineation of the pattern of lung involvement. On occasion, an electromyography or nerve conduction study may be needed to identify findings consistent with mononeuritis multiplex. Tissues that might be biopsied, according to pattern of involvement, are kidney, skin, nerve, muscle and lung. Positive MPO-ANCA is a strong evidence for MPA and renal biopsy and histopathology reveals glomerular crescents (found in 90% MPA cases) with pauci-immune glomerulonephritis.[2,3] which favor the diagnosis.

Treatment consists of two phases: induction and maintenance of remission. The choice of drugs should be guided by the degree of inflammation, the extent of disease, the rate of progression, and comorbidities. The quintessential combination of medications for induction includes a steroid (preferably prednisolone- at 1 mg/kg/day for 1 month, followed by gradual tapering with discontinuation after ~6-9 months), along with daily cyclophosphamide or rituximab. When remission is achieved (usually after around 4-6 months of starting treatment)[1], maintenance is continued with tapering dose of steroid and cyclophosphamide is usually replaced with another less-toxic drug (rituximab, methotrexate, azathioprine, or mycophenolate mofetil). The optimal duration of maintenance therapy is uncertain, and medications are needed for at least 2 years past remission, after which tapering over 6-12 month might be considered before discontinuation of drugs. Relapse rate is high (at least 34%) and needs same drug treatment as induction phase.[1,3]

REFERENCES

1. Johns Hopkins Vasculitis Center. Microscopic Polyangiitis. [online] Available from https://www.hopkinsvasculitis.org/types vasculitis/microscopic-polyangiitis/
2. Savage CO, Winearls CG, Evans DJ, Rees AJ, Lockwood CM. Microscopic polyarteritis: presentation, pathology and prognosis. Q J Med. 1985;56(220): 467-83.
3. Jameson JL, Kasper DL, Longo DL, Fauci AS, Hauser SL, Loscalzo J. Harrison's Principles of Internal Medicine. 20th ed. New York: McGraw Hill Education; 2018. pp. 2580-1.

CASE 7

YOUNG MALE WITH QUADRIPARESIS

CASE SUMMARY

A 26-year-old man was brought to hospital with weakness of all four limbs for 2 weeks. The man, who was previously healthy, developed calf muscle cramp followed by ascending weakness of lower limbs which progressively involved the upper limbs over the course of 2 days. Gradually, he found himself unable to stand and walk. There was no history of recent fever, back or neck pain, bowel and bladder disturbance, or association with intake of heavy carbohydrate meal. There was no similar illness in the past. Patient gave history of acute onset of severe right knee joint pain and swelling about 2 years back, which subsided with treatment prescribed by a local physician.

Examination revealed a well-oriented man having blood pressure (BP) 85/50 mm Hg, pulse rate 78 bpm, and respiratory rate 18 breaths/min, with no features of dehydration. Nervous system examination revealed bilateral flaccid quadriplegia [Medical Research Council (MRC) grade 2/5] and diminished ankle jerks. Plantar responses were flexor bilaterally and all modalities of sensation were intact.

Initial laboratory investigations revealed serum sodium (Na) 136 mmol/L, serum potassium (K) 1.67 mmol/L, serum chloride (Cl) 94 mmol/L, HCO_3 28 mmol/L, serum phosphate 1.67 mmol/L (low), serum magnesium (Mg) 1 mg/dL (low) and serum creatinine 0.8 mg/dL. Arterial blood gas (ABG) partially compensated metabolic alkalosis. A 24-hour urine examination revealed: total volume 2,800 mL/d, urine sodium (Na) and chloride (Cl) excretion was normal but potassium (K) excretion was high. Calcium excretion was within normal range and plasma renin activity was high. Urinary calcium/creatinine (Ca/Cr) ratio was 0.011. Ultrasonography (USG) of W/A was normal.

QUESTIONS

1. What is the underlying diagnosis?
2. How to confirm the diagnosis?

3. How can you explain the past history of right knee arthritis?
4. Can you mention some acquired causes?

DISCUSSION

Considering hypokalemia, a good number of differentials needed exploration. Evaluation of renal causes of hypokalaemia should be done based on presence or absence of hypertension. Hypokalaemia with hypertension may result from increased aldosterone secretion in Conn's syndrome, or a genetic defect called Liddle's syndrome.[1] Our patient had blood pressure of 85/50 mm Hg- in which setting hypokalaemia needed to be classified according to the associated change in acid–base balance. Hypokalemia with metabolic alkalosis points towards the differentials of Bartter's syndrome (BS) and Gitelman's syndrome (GS)- both of which have common characteristics of hypokalemia-hypomagnesemia. These two differentials could be sorted by measuring urinary calcium excretion which is increased in BS (hypercalciuria) leading to nephrocalcinosis and decreased (hypocalciuria) in GS.[1,2] Though hypocalciuria is the expected finding in GS, there are few other case reports from Asia which demonstrate that normocalciuria can rarely be present.[3] Our patient had normocalciuria, but his urinary Ca/Cr ratio was less than 0.20, which is suggestive of Gitelman's syndrome. In this case, there was also hypophosphatemia, which is not uncommon in GS. Patients with GS may suffer from chondrocalcinosis, an abnormal deposition of calcium pyrophosphate dihydrate (CPPD) in joint cartilage.[2] Our patient's past history of acute right knee arthritis might have been due to chondrocalcinosis mediated pseudogout. He was treated with potassium and magnesium sulfate which resolved his symptoms gradually.

Final Diagnosis: Gitelman's Syndrome

Gitelman's syndrome is an autosomal recessive renal tubular disorder causing defective ion transport in the distal convoluted tubule (DCT), and is linked to the gene encoding the thiazide sensitive Na-Cl-cotransporter located on chromosome 16q.[4]

As per the Kidney Disease Improving Global Outcomes (KDIGO) consensus and guidance, criteria for suspecting Gitelman's syndrome:[5]

- Chronic hypokalemia (<3.5 mmol/L) with inappropriate renal potassium wasting [spot potassium–creatinine ratio >2.0 mmol/mmol (>18 mmol/g)].
- Metabolic alkalosis and hypomagnesemia [<0.7 mmol/L (<1.70 mg/dL)] with inappropriate renal magnesium wasting (fractional excretion of magnesium >4%).
- Hypocalciuria [spot calcium–creatinine ratio <0.2 mmol/mmol (<0.07 mg/mg)] in adults.

- A high plasma renin activity or levels of fractional excretion of chloride more than 0.5% low or normal-low blood pressure, and normal renal ultrasound.

Criteria for establishing a diagnosis of Gitelman's syndrome:[5]
- Identification of biallelic inactivating mutations in *SLC12A3*
- Acquired Gitelman's syndrome is due to autoantibody against sodium chloride cotransporter (NCC) channel. It can be seen in Sjögren's syndrome, following renal transplantation. Thiazide diuretic can also produce similar biochemistry, which can be excluded by urinary assay for diuretic.

There is no cure for GS, and management is mainly symptomatic. The mainstay of treatment is a high salt diet with oral potassium and magnesium supplements; with the goal to improve symptoms- not to normalize electrolyte abnormalities. Dried fruits rich in potassium are helpful. Potassium-sparing diuretics could be used to improve hypokalemia. Magnesium supplements should be taken in small frequent doses (4-6 times/day) to avoid magnesium associated diarrhea which may worsen hypokalemia. For many individuals, lifelong daily supplementation with magnesium is recommended. In cases with severe muscle cramps, magnesium may be given intravenously. In presence of symptomatic chondrocalcinosis- magnesium supplementation, pain medications and/or nonsteroidal anti-inflammatory drugs (NSAIDs) such as ibuprofen may be beneficial.[6]

REFERENCES

1. Ralston SH, Penman ID, Strachan MWJ, Hobson RP. Davidson's Principles and Practice of Medicine. 23nd ed. Edinburgh: Churchill Livingstone/Elsevier; 2018. pp. 361-2.
2. Jameson JL, Kasper DL, Longo DL, Fauci AS, Hauser SL, Loscalzo J. Harrison's Principles of Internal Medicine. 20th ed. New York: McGraw Hill Education; 2018. p. 306.
3. Lin SH, Shiang JC, Huang CC, Yang SS, Hsu YJ, Cheng CJ. Phenotype and Genotype Analysis in Chinese Patients with Gitelman's Syndrome. J Clin Endocrinol Metab. 2005;90(5):2500-7. Epub 2005 Feb 1. https://doi.org/10.1210/jc.2004-1905.
4. Gjata M, Tase M, Gjata A, Gjergji ZH. Gitelman's syndrome (familial hypokalemia-hypomagnesemia). Hippokratia. 2007;11(3):150-3.
5. Blanchard A, Bockenhauer D, Bolignano D, Calò LA, Cosyns E, Devuyst O, et al. Gitelman syndrome: consensus and guidance from a Kidney Disease: Improving Global Outcomes (KDIGO) Controversies Conference. Kidney Int. 2017;91(1):24-33. doi: 10.1016/j.kint.2016.09.046.
6. Gitelman syndrome. Available from: https://rarediseases.org/rare-diseases/gitelman-syndrome/. Accessed on June 10, 2019.

CASE 8

MIDDLE-AGED MAN WITH VOMITING AND WEIGHT LOSS

CASE SUMMARY

A 60-year-old, normotensive, nondiabetic man with shortened left lower limb presented with persistent daily vomiting for last 1 month. Vomiting occurred 4–5 times a day, almost immediately after taking food, containing undigested food particles, color was nonbilious. Vomiting was not projectile in nature. There was history of hematemesis for two episodes since the symptoms started. On occasion, to get relief from discomfort- he was compelled to induce vomiting. Later, it became so severe that he refused to take food due to fear of vomiting. Sometimes he noticed a mobile mass in his abdomen passing from above downwards. His appetite also decreased progressively. All these led to about 6 kg weight loss over last 1 month. On query, he gave history of loose motion about 1 month ago, which persisted for 7–8 days, occurred almost 10–12 times in a day, the content of stool was tarry-black in color with very small amount of fecal matter. When asked about his visible shortening of left lower limb than the right one, he said that this developed insidiously over last several years and he faced problems in walking, but could manage to walk with aid. On repeated query he stated that he used to take tab prednisolone 10 mg for almost 10 years without consultation with physician. He used to feel better with this treatment, so he continued to take this drug. There was no history of early morning vomiting, head injury, chest pain, tinnitus, vertigo, fever, jaundice, itching, abdominal pain, bladder disturbance, cough, night sweat, palpitation, preference to hot and cold environment, alcohol or other substance abuse.

On examination, patient was ill-looking, angular stomatitis was present. Pulse rate: 72 beats/min. Blood pressure: 110/70 mm Hg, no postural drop. He was mildly anemic. No lymph node was palpable. Abdominal examination was unremarkable except visible peristalsis. Detailed findings on musculoskeletal system examination were- there was a hard bony swelling in the anterolateral aspect of left hip which was non-tender, with normal overlying skin and no rise of temperature. Left limb was shortened than right one by approximately 3 cm. Active movements of left hip were restricted in all direction, but passive movements were possible except extension. Range of movements in all other joints of upper and lower limbs and spine were within normal limit. Other systemic examinations revealed no abnormality.

Investigations showed, complete blood count (CBC): Hb level was 9.8 g/dL. MCV 73.8 fL, MCH 25.7 pg, MCHC 34.9 g/dL. RDW-CV 18%. WBC count was 8.43 K/μL, N 31.8%, L: 43.2%, M: 4.6%, E: 20.3%, platelet: 401 K/μL. ESR was 15 mm in first hour. PBF showed microcytic hypochromic anemia with eosinophilia. RBS was 6.5 mmol/L. X-ray chest P/A view was apparently normal (Fig. 1). X-ray left hip joint showed features consistent with avascular necrosis of the head of left femur (Fig. 2). Urine routine

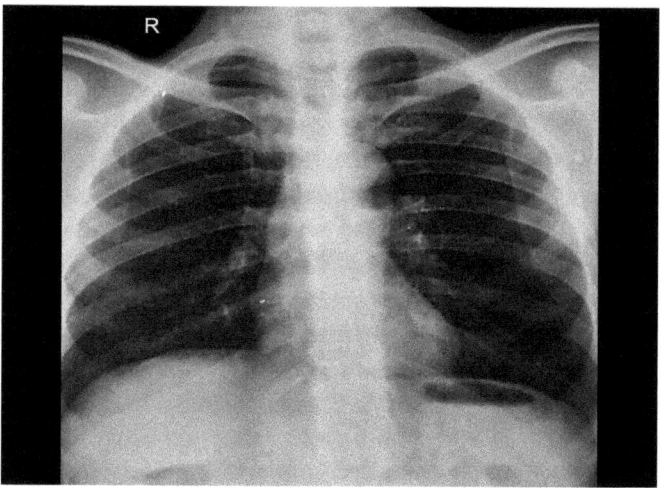

Fig. 1: Chest X-ray PA view showing normal study.

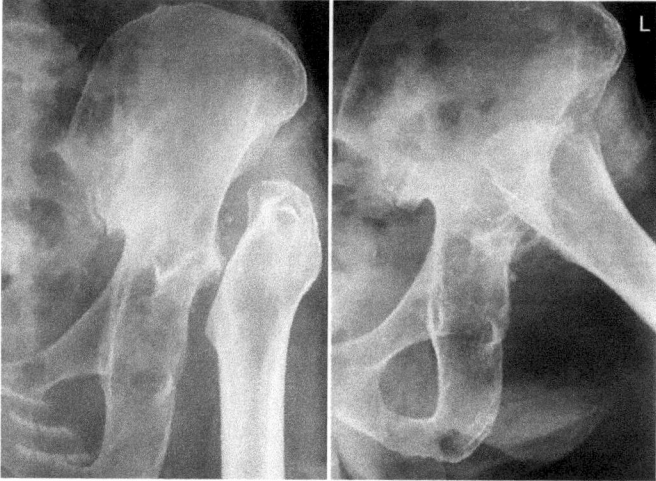

Fig. 2: X-ray of left hip joint showing features consistent with avascular necrosis of the head of left femur.

microscopic examination showed hazy appearance with pus cell 3–5/HPF. Serum electrolyte showed Na 122, K 3.61, Cl 92 mmol/L; serum creatinine: 0.68 mg/dL. USG of whole abdomen: distended gallbladder with sludge.

QUESTIONS

1. What is your provisional diagnosis?
2. What are your differentials?
3. What investigations will you do to reach your final diagnosis?

DISCUSSION

For this middle-aged gentleman presenting with obvious history of gastric outlet obstruction (GOO) and melena, our provisional diagnosis was bleeding peptic ulcer disease with GOO. Our differentials for the cause of GOO were:
- Gastric carcinoma
- Gastric lymphoma.

Following investigations were carried out to reach the diagnosis: Endoscopy of upper GIT showed reflux esophagitis (multiple linear lesions in lower end), gastric ulcer (extensive antral ulceration involving pyloric ring and incisura), duodenal ulcer (bulb was edematous, congested and contained few ulceration).

Biopsy from the gastric ulcer showed ulceration and dense infiltration of acute and chronic inflammatory cells along with extensive intestinal metaplasia. There were tiny helminthic bodies within the mucosal glands and on the surface consistent with *Strongyloides stercoralis* (Figs. 3A to F).

Stool microscopic examination confirmed the presence of larvae of *Strongyloides stercoralis* along with moderate yeast.

Computed tomography (CT) scan of chest: normal; MRI of brain: normal.

Final Diagnosis: ***Strongyloides Stercoralis* Infection Leading to Peptic Ulcer Disease (PUD) Complicated with Gastric Outlet Obstruction with Steroid-induced Avascular Necrosis of the Head of Femur (Left)**

Global prevalence of *Strongyloides stercoralis* infection is unknown, but it is estimated that more than 3 million people are infected worldwide.[1] Infected patients usually remain asymptomatic with peripheral eosinophilia or may complain of myriad of symptoms including skin rash due to larval penetration, cough, wheezing, dyspnea, upper abdominal pain, nausea, vomiting or diarrhea. *Strongyloides stercoralis*-induced gastrointestinal ulcer disease in immunocompromised patients has been well described in the literature. Our patient was immunocompromised due to prolonged steroid intake. Though strongyloidiasis-induced gastric ulcer is very rare yet strong suspicion should be there especially in immunocompromised patients.[2]

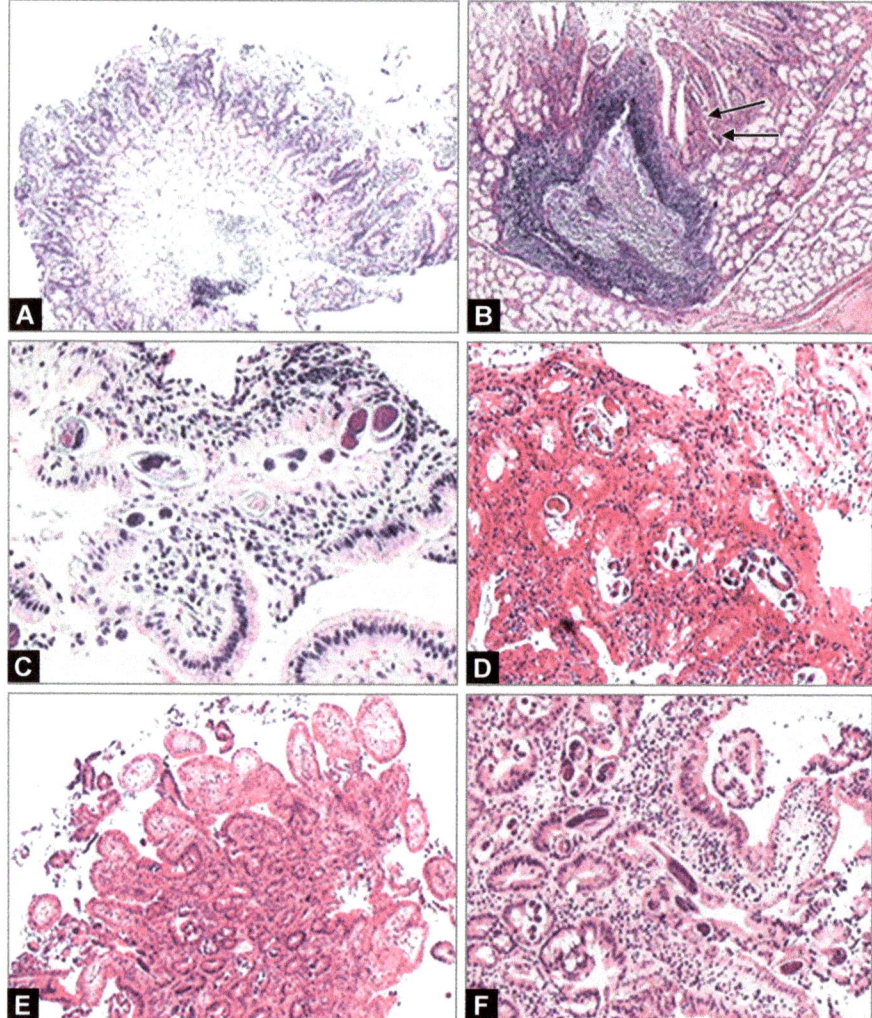

Figs. 3A to F: Photomicrograph of histopathology of gastric ulcer showing tiny helminthic bodies within the mucosal glands and on the surface.

REFERENCES

1. Beknazarova M, Whiley H, Ross K. Strongyloidiasis: a disease of socioeconomic disadvantage. Int J Environ Res Public Health. 2016;13(5):517. doi:10.3390/ijerph13050517.
2. Keiser PB, Nutman TB. *Strongyloides stercoralis* in the immunocompromised population Clin Mic Rev. 2004;17(1):208-17.

CASE 9

HYPERPIGMENTED GENTLEMAN WITH LIMB WEAKNESS AND HEMATEMESIS

CASE SUMMARY

A 46-year-old gentleman, permanent resident of Rajbari, Faridpur (southern part of Bangladesh) came to us with the complaints of flaccid paraparesis and paresthesia for 6 months; irregular low-grade fever for 2 months; swelling of body and hyperpigmentation for 1.5 months. The flaccid paraparesis was gradual in onset and progressive. The paresthesia was initially present on the soles of both feet, then gradually involved the lower limbs and was associated with moderate, persistent myalgia. He also had low-grade, intermittent fever that was associated with nausea, anorexia and weight loss. Later, patient had developed hyperpigmentation of the skin, which was diffusely scattered throughout the body, including trunk, all four limbs, face, palmar creases and soles of the feet, gum and hard palate. There was no history of jaundice, itching, pale stool, hematemesis, melena, joint pain, oral ulceration, skin rash, cough, breathlessness, vomiting, abdominal pain, impaired consciousness or seizure. He was nonsmoker and nonalcoholic.

On examination, patient was anemic, ill-looking; and body built was poor. Leukonychia and bilateral pitting edema were present. Medial group of axillary lymph nodes and inguinal lymph nodes were palpable bilaterally which were of variable sizes, smooth surfaced, firm, nontender with no fixity and no discharging sinus. There was hyperpigmentation of the whole body in the forms of mixed hypopigmented and hyperpigmented macules in the trunk and limbs, and diffuse darkening of the skin of the face and hands (most prominent) (Figs. 1A to C). He had palmar and solar keratosis. Alimentary system examination revealed smooth tongue with loss of papilla and there was hyperpigmentation on gum and hard palate (Fig. 1D). Liver was just palpable, firm with no bruit. Ascites was evidenced by positive fluid thrill. Testes were bilaterally small, soft and symmetrical. Nervous system examination revealed intact cranial nerves with features of bilateral symmetrical sensory motor polyneuropathy on both lower limbs which was

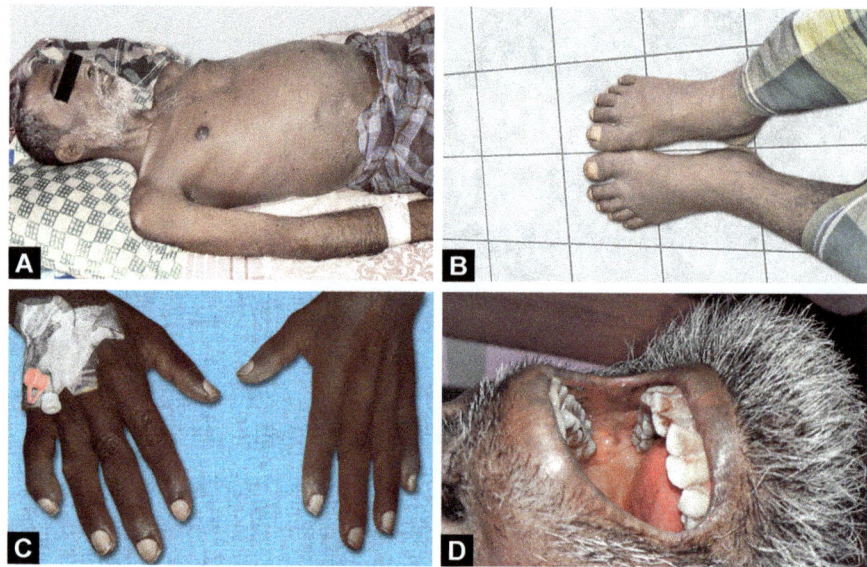

Figs. 1A to D: (A and B) Mixed hypopigmented and hyperpigmented macules on trunk and limbs with distended abdomen; (C) Diffuse darkening of the skin of hands; (D) Hyperpigmentation of buccal mucosa.

evident by muscle power 4/5 distally, diminished deep tendon reflexes and impairment of pain and touch sensation on feet up to ankles. Coordination and gait were normal. Respiratory system examination revealed bilateral pleural effusion with end inspiratory crackles in mid-zone of right lung. Other systemic examinations revealed no abnormality.

Investigation showed: hemoglobin (Hb): 9.3 g/L (MCV: 71 fL, MCH: 22 pg, MCHC: 30 g/dL); white blood cell (WBC):10,500/mm^3 (N 68%, L 26%), platelet: 340,000/mm^3, erythrocyte sedimentation rate (ESR): 41 mm; peripheral blood film (PBF): microcytic hypochromic anemia. Iron profile: serum iron: 17 μg/dL (60–150 μg/dL), serum ferritin: 109 ng/mL (20–300 ng/mL), TIBC: 210 μg/dL (250–400 μg/dL), transferrin saturation: 8% (20–50%). Urine R/M/E: albumin+, 24 hours urinary total protein: 0.21 g (0.028–0.141 g), serum creatinine: 1.6 mg/dL; liver function test (LFT): serum bilirubin: 0.4 mg/dL, alanine aminotransferase (ALT): 15 U/L, aspartate aminotransferase (AST): 15 U/L, ALP: 224 U/L, PT: 17.6 sec, serum albumin: 2.5 g/dL, serum globulin: 3.5 g/dL; A:G ratio: 0.71. Oral glucose tolerance test (OGTT): FBS: 3.44 mmol/L, 2 hours after 75 g glucose: 8.89 mmol/L; HbA1C 5.2%. Serum electrolytes, serum urea, fasting lipid profile: normal; ultrasonography (USG): mild hepatomegaly with distended gallbladder, gross ascites and right-side minimal pleural effusion. Ascitic fluid study: cell count: 558/mm^3 (neutrophil: 19%, lymphocyte, mesothelial cells and others: 81%), protein: 3.1 g/dL, glucose: 4.1 g/dL, staining: no

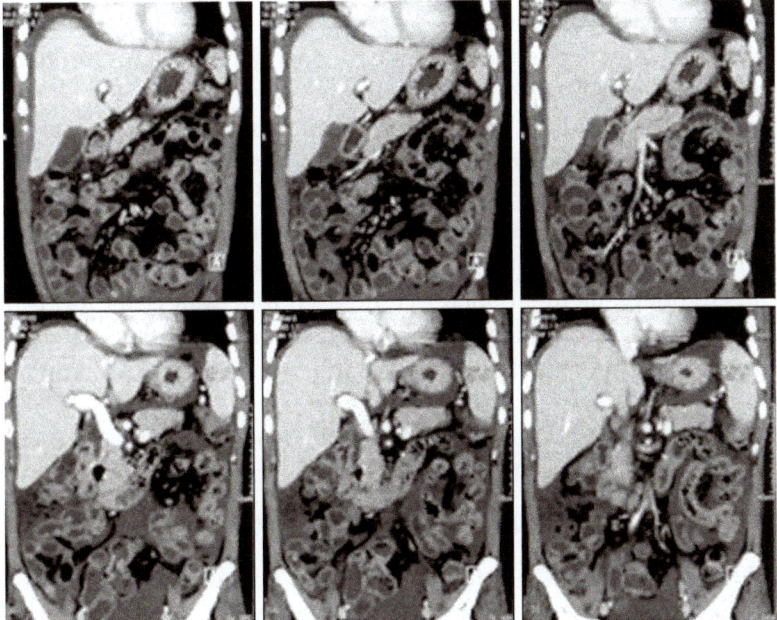

Fig. 2: Computed tomography (CT) abdomen of the patient showing intra-abdominal lymphadenopathy and heavy metal infiltrate in the mucosal layer of a large portion of gut.

acid-fast bacilli (AFB) or Gram-reactive organism found, adenosine deaminase (ADA): normal, serum ascites albumin gradient (SAAG): 1.4, GeneXpert: *Mycobacterium tuberculosis* DNA not detected. Lymph node biopsy showed no granuloma or malignancy. Nerve conduction study (NCS) findings were consistent with sensory-motor polyneuropathy predominantly affecting the lower limbs. Computed tomography (CT) scan of abdomen revealed mild to moderate amount of ascites and multiple enlarged retroperitoneal and mesenteric lymphnodes. The striking feature was the evidence of heavy metal infiltrate in the mucosal layer of a large portion of gut (Fig. 2).

QUESTIONS

1. What are the possible differential diagnoses?
2. What further history and investigation will you consider to reveal the diagnosis?

DISCUSSION

For this case, our differentials were:
- Chronic liver disease (CLD) (decompensated) with peripheral neuropathy
- Lymphoma with paraneoplastic syndrome
- Disseminated tuberculosis with peripheral neuropathy

- Malignancy with metastasis
- Polyneuropathy, organomegaly, endocrinopathy, monoclonal gammopathy and skin changes (POEMS) syndrome.

Patient's unexplained peripheral neuropathy, organomegaly, and abdominal CT scan showing gut mucosa infiltration led us to think of a heavy metal accumulation in different organ systems of the body, which is most commonly explainable by arsenicosis in perspective of our country. To correlate all the symptoms together, then we took targeted history from the patient. On query, he mentioned that he used tube well water for drinking and domestic purpose; though arsenic had been detected above normal level in that tube well water and had been declared unsafe for use with red mark 1 year back.

Then we tested arsenic concentration in nail of the patient and the result was 0.45 mg/kg which was higher than normal.

Final Diagnosis: Chronic Arsenicosis with Multisystem Involvement

Chronic arsenicosis due to drinking of arsenic contaminated ground water is a major environmental health hazard throughout the world including Bangladesh. The safe dose of arsenic in drinking water in Bangladesh is 0.05 mg/L.[1,2]

For a case to be called chronic arsenicosis, two major criteria are to be met:[1]
- Pigmented and keratotic skin lesions
- Evidence of elevated levels of arsenic exposure; established by history of arsenic contaminated water consumption, or by arsenic concentration in hair or nails.

Skin lesions are the hallmark signs of chronic arsenic exposure. Most common health effects in populations consuming arsenic-contaminated drinking water are hyperpigmentation and keratotic lesions. Nonhealing ulcers may also develop which could progress to malignancies. In our patient, the skin manifestations were increased pigmentation in the form of characteristic raindrop pigmentation, and diffuse hyperpigmentation; and skin hardening, which results from melanosis and keratosis.

Chronic aresenicosis also produces systemic manifestations:
- *Lung involvement:* Chronic bronchitis, chronic obstructive pulmonary disease and bronchiectasis
- *Liver involvement:* Noncirrhotic portal fibrosis
- *Vascular involvement:* Peripheral vascular disease, hypertension and ischemic heart disease
- *Others:* Polyneuropathy, diabetes mellitus, nonpitting edema of feet or hands, weakness and anemia
- *Malignancy:* Skin, lung and urinary bladder.

Our patient had several systemic manifestations (involving lungs, liver, intestines, peripheral nerves, and skin) of this deadly poison.

The mainstay in the management of arsenicosis is stoppage of drinking of arsenic-contaminated water. Specific chelation therapy has limited value. Early skin cancer, detectable by regular active surveillance, is curable.

We have educated the patient regarding the harmful effects of arsenic on his different organ systems and their possible outcomes, as well as asked him to use safe drinking water and to install a new arsenic-free tube well. Patient was advised for regular follow-up to assess disease progression.

REFERENCES

1. Caussy D. A field guide for detection, management and surveillance of arsenicosis cases. WHO SEARO. 2005. Available from: http://apps.searo.who.int/PDS_DOCS/B0301.pdf
2. Ahmad SA, Khan MH. Ground water arsenic contamination and its health effects in Bangladesh. Handbook of Arsenic Toxicology. USA: Academic Press Publishers; 2015. pp. 51-72.

CASE 10

YOUNG LADY WITH MULTIPLE BLISTERS AND EROSIONS

CASE SUMMARY

A 25-year-old housewife presented with nonhealing oral ulcer for 3 weeks, and multiple blisters and erosions over the whole body for 1 week. At the beginning, she noticed reddish discolorations over her both cheeks and developed severely painful oral ulcer confined only to the palate, making her unable to take any solid food. She consulted a general practitioner (GP) and completed an antibiotic course (cefixime and clindamycin), but there was no improvement. Meanwhile she developed multiple blisters of different sizes and shapes all over the body, first appearing in the right ear, then the face, and later spreading to scalp of head, skin of trunk, and upper and lower extremities. The blisters were initially small with reddish surrounding area, gradually increasing in size and later became eroded. She complained of excessive menstrual bleeding for two times within last 6 months with history of one unit whole blood transfusion. She was a mother of one child, took oral contraceptive pills, and had no bad obstetric history. There was no history of pruritus, involvement of conjunctival mucosa, genital mucosa, epistaxis, dysphagia, malaise, fever, weight loss, arthralgia, photosensitivity, headache, leg edema, abdominal pain or any history of hepatitis. She was nonsmoker and nonalcoholic without any family history of similar skin changes.

On general examination, she was anxious, mildly anemic and vital signs were stable. Integumentary system examination revealed multiple vesiculobullous lesions with denuded area, some tense and flaccid blisters containing clear fluid also with some crust. Bulla-spread sign was positive (extension with regular, rounded border). Mucous membrane of the hard palate had a tender eroded lesion. There was diffuse loss of scalp hair with scarring but nails of all four limbs appeared normal. Other systemic examinations revealed unremarkable findings.

Investigations showed: hemoglobin (Hb)—10.1 g/dL, erythrocyte sedimentation rate (ESR)—15 mm in first hour, white blood cell

(WBC)—14,900/mm^3 (N—70.5%, L—22.7%, M—6.1%), platelet count—242,000/mm^3, PBF—normocytic anemia with fair number of elliptocytes with neutrophilic leukocytosis; Coomb's test- negative; serum creatinine—0.63 mg/dL, serum electrolytes—normal, urine routine examination (RE): pus cell—0-2/hpf, red blood cell (RBC)—nil/hpf, albumin—nil. Liver function tests were normal.

QUESTIONS

1. What could be the clinical diagnosis?
2. What next investigations could be done to reach a diagnosis?

DISCUSSION

After admission, initially the patient was clinically diagnosed and treated as a case of "Stevens–Johnson syndrome" and was referred for dermatological opinion. Dermatologists clinically diagnosed the case as "pemphigus vulgaris" and advised to do a skin biopsy for histopathology and direct immunofluorescence (DIF). Skin biopsy on microscopic examination showed subepidermal bulla with chronic inflammatory reaction in upper dermis. On skin DIF there was linear deposition of C3 in the basement membrane zone without any immunoglobulin G (IgG), IgA or IgM deposition. The histological diagnosis was "bullous pemphigoid." Though the patient was treated according to the diagnosis (with very potent topical steroid), but there was no improvement of her skin condition.

The patient was reviewed and considering the important findings such as reddish discoloration of both cheeks and painful palatal ulcer with scarring alopecia, multiple nontender nonitchy vesiculobullous lesions involving the whole body; it was thought be a connective tissue or autoimmune disorder. Next, autoantibody profiles were done which revealed positive antinuclear antibody (ANA) [both indirect immunofluorescence (IIF) and enzyme-linked immunosorbent assay (ELISA)] and anti-double stranded deoxyribonucleic acid (anti-dsDNA). Extractable nuclear antigen (ENA) profile (immunoblot assay) showed positive anti-Sjögren's syndrome type B (SSB) antibody and anti-small nuclear ribonucleoprotein (snRNP). Antiphospholipid antibody (IgM) was positive and complements were grossly reduced. 24 hours urinary total protein (UTP) was 0.1 g/day.

Final Diagnosis: Bullous Systemic Lupus Erythematosus

Bullous systemic lupus erythematosus (BSLE) is a rare variety of SLE characterized by the rapid development of a widespread vesiculobullous eruption accompanied by pruritus and painful mucosal lesions. Clinically, it is characterized by subepidermal blisters with a predilection for face, upper trunk, and proximal extremities. Lesions can mimic bullous pemphigoid, inflammatory variant of epidermolysis bullosa acquisita, and linear IgA disease.[1]

As BSLE occurs in the setting of SLE-ANA, anti-dsDNA and other ENA profile results generally are positive. Other laboratory abnormalities include low levels of complement (C3, C4 and CH50), Hb, white blood cells and platelets with elevated ESR and proteinuria or cellular casts in urinalysis; some of these were consistent with the laboratory findings of our patient.[2,3]

The therapeutic options for SLE usually do not work well for BSLE; rather the eruptions might flare after systemic corticosteroid administration for SLE. For treatment of BSLE, dapsone is the effective basic therapy, and it often induces a dramatic response: new blister formation ceases in 1-2 days and existing lesions heal within several days. In cases with inadequate response, or when the SLE disease activity index is high, other immunosuppressants, such as prednisolone, methotrexate, and azathioprine, pulse cyclophosphamide, or mycophenolate mofetil can be used. In special cases, where dapsone or other chemical drugs induce serious side effects (hemolysis, hepatotoxicity or nephrotoxicity), or in pregnant ladies (as dapsone is a pregnancy category C drug) biologic agents (infliximab, rituximab, and anakinra) might be chosen for BSLE.[4-6]

REFERENCES

1. Vassileve S. Bullous systemic lupus erythematosus. Clin Dermatol. 2004;22: 129-38.
2. Fujimoto W, Hamada T, Yamada J, Matsuura H, Iwatsuki K. Bullous Systemic Lupus Erythematosus as an Initial Manifestation of SLE. J Dermatol. 2005; 32(12):1021-7.
3. Lee HJ, Yun SJ, Lee SC, Lee JB. A Case of Linear IgA Bullous Dermatosis Associated with Systemic Lupus Erythematosus. Ann Dermatol. 2016;28(5): 660-2.
4. Grover C, Khurana A, Sharma S, Singal A. Bullous systemic lupus erythematosus. Indian J Dermatol. 2013;58(6):492. doi: 10.4103/ 0019-5154.119973.
5. Lalova A, Pramatarov K, Vassileva S. Facial bullous systemic lupus erythematosus. Int J Dermatol. 1997;36:369-71.
6. Duan L, Chen L, Zhong S, et al. Treatment of Bullous Systemic Lupus Erythematosus. J Immunol Res. 2015;2015:167064. doi:10.1155/2015/167064.

CASE 11

YOUNG LADY WITH FEVER AND POLYARTHRITIS

CASE SUMMARY

A 26-year-old woman, primigravida with 18-weeks of pregnancy presented with asymmetrical, migratory polyarthritis for 15 days; low-grade, continued fever for the same duration and generalized weakness for 1 month. Initially her left ankle was involved, then sequentially left knee, right knee, both elbows and multiple small joints of both hands were involved. The pain persisted throughout the day. There was no morning stiffness or back pain. She had low-grade (temperature 99–100 °F), continued fever along with joint pain, not associated with chills, rigors and sweating. There was no recent history of sore throat, rash, oral ulceration, photosensitivity, skin nodule, respiratory, cardiac or urinary complaints. On query, she stated that 15 days back she had watery diarrhea (4-5 times) for 1 day.

On examination, she was found to be febrile (temperature—100°F). A musculoskeletal system examination revealed the presence of inflammatory signs in the left wrist, second and third metacarpophalangeal (MCP) joints of both hands, left first metatarsophalangeal and left knee joint, and only tenderness was present over right wrist, second and third proximal interphalangeal (PIP) joints of the left hand. On left knee joint examination, fluctuation test was positive and movement was restricted.

Investigations showed Hb%—70%, white blood cells (WBCs)—11,500/cumm (N—70%), platelet (PLT)—180,000/cumm, erythrocyte sedimentation rate (ESR) in first hour—60 mm, urine R/M/E: pus cells—12-15/HPF, albumin—trace, urine culture and sensitivity (C/S)—no growth, C-reactive protein (CRP)—133 u/L, rheumatoid factor—negative, anti-cyclic citrullinated peptide (anti-CCP) antibody—negative, human leukocyte antigen (HLA)

B27—negative, electrocardiogram (ECG)—normal study, ultrasonography (USG) of pregnancy profile—12 weeks' pregnancy, serum extractable nuclear antigen (ENA) profile—negative, antistreptolysin O (ASO) titer—400 and 214 (done twice), throat swab for C/S—no growth.

QUESTIONS

1. What is the final diagnosis?
2. What would be the management?

DISCUSSION

Our patient had one major plus two minor criteria which were sufficient to make the diagnosis of rheumatic fever (RF) (Table 1).

She was put on high-dose tablet aspirin (300 mg) four times a day and tablet prednisolone 30 mg daily. After 5 days, she had significant improvement.

Her swelling and pain subsided. She was discharged with tablet penicillin (250 mg) twice daily and asked to have regular follow-ups. The patient's response to high dose aspirin and steroid gave us additional support regarding diagnosis.

Final Diagnosis: Acute Rheumatic Fever

Acute rheumatic fever (ARF) is a sequela of streptococcal infection—typically following 2–3 weeks after Group A streptococcal pharyngitis in a genetically susceptible host. It affects the heart, joints, brain and subcutaneous tissue; however, when affected, heart valves bear the brunt of rheumatic fever (RF).

Like other developing countries, Bangladesh has most of the recognized risk factors, making it a fertile soil for RF and rheumatic heart disease (RHD). Its geographical condition, climate, socioeconomic condition and prevalence of streptococcal infection, are as marked as any other country, where RF is known to be prevalent.

The initial attack of ARF occurs most frequently in persons aged between 6 years and 20 years and rarely occurs in persons older than 30 years.

Physicians have a great role in terms of accurate diagnosis in countries where the disease is prevalent. It is very important that physicians make an accurate diagnosis in ARF patients with their own logic and assessments in addition to using the diagnostic criteria proposed for ARF.

Table 1: Diagnosis of acute rheumatic fever, modified Jones criteria, 2015.[1]	
A. For all patient populations with evidence of preceding group A streptococcal infection (other than chorea)	
Diagnosis: initial ARF	Two major or one major plus two minor manifestations
Diagnosis: recurrent ARF	Two major or one major and two minor or three minor manifestations
B. Major criteria	
Low-risk populations[a]	Moderate- and high-risk populations
Carditis[b] (clinical and/or subclinical)	Carditis[b] (clinical and/or subclinical)
Arthritis (polyarthritis only)	Arthritis (monoarthritis or polyarthritis or polyarthralgia[c])
Chorea	Chorea
Erythema marginatum	Erythema marginatum
Subcutaneous nodules	Subcutaneous nodules
C. Minor criteria	
Low-risk populations[a]	Moderate- and high-risk populations
Polyarthralgia	Monoarthralgia
Fever (≥38.5°C)	Fever (≥38°C)
ESR ≥60 mm/h and/or CRP ≥3 mg/dL[d]	ESR ≥30 mm/h and/or CRP ≥3 mg/dL[d]
Prolonged PR on ECG (for age) (unless carditis is a major criterion)	Prolonged PR on ECG (for age) (unless carditis is a major criterion)

[a] Low-risk populations are those with ARF incidence ≤2/per 100,000 school-aged children or all-age rheumatic heart disease prevalence of ≤1/per 1,000 population per year.
[b] Subclinical carditis is pathological echocardiographic valvulitis.
[c] Polyarthralgia should only be considered as a major manifestation in moderate- to high-risk populations after exclusion of other causes. As in past versions of the criteria, erythema marginatum and subcutaneous nodules are "stand-alone" major criteria. Additionally, joint manifestations can only be considered in either the major or minor categories but not both in the same patient.
[d] CRP value must be greater than upper limit of normal for the laboratory. Also because ESR may evolve during the course of ARF, peak ESR values should be used.
ARF, acute rheumatic fever; CRP, C-reactive protein; ESR, erythrocyte sedimentation rate.

REFERENCE

1. Gewitz MH, Baltimore RS, Tani LY. Revision of the Jones criteria for the diagnosis of acute rheumatic fever in the era of Doppler echocardiography. A scientific statement from the American Heart Association. Circulation. 2015;131:1806-18.

CASE 12

YOUNG BOY WITH RECURRENT ANGIOEDEMA

CASE SUMMARY

A 15-year-old young boy presented with recurrent swelling of the lips for 1.5 years, recurrent dyspnea mostly when sleeping for 1 year and unintended weight gain over the last 1 year (from 70 to 90 kg). He noticed gradual swelling of the lips (predominantly lower lip). It was not associated with swelling in any other part of the body. It was not associated with hives and was also not related with the use of any implicated medications [angiotensin-converting enzyme inhibitors (ACEI) or calcium channel blocker (CCB)]. Later on, he had facial swelling along with lip swelling for which he sought medical attention and was treated with injection hydrocortisone, ranitidine and antihistamine tablets, and was discharged with dexamethasone tablet on a weaning dose for 3 months and was asked to follow up. On follow-up, as improvement was observed, he was asked to continue taking dexamethasone tablets for another 3 months and follow-up. After stopping the medication, his swelling reappeared and he was again admitted in the medicine unit. He had a past history of motor vehicle accident with traumatic brain injury resulting in left-sided weakness and secondary seizure. He received carbamazepine and clobazam tablets, and physiotherapy which allowed good recovery from motor deficit. He was admitted to the hospital in 2013 for respiratory distress and fever, and was labeled as encephalomalacia (post-head injury), epilepsy and bronchial asthma and was managed accordingly. He was not able to go back to school to complete education after the accident. There was no history of similar illness in his family.

On examination, he was overweight having a body mass index (BMI) of 32 kg/m^2 with a noticeable swelling around lips and fissured tongue (Figs. 1A and B). His thyroid and lymphnodes were impalpable. Skin condition was normal except few striae on the abdomen. Nervous system examination revealed that he was oriented to time, place and person. All cranial nerves

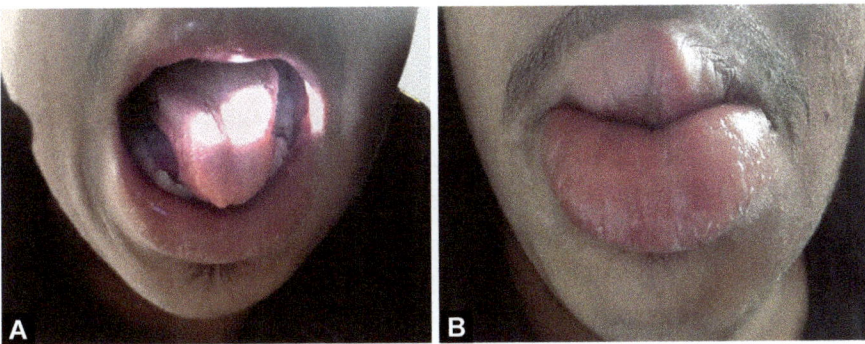

Figs. 1A and B: Fissure in tongue (A) and lip swelling (lower predominant than upper) (B).

were intact. On motor examination muscle bulk and power were normal bilaterally, but tone was increased on left side. All deep tendon reflexes (biceps, triceps, knee, ankle, etc.) were exaggerated, along with extensor plantar response on left side. Patient had hemiplegic gait, and all sensory modalities were intact. Other systemic examinations were unremarkable.

Investigation showed Hb level—14.1 g/dL, white blood cells (WBC)—9,000/cumm (N: 83%), platelet (PLT)—370,000/cumm, erythrocyte sedimentation rate (ESR) in first hour—60 mm, peripheral blood film (PBF)—nonspecific findings, urine R/M/E—normal, immunoglobulin E (IgE)—865 IU/mL (ref: <200), C3—1.28 g/L, C4—0.286 g/L, sputum for Gene Xpert—negative, chest X-ray (CXR) posteroanterior view—normal, immunochromatographic (ICT) for filarial antigen—negative, serum calcium—9.1 mg/dL, angiotensin-converting enzyme (ACE) level—27 U/L, serum cortisol—27 U/L (8-65), thyroid-stimulating hormone (TSH)—6.53 mU/mL, FT3—127.53 ng/dL, FT4—7.10 mU/mL. Video bronchoscopy was done and the findings included edematous epiglottis and laryngeal wall. The pathway was extensively narrow and distorted. Magnetic resonance imaging (MRI) of brain—large encephalomalacic change was noted as evidenced by dilatation of lateral ventricle resulting in atrophy of frontal and right parietal region. Other scanned parts of the brain were unremarkable.

QUESTIONS

1. What are the differential diagnoses?
2. Would you suggest any other investigation?
3. What should be the management?

DISCUSSION

For this boy with encephalomalacia (post-head injury) with secondary epilepsy, our differentials for lip swelling were:

- Recurrent hypersensitivity
- Sarcoidosis
- Vasculitis.

Further investigations included, biopsy of tissue of the upper lip showing non-caseating granulomatous cheilitis, but biopsy from tissue of deltoid muscle showed no granuloma or malignancy.

Final Diagnosis: Melkersson-Rosenthal Syndrome (Orofacial Granulomatosis) with Encephalomalacia (post-head injury) with Secondary Epilepsy

Melkersson-Rosenthal syndrome (MRS) is a rare, inherited neurocutaneous syndrome which may be characterized by three main features: recurrent facial nerve palsy, episodes of swelling of the face and lips, and fissuring of the tongue (formation of deep grooves). The majority of people with MRS only have one or two of these features, rather than all three, leaving the diagnosis difficult.[1] Frequent exacerbations and recurrences are common.

The orofacial swelling is characterized by fissured, reddish-brown, swollen, nonpruritic lips or firm edema of the face. The facial palsy is indistinguishable from Bell's palsy.[2] However, the characteristically important fissured tongue is seen only in one-third to one-half of the patients.

Though MRS is linked genetically as it is an autosomal dominant disease, it is diagnosed mainly clinically. A biopsy of the lips may be needed to confirm the diagnosis in some cases. The histologic findings include noncaseating granulomas.[2] These granulomas are not invariably present, and their absence does not exclude the diagnosis of the MRS.[2]

Differential diagnosis of MRS might be thyroid orbitopathy, allergy, atopy, angioedema, bacterial, viral or filarial infections, systemic lupus erythematosus, dermatomyositis, Bell's palsy, leprosy and rosacea. This syndrome of oral lesions with noncaseating granulomas has also been associated with many connective tissue or inflammatory diseases like Crohn's disease, sarcoidosis, etc.[3]

Treatment for MRS aims to relieve symptoms, but the effectiveness of current treatment options has not been well established.[4] Treatment options may include medications to reduce swelling (such as nonsteroidal anti-inflammatory drugs and corticosteroids), antibiotics, immunosuppressants, surgery (to relieve pressure on the facial nerves and reduce swelling) and facial rehabilitation (which may involve physiotherapy and speech-language therapy).[5]

We treated our patient with intralesional triamcinolone along with oral minocycline and metronidazole and observed significant improvement (Fig. 2).

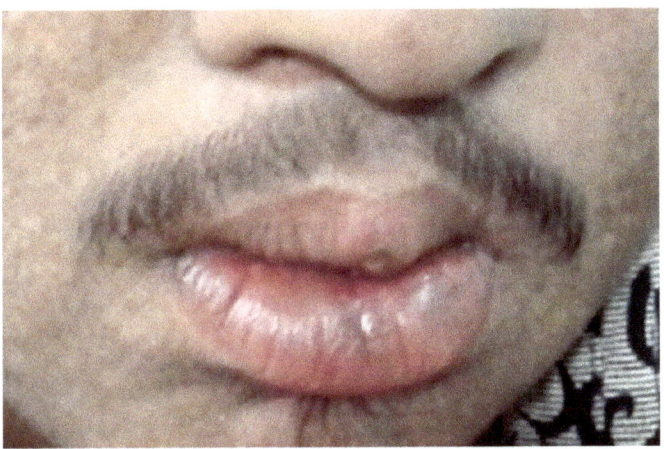

Fig. 2: Significant improvement of lip swelling after the treatment.

REFERENCES

1. Pei Y, Beaman GM, Mansfield D, Clayton-Smith J, Stewart M, Newman WG. Clinical and genetic heterogeneity in Melkersson-Rosenthal syndrome. Eur J Med Genet. 2018 Sep 11 [Epub ahead of print]. Available from: https://www.sciencedirect.com/science/article/pii/S176972121830394X.
2. Rogers RS 3rd. Melkersson-Rosenthal syndrome and orofacial granulomatosis. Dermatol Clin. 1996;14(2):371-9.
3. Desai SD, Dumraliya P, Mehta D. Melkersson-Rosenthal syndrome. J Neurosci Rural Pract [Serial online]. 2014 [cited 2018 Oct 16];5(Suppl S1):112-4. Available from: http://www.ruralneuropractice.com/text.asp?2014/5/5/112/145258.
4. Wehl G, Rauchenzauner M. A systematic review of the literature of the three related disease entities cheilitis granulomatosa, orofacial granulomatosis and Melkersson-Rosenthal syndrome. Curr Pediatr Rev. 2018 May 14 [Epub ahead of print]. Available from: https://www.ncbi.nlm.nih.gov/pubmed/29766816.
5. Melkersson-Rosenthal syndrome. Facial Palsy UK [online]. Available from: https://www.facialpalsy.org.uk/causesanddiagnoses/melkersson-rosenthal-syndrome/ [Accessed Apr 4 2017].

CASE 13

YOUNG BOY WITH BIZARRE-LOOKING CHEST AND ABDOMEN

CASE SUMMARY

An 18-year-old boy presented with a history of progressive nodular swellings over anterior and posterior thoracic wall, and upper abdomen for 4 years. The nodules transformed to painful pustules and spread circumferentially in the chest wall and abdomen, and started draining purulent, non-sanguineous fluid. Crops of pustules healed with ulceration but eruption of new pustules occurred across the periphery. He visited multiple care settings and received a course of oral doxycycline and cefadroxil with no significant improvement. He was also given vitamin C and acetaminophen for his pain. Approximately 4 months prior to his admission in our care, he developed acute lower limb edema, jaundice and abdominal pain with distension.

On examination, he was cachexic, anemic, icteric, febrile (temperature 102 °F), with tachycardia, bipedal pitting edema. There was a diffuse patch of extensive tender nodules with purulent discharge over the anterior, right thoracic region, extending to the back and upper abdomen above the umbilicus. The older crop of pustules were ulcerated. Skin thickening was present. Scanty, purulent discharge was noted from the newer, peripheral lesions (Fig. 1). A few crops of similar pustular lesions were also observed in bilateral shin area. On abdominal examination, diffuse tenderness was present. There was evidence of ascites. There were no stigmata of chronic liver disease. Respiratory system examination revealed diminished breath sound in lower part of the chest bilaterally.

The patient had microcytic hypochromic anemia with Hb%—9.8 g/dL, white blood cells (WBCs)—23,000/cumm (N: 85%, L: 8%), platelet (PLT)—230,000/cumm, erythrocyte sedimentation rate (ESR) in first hour—20 mm, urine R/M/E—trace albumin, sugar—nil, serum electrolytes were normal, except serum potassium which was 2.9 mmol, albumin—15 g/L, serum bilirubin—8.62 mg/dL, alanine aminotransferase (ALT)—91 IU/L, aspartate aminotransferase (AST)—30 IU/L, alkaline phosphatase—442 IU/L,

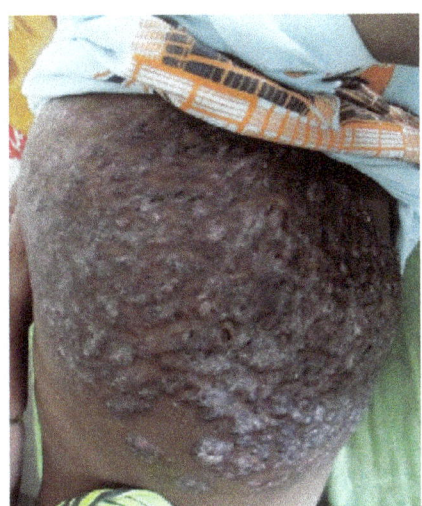

Fig. 1: Inspection of chest and upper abdomen revealed diffuse nodules, pustules, ulceration and scanty purulent discharge.

prothrombin time (PT)—18.99 seconds, international normalized ratio (INR)—1.59, chest X-ray (CXR) posteroanterior view—bilateral pleural effusion with pulmonary venous congestion. Fibrotic ring on the right middle lobe with patchy opacification and volume loss. Blood C/S—negative, antinuclear antibody (ANA)—negative, ascitic fluid study showed WBC—150/uL [polymorphonuclear neutrophils (PMN)—40%, L-60%], few red blood cells (RBCs), Gram stain was negative for any organism, negative for acid-fast bacilli (AFB). Ultrasonography (USG) of W/A—extensive free fluid collection in the peritoneal cavity, with the liver pushed caudally. Liver span was 7 cm, liver parenchyma was coarse and nonhomogeneous with no focal lesions present. Spleen size was 12.6 cm, parenchyma of both kidney was echogenic with poor corticomedullary differentiation. Gallbladder was thick-walled and contracted. Hepatic elastography showed a fibrosis score 25.7 kPA (>9.3 is indicative of fibrosis and >12.3 indicates cirrhosis). The patient was diagnosed with stage F4 cirrhosis (predominantly fibrosis) by elastography. The upper gastrointestinal (GI) endoscopy was normal. Computed tomography (CT) scan of chest showed focal consolidation in the right lower lobe with surrounding pleural thickening with subpleural fat infiltration, septal wall thickening and chest wall infiltration with compression of right lung parenchyma. Sputum culture and sensitivity revealed presence of *Enterobacter*.

QUESTIONS

1. What should be the next investigation?
2. What is the final diagnosis?

DISCUSSION

This young boy with progressive purulent discharging sinus followed by skin fibrosis with involvement of chest and abdominal wall, respiratory system, and liver had a strong possibility of having systemic deep fungal infection, or systemic bacterial infection like melioidosis or polymicrobial infection. To reach a definite diagnosis, we planned for skin biopsy.

An initial biopsy of the skin pustule showed neutrophils in the stratum corneum. Subepithelium showed granulation tissue infiltrated by acute and chronic inflammatory cells and colonies of actinomyces. Few giant cells were present. A repeat skin biopsy showed abscess cavity in the dermis lined by granulation tissue. Abscess contained colonies of actinomycetes surrounded by suppuration. A third and final biopsy of the dermis at different sites on the thorax showed sinus tract with granulation tissue, dense acute and chronic inflammatory cells. No granuloma or malignancy was seen.

Final Diagnosis: Disseminated Actinomycosis (Pulmonary, Chest Wall, Skin and Subdiaphragmatic Extension Leading to Hepatic Involvement)

Actinomycosis is a rare, slowly progressive disease caused by various species of the *Actinomyces* genus, most commonly *Actinomyces israelii*, a filamentous, microaerophilic, gram-positive bacterium. After cervicofacial actinomycosis, pulmonary infection is the second most common manifestation of this disease accounting for 15-45% of all cases.[1] Thoracic, abdominal and cardiac involvements are also seen but are exceedingly rare in incidence. It can mimic malignancy.

Actinomycosis presents with a bimodal age distribution with a peak between ages 11 and 20, and a second peak in the fourth and fifth decades. Incidence is 2-4 times greater in males compared with females, possibly due to higher incidence of facial trauma and poorer oral hygiene in males.[1]

Depending on the site of infection, most cases of actinomycosis are accompanied by multiple other microorganisms found on culture which do not necessarily need to be treated separately. Actinomycosis can also coexist with lung cancer as the bacteria preferentially colonize devitalized tissue that can be present in necrotic neoplasms. In liver, actinomycosis causes extensive fibrosis which can be seen as stage 4 in elastography.

Diagnosis thus requires a combination of physical findings of fever, weight loss, cachexia, chest pain, dyspnea and jaundice; imaging; lab work and biopsy from involving sites.

Recommended treatment with clinically proven efficacy includes intravenous (IV) penicillin G 150,000 U/kg/day to 200,000 U/kg/day divided three times a day or four times a day for 4-6 weeks. This is followed by a prolonged PO penicillin V 2 g/day to 4 g/day course divided 3-4 times daily for an additional 6–12 months. The tetracycline/doxycycline, erythromycin and clindamycin may also be used if there is a penicillin allergy.[1]

As the penicillin was not available at the time of diagnosis, the selection of antibiotics in our case was a combination of amoxicillin–clavulanic acid and clindamycin, both were shown to have clinical efficacy and success in clinical trials in the past. After initiation of antibiotics, there was a sustainable response of reduction in liver enzymes and bilirubin came back to normal. Although hepatic actinomycosis commonly presented with hepatic abscess on presentation, in this case we found extensive fibrosis (confirmed on fibroscan) indicating prolonged involvement of hepatic parenchyma mimicking cirrhosis.

Surgery remains an important therapeutic adjunct with antibiotics and may be required if complications are present, including well-defined abscess, empyema, life-threatening hemoptysis or in blocked discharging fistulas that need surgical opening.

Prognosis of disseminated actinomycosis involving pulmonary and hepatic tissue is usually less favorable compared with the cervicofacial and abdominal forms.

REFERENCE

1. Valour F, Sénéchal, Dupieux AC, Karsenty, JK, Lustig, Breton PS, Ferry, T. Actinomycosis: etiology, clinical features, diagnosis, treatment, and management. Infect Drug Resist; 2014. pp. 183–97. doi:10.2147/IDR.S39601.

CASE 14

YOUNG MAN WITH RECURRENT EPISODES OF LEFT-SIDED WEAKNESS

CASE SUMMARY

A 38-year-old man got admitted with complaints of sudden left-sided weakness for the last 20 days, slurring of speech for the same duration and history of low-grade intermittent fever before the development of weakness which lasted for 3 days. Following complete resolution of fever, he developed left-sided weakness predominantly in the upper limb which was gradually progressive, associated with mild pain which improved after taking analgesics and application of hot compression. He faced difficulties in performing daily activities with his left upper limb, for example, lifting up objects, dressing up, etc. He also complained of slurring of speech and difficulty in walking but could walk by himself without the aid of others. On query, he gave history of urge incontinence, mild burning sensation and increased frequency of micturition which persisted for a week along with weakness. With these complaints, he was diagnosed as a case of stroke by a local doctor, was treated accordingly; and was referred to a tertiary care hospital. He had history of similar type of illness 4 years back (fever followed by left-sided weakness, slurring of speech, and tendency to fall). For this reason, he was immediately hospitalized. Later, he developed disorientation followed by irrelevant talk and aggressive behavior. A computed tomography (CT) scan was done (the reports of which the patient's attendants could not provide). With treatment, his condition gradually improved and he could walk on his own. His illness was not associated with convulsion, visual problem, nasal regurgitation, dysphagia, muscle wasting, and tingling, numbness.

On examination, the vitals were normal. Nervous system examination revealed dysarthric speech and intact cranial nerve, muscle power was 3/5 in the left lower limb, knee jerk was absent bilaterally with normal ankle jerk, plantar responses were bilaterally equivocal without any clonus. The rest of the neurological examinations including the fundoscopic examination were normal. All other systemic examinations revealed normal findings.

Investigations showed Hb —13.70 g/dL; white blood cells (WBCs)—20,000/cumm (N: 90%, L: 10%); platelet (PLT)—190,000/cumm; erythrocyte sedimentation rate (ESR) in first hour—20 mm; urine R/M/E—normal; fasting blood sugar (FBS)—6.8 mmol/L; lipid profile: total cholesterol—235 mg/dL, TG—199 mg/dL, HDL_c—49 mg/dL, LDL_c—146.2 mg/dL. Serum creatinine, electrolytes, C-reactive protein (CRP) levels were within normal limit. Electrocardiography (ECG) and chest X-ray (CXR) posteroanterior view were also normal. CT scan of head showed bilateral acute cerebral infarct; cerebrospinal fluid (CSF) study revealed total WBC—2/cumm (L: 100%), protein—39 mg/dL, sugar—145.62 mg/dL; adenosine deaminase (ADA)—1.67 U/L.

QUESTIONS

1. What further investigation should be done?
2. What is the final diagnosis?

DISCUSSION

We performed the following investigations:
- Magnetic resonance imaging (MRI) of brain—few variable-sized (3–1.5 cm) T1 hypo and fluid-attenuated inversion recovery (FLAIR) hyperintense areas seen in paraventricular and subcortical fronto-parieto-temporal regions. The lesions show restricted diffusion in diffusion-weighted imaging (DWI) and high signal in corresponding apparent diffusion coefficient (ADC) map (Fig. 1).
- An MRI of the cervical spine with screening of the whole spine was insignificant.
- CSF was sent for oligoclonal band—no oligoclonal band was seen.
- Visual evoked potential was found to be negative.

On the basis of his signs and symptoms, and MRI findings, a diagnosis of **multiple sclerosis** was made. He was given injection methylprednisolone (1 g) daily for 5 days and his condition dramatically improved after the course of treatment. There was no residual neurological deficit.

Final Diagnosis: Multiple Sclerosis (MS)—Relapsing and Remitting Type

Multiple sclerosis is an autoimmune demyelinating disorder of the central nervous system (CNS).

There are several common presentations of MS, and relapsing-remitting MS is one of them.

Diagnostic criteria for MS include both clinical, radiological and laboratory assessments emphasizing the need to demonstrate dissemination of lesions in space (DIS) and time (DIT) and to exclude alternative diagnoses.

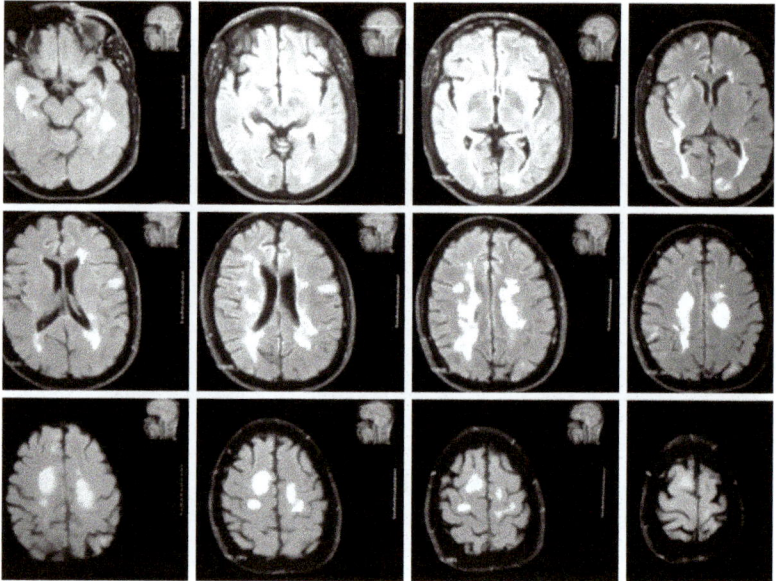

Fig. 1: MRI of brain showing hyperintense lesions in cortex, periventricular area and infratentorial area.

Although the diagnosis can be made on clinical grounds alone, MRI of the CNS can support, supplement or even replace some clinical criteria.[1]

The MS is not a curable disease. During the acute attacks, administration of high doses of intravenous corticosteroids, such as methylprednisolone, is the usual therapy. Several disease-modifying treatments have an important role. However, physiotherapy and other supportive therapy are often necessary.

REFERENCE

1. Polman CH, Reingold SC, Banwell B, et al. Diagnostic criteria for multiple sclerosis: 2010 revisions to the McDonald criteria. Anal Neurol. 2011;68:292-302.

CASE 15

YOUNG BOY WITH ARTHRALGIA AND ABDOMINAL PAIN

CASE SUMMARY

A 16-year-old immunized boy, fifth child of non-consanguineous marriage presented with complaints of recurrent abdominal pain, and fever for 8 months, and polyarthralgia for the last 6 months. The pain was in the upper abdomen, moderate in intensity, dull-aching, without any radiation, aggravated after taking meal. But there was no specific relieving factor. He had low-grade relapsing fever for same duration. The maximum recorded temperature was 100°F without chills and rigors, and subsided with paracetamol. Fever persisted for 4–5 days followed by a gap of 10–14 days in between two bouts. It was associated with anorexia and generalized weakness which was gradually increasing in severity. He experienced asymmetric joint pain, predominantly involving wrist, elbow and knee involvement for last 6 months. There was no history of headache, convulsion, skin rash, Raynaud's phenomenon, weight loss, bowel or bladder abnormality. He mentioned traveling to Sirajganj (in north-central part of Bangladesh) 2–3 times per year. He used to live in tin-shed muddy house. There was a cowshed beside his house.

On examination, he was undernourished having body mass index (BMI): 14.2 kg/m^2, moderately anemic, non-icteric, pyrexic (temperature—100°F). No lymphadenopathy was found. On systemic examination, there was an evidence of non-tender hepatomegaly, which was 4 cm from right costal margin, firm in consistency, surface was smooth, liver span was 14 cm, no hepatic bruit; also there was non-tender splenomegaly about 4 cm from the left costal margin toward right iliac fossa, firm in consistency. Other systemic examinations were unremarkable.

Investigations showed: Hb level—7.6 g/dL; white blood cells (WBCs)—3,000/cumm (N: 57%, L: 34%); platelet (PLT) count—160,000/cumm; erythrocyte sedimentation rate (ESR) in first hour—25 mm; peripheral blood film (PBF)—hypochromasia, aniso-poikilocytosis, target cells, tear drop cells and leptocytes; iron profile: serum ferritin—535.13 mcg/L, total iron-binding capacity (TIBC)—175 mcg/dL, iron—28 mcg/dL; thyroid-stimulating hormone (TSH)—2.54 U/mL; urine R/M/E—normal; serum creatinine—0.67 mg/dL; serum bilirubin—0.4 mg/dL; alanine aminotransferase (ALT)—20 U/L; prothrombin time (PT)—14.2 sec; international normalized ratio (INR)—1.22; MT—negative; immunochromatographic test (ICT) for kala-azar—negative; rk39—negative; ICT for malaria—negative; rheumatoid factor (RA) test—negative; antinuclear antibody (ANA) and Coombs test (direct and indirect)—negative; chest X-ray (CXR) posteroanterior view—normal; ultrasonography (USG) of W/A—hepatosplenomegaly; contracted gallbladder with cholelithiasis.

QUESTIONS

1. What are the possible differential diagnoses?
2. How would you proceed to reach diagnosis?
3. Mention one investigation which will give the diagnostic clue.
4. How would you manage this case?

DISCUSSION

Since this boy with fever and hepatosplenomegaly had history of travel to kala-azar endemic zone (Sirajganj), we searched for kala-azar first. But as rk39 was negative, we considered several other differentials: hemolytic anemia—hereditary or acquired, disseminated tuberculosis, juvenile idiopathic arthritis (systemic onset).

For further evaluation of the PBF finding, we went for Hb electrophoresis- which came up with the following findings:

- *Hemoglobin (Hb) electrophoresis:* HbF: 20.4%, Hb S/D: 76.7%, HbA2: 2.9%; final comment: Hb S/D Punjab.
- *Repeat Hb electrophoresis:* HbF: 17.4%, Hb S/D: 79.7%, HbA2: 2.9%; comment: Homozygous hemoglobin S disease.
- *Sickling test:* Under controlled hypoxic condition smear showed >90% sickle cells (Fig. 1).

These tests were conclusive to put the diagnosis of sickle cell disease in our index patient. But as there was no consanguinity between parents, we decided to go for DNA test for unequivocal confirmation of cases and trait.

- *DNA analysis of patient:* Homozygous for codon 6 mutation (GAG > GTG). This mutation produces single base substitution at the 17th nucleotide of the first exon of beta globin gene converting a codon for glutamic acid (GAG) to a codon for valine (GTG). The individual was therefore predicted to be affected by sickle cell anemia.
- *Parent's screening:* Both parents were sickle cell (HbS) trait.

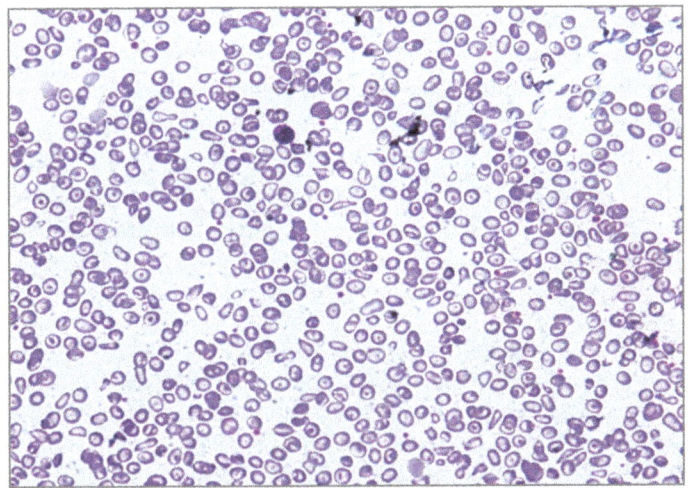

Fig. 1: Peripheral blood film (PBF) showing sickle cells in sickling test.

Final Diagnosis: Sickle Cell (HbSS) Anemia with Cholelithiasis

We treated the case with hydroxyurea tablet, and his condition improved symptomatically.

Sickle cell disease (SCD) typically originates from the substitution of a valine for glutamic acid at position 6 in the beta-subunit of Hb. The predominant clinical presentations of SCD include chronic hemolytic anemia and vaso-occlusive crisis. However, other manifestations may include aplastic crisis and multiple organ infarctions resulting from widespread vascular occlusion. A vaso-occlusive crisis results from the obstruction of microcirculation by sickled red blood cells (RBCs), leading to ischemic injury and resultant pain. The pain can affect any body part. The acute chest syndrome is a vaso-occlusive crisis of the pulmonary vasculature commonly seen in people with sickle cell anemia. Renal papillary necrosis is typically associated with vaso-occlusion, leading to isosthenuria (i.e., inability to concentrate urine). Involvement of the central nervous system can have devastating consequences in SCD patients. For instance, the most severe manifestation is stroke, resulting in varying degrees of neurological deficit. The heart is involved due to chronic anemia and microinfarcts. Cholelithiasis is a common manifestation in children with SCD, as chronic hemolysis with hyperbilirubinemia is associated with the formation of bile stones. The other important clinical features might be leg ulcer and priaprism which lead to male impotency. Universally, as anemia is chronic and hemolytic in nature, it is usually well tolerated but infection caused by parvovirus B-19 (B19V) can potentially lead to aplastic crisis. Splenic sequestration may occur independent of age of the individuals with other sickle syndromes.[1] Sickle cells block blood flow to spleen causing scarring and eventual atrophy of the organ.

Electrophoresis confirms the diagnosis with the presence of homozygous HbS and can also document other hemoglobinopathies (e.g., HbSC, Hb S-beta+ thalassemia). Blood transfusions are reserved for sudden, severe anemia due to acute splenic sequestration, parvovirus B19 infection or hyperhemolytic crises. SCD may be treated with multiple medications. Stem cell transplantation can be curative.[2]

REFERENCES

1. Saad AA, Beshlawi I, Al-Rawas AH, Zachariah M, Nazir HF, Wali Y. Human parvovirus B19 in children with sickle cell disease; poking the spleen. Oman Med J. 2017;32(5):425-8. doi: 10.5001/omj.2017.79.
2. Archer N, Galacteros F, Brugnara C. Clinical trials update in sickle cell anemia. Am J Hematol. 2015;90:934-50.

CASE 16

YOUNG MAN WITH HARD MASS IN ABDOMEN

CASE SUMMARY

A 23-year-old gentleman presented with upper abdominal pain and fullness in the right side for 2½ months. The pain was gradual in onset, intermittent, cramping, more during night with radiation to back (right side). It was aggravated with movement and partially relieved by taking pain killer. He also complained of anorexia and weight loss about 12 kg in 2 months. He experienced right sided, continued, band-like headache without having any radiation. There was no specific aggravating factors but it was partially relieved by pain killer. He also complained of occasional palpitation and feverish feeling although it was not documented. His bowel and bladder habit was normal.

On examination, his blood pressure was found to be persistently high on multiple times but there was no postural drop. There was evidence of tender hepatomegaly which was about 4.5 cm from the right costal margin, firm-hard in consistency, surface was nodular, margin was irregular, upper border of liver dullness was found in right fourth intercostal space, with no hepatic bruit. Another slightly tender mass was found in the right lumbar region about 3 × 3 cm, hard in consistency, surface was smooth, did not move with respiration. Respiratory system examination revealed dullness from right fourth intercostal space to downward with diminished breath sound. Other findings were unremarkable.

Investigations showed, hemoglobin (Hb%)—11.4 g/dL, WBC—9,000/mm^3 (N—78%, L—12%, E—1%), platelets—340,000/mm^3, ESR in first hour—120 mm, PBF showed microcytic hypochromic anemia, urine R/M/E—occasional RBC/HPF, serum creatinine—0.7 mg/dL, serum bilirubin—0.6 mg/dL, serum albumin—22 g/L, SGPT—10 U/L, SGOT—75 U/L, PT with INR 20.60 sec, 1.73, alkaline phosphatase—59 U/L, AFP—1.24 ng/mL, HBsAg—negative, anti-HCV—negative, serum CA 19.9—11.9 U/mL, serum CEA—0.62 ng/mL, USG of whole abdomen illustrated—mass in the right lobe of liver suggestive of hepatoma.

QUESTION

1. What are the possible diagnoses?
2. What further investigation can be done to reach final diagnosis?

DISCUSSION

Initially it seemed to be a case of hepatic malignancy (primary or secondary). Further investigations showed:
- *Computed tomography (CT) scan of whole abdomen with contrast:* Right-sided adrenal mass with hepatic invasion.
- *Fine-needle aspiration cytology (FNAC) from right suprarenal gland:* Positive for malignant cells suggestive of neuroblastoma.
- *FNAC from liver mass:* Positive for malignant cells suggestive of metastatic neuroblastoma.
- *24 hours metanephrine in urine:* 1,150 nmol/day (normal).

Final Diagnosis: Adrenal Neuroblastoma with Hepatic Metastasis

The patient received one cycle of chemotherapy. But his condition deteriorated rapidly and he expired before starting the second cycle.

Neuroblastomas are aggressive, malignant tumors derived from primitive neural crest cells. Although it is a childhood tumor occurring in infants and young children, few cases have also been found in adolescence period. The tumors are still classed as a medical rarity in adulthood (20 years of age or older). The most common locations for primary diseases in adult are abdomen (about 40% in adrenal gland and 25% in paraspinal glands), followed by the thorax, pelvis, occasionally head and neck and extremities.[1]

Clinical presentation depends on the location of the primary tumor and extent of tumor. It comprises asymptomatic abdominal mass, various neurological features like paralysis, bowel and bladder dysfunction if arising from paraspinal sympathetic ganglia, Horner's syndrome if located in the posterior mediastinum. It can produce paraneoplastic features like watery diarrhea, opsoclonus, myoclonic jerk, rapid eye movement. Metastasis especially to the liver, skin and bone marrow can be a presenting feature. Fever, anemia, weight loss and fatigue are less common.[2]

Our patient had metastatic lesion in the liver with anorexia and weight loss. In addition there was an ill-defined abdominal mass. Hypertension is not that common however was present in our case, which is thought to be caused by compression of renal arteries by the mass.

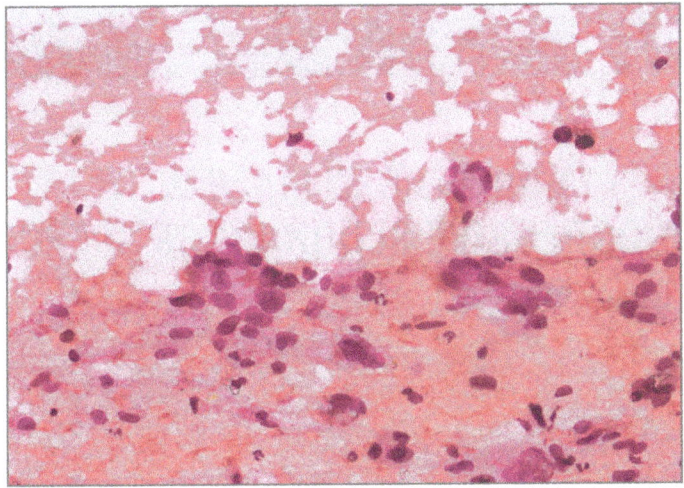

Fig. 1: Pseudorosettes pattern of neuroblastoma.

Diagnosis depends on abdominal imaging and laboratory markers. Histopathology and immunohistochemistry are the gold standard for the diagnosis of neuroblastoma. Microscopic appearances vary but synchronous differentiation of nucleus and abundant, eosinophilic/amphophilic cytoplasm along with Homer-Wright pseudorosettes pattern are characteristics of neuroblastoma.[2] This striking pseudorosettes pattern was found in our case (Fig. 1).

Careful observation, surgery, chemotherapy, radiotherapy or stem cell transplantation are different modalities which can be employed in the treatment.

REFERENCES

1. Das A, Datta A. Adult onset neuroblastoma, presenting as pleural effusion: a rare entity. J Assoc Chest Physicians [serial online] 2014;2:43-6.
2. Franks, Loraine M, Bollen, Andrew, Seeger, Robert C, Stram, Daniel O; Matthay, Katherine K. "Neuroblastoma in adults and adolescents". Cancer. 1997;79(10):2028-35.

CASE 17

MIDDLE-AGED MALE WITH PROGRESSIVE SLURRING OF SPEECH

CASE SUMMARY

A 55-year-old male presented with progressive slurring of speech for 2.5 years and tremor in the hands for 2 years. His speech was indistinct, rapid, low volume and difficult to understand but it was not associated with dribbling of saliva, nasal regurgitation, hoarseness of voice or swallowing difficulty. There was no history of fever, headache, vomiting, head injury, unconsciousness and seizure disorder; no limb weakness or visual impairment. Six months later, he experienced action tremor in both hands and also noticed clumsiness of his daily activities like eating, drinking, combing, writing, etc. For the same duration, he had been suffering from pain in the lower back which was dull aching in nature, nonprogressive and localized. There was no associated lower limb weakness or paresthesia; bowel and bladder habits were normal. Later he consulted with a neurologist and was treated as a case of ischemic stroke with newly detected hypothyroidism. Patient was nondiabetic, normotensive, with unremarkable past medical history.

On examination, he was well behaved, cooperative with average body build. His pulse rate was 76 beats/min and blood pressure was 120/70 mm Hg. On nervous system examination, his higher psychic function was normal except non-specific slurring of speech. Mini-mental state examination score was 28 out of 30. Bulk and power of the muscle was normal but tone of the muscle was increased in both upper and lower limbs. All reflexes were exaggerated and plantar was bilaterally extensor. Action tremor was present in both hands. Sensory modalities were intact, cerebellar function was normal with no sign of meningeal irritation. Examination of spine was unremarkable and there was no feature of nerve root compression. All other systemic examination revealed no abnormality.

Investigations showed Hb: 15.40 g/dL, erythrocyte sedimentation rate (ESR) 07 mm in first hour, red blood cell (RBC), white blood cell (WBC) and platelets were normal in amount and distribution. His creatinine and electrolytes were within normal range. Serum calcium was 9.93 mg/dL; inorganic phosphate was 2.90 mg/dL and serum albumin was 4.82 g/dL. Intact parathyroid hormone (PTH) was 43.80 pg/mL; vitamin D level was 18.50 ng/mL; thyroid stimulating hormone (TSH) was 82.40 IU/mL; free T3—2.18 pg/mL and T4—0.62 ng/mL; antithyroid peroxidase (TPO) antibody was negative; serum ceruloplasmin—200 mg/L; 24 hours urinary copper less than 20.2 µg/L. His antinuclear antibodies (ANA), cytoplasmic antineutrophil cytoplasmic antibodies (cANCA), perinuclear antineutrophil cytoplasmic antibodies (pANCA) were all negative; chest X-ray posteroanterior (P/A) view and ECG were normal. Magnetic resonance imaging (MRI) screening of whole spine showed extruded disk with posterolateral osteophytosis at L4/5 levels which was the reason for thecal sac indentation and ultimately caused spinal canal stenosis. Computed tomography (CT) scan of head revealed extensive bilateral and symmetrical calcification in both paraventricular white matter, basal ganglia, cerebellum (dentate nucleus), pons and midbrain (Figs. 1 to 4).

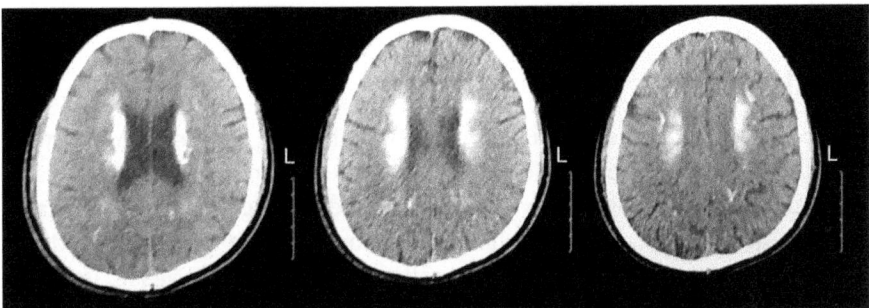

Fig. 1: Calcification in paraventricular white matter.

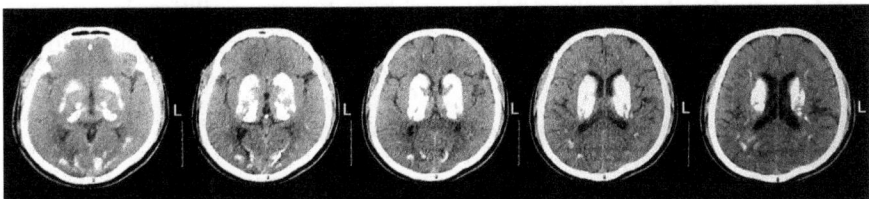

Fig. 2: Calcification in basal ganglia.

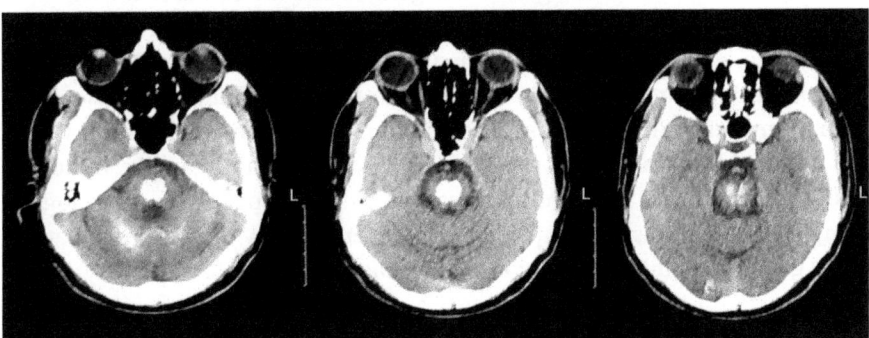

Fig. 3: Calcification in pons and midbrain.

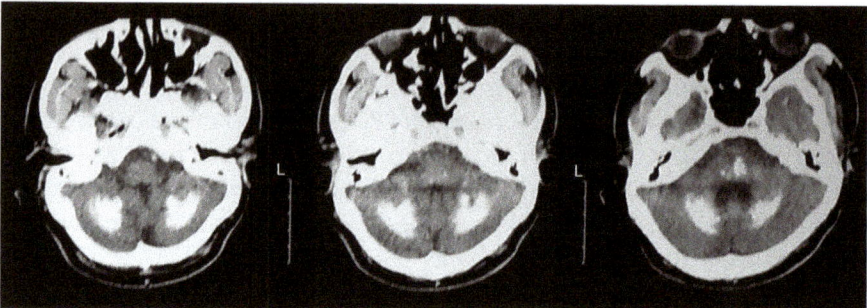

Fig. 4: Calcification in cerebellum.

QUESTIONS

1. What would be the most appropriate explanation of calcification?
2. How can we reach a clinical diagnosis?

DISCUSSION

Clinically we diagnosed our case as Parkinson's plus syndrome with hypothyroidism, and our differentials were metabolic encephalopathy and multiple sclerosis (progressive variant). But after seeing investigations that is CT scan showing extensive calcification we considered hypoparathyroidism, pseudohypoparathyroidism, hyperparathyroidism, Fahr's disease, and calcification in HIV encephalopathy. Though patient was 55 years old, senile calification is usually not this much extensive, and our patient did not have any feature of HIV infection- ruling out these two possibilities. In our case serum calcium and serum PTH level were completely normal which excluded hypo- or hyperparathyroidism.

Final Diagnosis: Fahr's Disease with Hypothyroidism

Fahr's disease is a rare, autosomal dominant, inherited neurological disorder characterized by abnormal deposits of calcium in areas of the brain that control movement, including the basal ganglia and the cerebral cortex.[1]

The diagnosis of Fahr's disease is complex and requires both clinical and radiological evidence. The criteria include bilateral calcification of the basal ganglia with neuropsychiatric and/or extrapyramidal features associated with normal calcium and phosphate metabolism.[2] These calcifications which are usually idiopathic occur most commonly at the basal ganglia, but other structures may also be affected.[2] Patients exhibit progressive neurological symptoms such as seizures, rigidity, and dementia with classical bilateral basal ganglia calcification shown on CT imaging.[3]

Exclusion of infective, metabolic, toxic, or traumatic causes is critical and a family history is commonly described. Laboratory examinations in the suspected cases of Fahr's disease should include tests for blood calcium and parathyroid hormone. This will help differentiate idiopathic Fahr's disease (unremarkable laboratory test results) from secondary cases especially due to hypoparathyroidism. Some authors have used the term Fahr's syndrome to describe the basal ganglia calcification, which is secondary to some other disorders such as hypoparathyroidism.[4,5]

The treatment for Fahr's disease targets symptomatic support and improvement in the quality of life.[6] Treatment of the underlying disease process may lead to a marginal improvement in neuropsychiatric features. Prognosis is variable, unpredictable, and is unrelated to the extent of calcification.[7] Use of haloperidol or lithium carbonate has been reported to help in patients with psychotic symptoms.[7]

REFERENCES

1. Otu AA, Anikwe JC, Cocker D. Fahr's disease: a rare neurological presentation in a tropical setting. Clin Case Rep. 2015;3(10):806-8. doi:10.1002/ccr3.349
2. Trautner RI, Cummings IL, Read SL. Benson DF. Idiopathic basal ganglia calcification and organic mood disorder. Am J Psychiatry. 1988;145:350-3.
3. Taxer F, Halter R. Konig P. Clinical early symptoms and CT-Scan findings in Fahr syndrome. Nervenarzt. 1986;57:583-8.
4. Guerreiro MM. Scotoni AE. Calcifications dosgânglios da base nainfância. Arq. Neuropsiquiatr. 1992;50:513-8.
5. Oliveira JR, Spiteri E, Sobrido MJ, Hopfer S, Klepper J, Voit T, et al. Genetic heterogeneity in familial idiopathic basal ganglia calcification (Fahr disease) Neurology. 2004;63:2165-7.
6. Senoglu M, Tuncel D, Orhan FO, Yuksel Z. Gokce M. Fahr's syndrome: a report of two cases. Firat Tip Dergisi. 2007;12:70-2.
7. Rastogi R, Singh AK, Rastogi UC, Chander Mohan C. Vaibhav Rastogi V. Fahr's syndrome: a rare clinico-radiologic entity. Med J Armed Forces India. 2011;67:159-61.

CASE 18

FEBRILE MIDDLE-AGED MAN WITH HIP AND ABDOMINAL PAIN

CASE SUMMARY

A 45-year-old man was admitted in the hospital with complaints of left-sided hip pain for 5 years, irregular fever for 2 years and upper abdominal pain for 2 months. His hip pain was gradual in onset, dull aching with radiation to back which was aggravated with daily activities and partially relieved by pain killers. Occasionally, he experienced pain in left lower part of the chest and right hip. The fever was initially low grade and irregular, and later on became high grade, which was relieved by taking antipyretic. He also experienced dull aching and intermittent upper abdominal pain, which was gradual in onset, and associated with nausea and vomiting. He complained of anorexia and weight loss. On query, he gave past history of thoracic surgery though he could not mention the underlying disease. Then we searched for medical documents, and the patient provided us previous reports of imagings of chest and abdomen which included chest X-ray posteroanterior view showing a mass arising from right third rib with extension in chest wall. Computed tomography (CT) guided fine needle aspiration cytology (FNAC) from right-sided bony (rib) swelling revealed giant-cell tumor. CT scan of chest including bony window was suggestive of neoplastic bone lesion (Fig. 1).

On examination, he was ill-looking, cachectic, severely anemic and febrile (101°F). Examination of abdomen revealed evidence of slightly tender hepatomegaly of about 2 cm from right costal margin, firm in consistency, with smooth surface, regular margin, without any hepatic bruit. Another ill-defined tender mass was found in the area involving left hypochondrium, part of epigastric and lumbar regions, which was soft in consistency and its surface was smooth. Examination of respiratory system revealed presence of a horizontal scar mark in the right upper part of the chest. The rest of the findings were normal. GALS (Gait, Arms, Legs, Spine) screening revealed limping gait, pain and restricted movement during flexion, external rotation and internal rotation of the left hip joint.

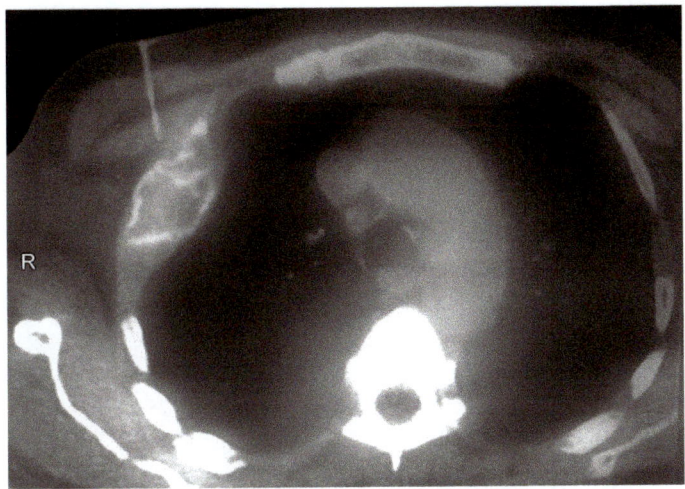

Fig. 1: CT scan of chest including bony window, suggestive of neoplastic bone lesion.

On investigation, complete blood count revealed hemoglobin (Hb): 7.80 g/dL, white blood cells (WBCs): 11,500/mm^3 (N: 76%, L: 20%), platelet (PLT): 430,000/mm^3, erythrocyte sedimentation rate (ESR) in first hour: 90 mm, C-reactive protein (CRP): 66 mg/L, serum creatinine: 1.08 mg/dL, serum alkaline phosphatase: 251 U/L. Urasonography (USG) of the whole abdomen revealed mild ascites, moderate hepatomegaly, cholelithiasis, septate cystic space-occupying lesion (SOL) in the retroperitoneal aspect left side of the lower abdomen, large cystic SOL in the left lumbar region, thickened pyloric antral wall and mildly enlarged prostate. CT scan of the abdomen with contrast showed features similar to ultrasonography with additional finding of- destructed left iliac bone with multiple cystic SOLs in left ilium and multiple small cystic SOLs in right ilium.

QUESTIONS

1. What further investigation should be carried out?
2. What could be the diagnosis?

DISCUSSION

Our patient had giant-cell tumor of anterior arc of rib which was diagnosed by FNAC. After surgical removal, he experienced left hip pain which was managed with analgesics but was not explored. After 5 years, he got admitted in our care with intra-abdominal abscess with systemic symptoms which was managed conservatively, but his hip pain persisted. After getting reports of imaging study we suspected **recurrent giant cell tumor**, this time in left iliac bone. So, we decided to do several further investigations.

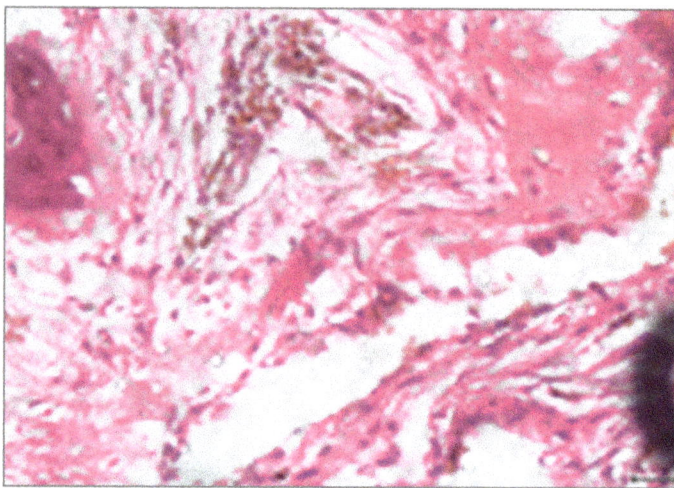

Fig. 2: Bone section showing curvilinear trabeculae of woven bone surrounded by moderately cellular fibroblastic proliferation. The shapes of trabeculae mimic chinese letters and bone lacks prominent osteoblastic rimming.

Ultrasound-guided aspiration from multicystic retroperitoneal mass yielded turbid fluid, and the mass appeared to have risen from left iliac bone. Under ultrasound guidance, turbid ascitic fluid was aspirated. During aspiration, the mass appeared to be arising from left iliac bone. A culture and sensitivity report revealed growth of *Bacteroides* species. FNAC from left iliac bone lesion showed number of inflammatory cells in a blood mixed fluid background, and no malignant cell was seen. Biopsy from left iliac bone lesion revealed curvilinear trabeculae of woven bone surrounded by moderately cellular fibroblastic proliferation. The shapes of trabeculae mimicked Chinese letters and the bone lacked prominent osteoblastic rimming. The findings were consistent with fibrous dysplasia (Fig. 2).

Final Diagnosis: Giant-cell Tumor with Fibrous Dysplasia (involving Right-sided Ribs, Right and Left Iliac Bones) with Intra-abdominal Abscess Due to *Bacteroides* spp.

Benign fibro-osseous lesions (BFOLs) such as fibrous dysplasia (FD) and giant cell lesions are dimorphic conditions having fibro-osseous component in common.

Giant cell tumor is a relatively uncommon tumor of the bone. There are multinucleated giant cells, commonly benign with unpredictable behavior. It follows variable clinical courses. It may remain as an asymptomatic mass or may become aggressive causing pain. It has a tendency to recur after surgical removal.[1]

When the components of different pathologies are present in one lesion, it is called "hybrid" lesions. Hybrid lesions comprising central giant-cell granuloma (CGCG) along with fibro-osseous lesions are very rare. A histopathological examination plays a pivotal role in diagnosing these specific types of conditions.[2]

Fibrous dysplasia mainly involves mandible with male predominance. The lesion described here was observed in the iliac bone which was unique.

The association between giant cell tumor and FD is still a subject of debate.

REFERENCES

1. Kurra S, Reddy DS, Gunupati SKS, Reddy MS. Fibrous dysplasia and central giant cell granuloma: a report of hybrid lesion with its review and hypotheticated pathogenesis. J Clin and Diag Res. 2013;7(5):954-8. doi:10.7860/JCDR/2013/5533.2987
2. Jawanda MK, Narula R, Shankari M, Gupta S. Hybrid lesions comprising central giant cell granuloma and fibrous dysplasia: A diagnostic challenge for pathologist. J Oral Maxillofac Pathol. 2015;19(3):408. doi:10.4103/0973-029X.174631.

CASE 19

YOUNG MAN WITH ARTHRALGIA, HYPERPIGMENTED SKIN LESIONS AND FEVER

CASE SUMMARY

A 26-year-old gentleman presented with the complaints of polyarthralgia for 17 months, hyperpigmented skin lesions for 10 months and high-grade fever for 1 month. Initially arthralgia started in large joints of lower limbs followed by small joints of hands and feet (bilateral asymmetrical). Pain persisted all through the day which was associated with feverish feeling. There was no history of morning stiffness, back pain, Raynaud's phenomenon, visual problems, skin changes, respiratory and cardiac or urinary complaints, alopecia, rash, oral ulceration, proximal myopathy or myalgia. Pain relieved to great extent after taking pain killers and oral steroid occasionally. He noticed maculopapular, painless, nonitchy, nondischarging skin lesions at first in the upper part of left arm, then left side of the cheek and afterwards right side of the cheek which gradually increased in size. He was prescribed multiple ointments/creams including topical steroids and retinoic acid derivatives which helped him to remain symptom free to some extent for 8 months. Later on he experienced high grade, continued fever, maximum recorded temperature was 102°F, associated with chills and rigor along with nausea and vomiting and significant weight loss (13 kg in 1 month). He also developed bilateral painful parotid swelling, bilateral painful neck swelling, gum swelling, halitosis and burning sensation in the tongue and gum. His prior symptoms of polyarthralgia and facial hyperpigmentation reappeared. Hyperpigmentation also involved trunk and left shoulder sparing the palmar creases, soles of the feet, gum and hard palate. He was diagnosed as mumps and sarcoidosis in different tertiary care hospitals in Bangladesh and was treated accordingly but without any improvement. During hospital stay in our care, he developed bilateral orchitis (right>left) and had dryness of mouth. He did not have any history of cough, hemoptysis, night sweats, and headache. His mother had bone tuberculosis (TB) 20 years back (completed

Young Man with Arthralgia, Hyperpigmented Skin Lesion and Fever

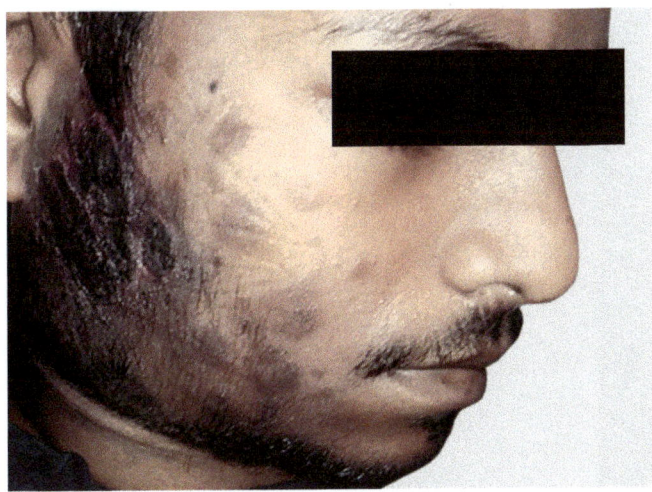

Fig. 1: Facial hyperpigmented lesions.

anti-TB for 9 months) and his grandmother had gland TB 3 years back (completed anti-TB for 9 months).

On examination, he was mildly anemic and febrile (102°F), BP 100/70 mm Hg without any postural drop, evidence of slightly tender cervical lymphadenopathy (both anterior and posterior chain), discrete, firm, variable size, with no discharging sinus. Hyperpigmented skin lesions were found over both side of the face measuring about 6.5 cm having ill-defined margin (Fig. 1). Few papule, nodule and ulcer present in the left arm and front and back of the chest. Parotid glands were bilaterally enlarged, which were tender, firm without any discharging sinus. Also there was oral thrush. All other findings were unremarkable.

Investigations showed hemoglobin (Hb%) was persistently low on several times (ranging from 10.0 g/dL to 10.90 g/dL), white blood cell (WBC) counts were also low [lowest one was 1,600/mm^3 (N—70%, L—25%), highest one was 3,660/mm^3 (N—84%, L—13.7%)], normal platelet count, ESR in first hour 21 mm, PBF normocytic normochromic anemia, leukopenia, platelets were adequate, S. creatinine— 0.6 mg/dL, S. electrolytes—Na 134 mmol/L, K 3.5 mmol/L, blood C/S— no growth, bone marrow study—hypercellular marrow, anti-HIV 1 and 2—negative, S. calcium—8.5 mg/dL, S. ACE level—14 U/L (ref: 12-68), ANA and anti-ds DNA—negative, ENA profile—negative, C3 and C4—normal, CXR P/A view—normal, USG of W/A—normal.

QUESTIONS

1. What special investigation is needed to reach diagnosis?
2. How will you treat the case?

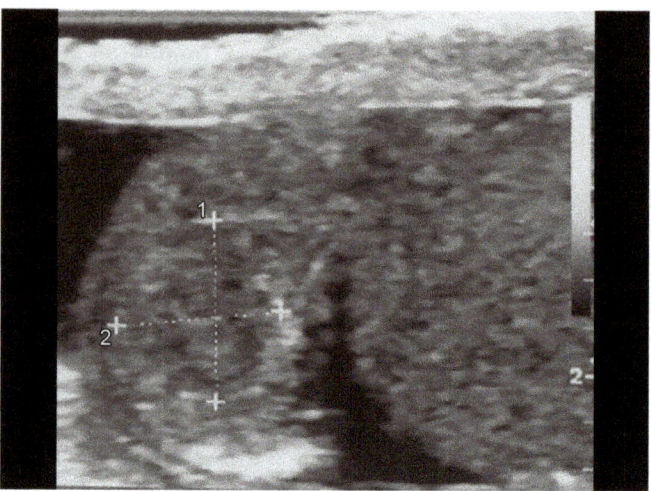

Fig. 2: USG of scrotum—right-sided epididymal mass.

DISCUSSION

Several investigations were considered for this case. Fine-needle aspiration cytology (FNAC) from lymph node depicted granulomatous inflammation (including caseous necrosis) histologically consistent with TB, FNAC from skin revealed chronic sinus tract with granulomatous inflammation, USG of scrotum showed-right sided epididymal mass (Fig. 2). FNAC from right epididymal lesion—no granuloma or malignant cell is seen and negative for malignant cell.

Final Diagnosis: Disseminated TB (TB Lymphadenitis with Lupus Vulgaris with Bilateral Parotid Gland TB with Tubercular Epididymo-Orchitis with TB Arthralgia) with Oral Moniliasis

He had excellent recovery following treatment with anti-TB chemotherapy for 6 months. The category I treatment was prescribed and as there was rapid onset of multiple organ involvement, he was also prescribed steroids (prednisolone 1 mg/kg body weight initially for 3 weeks followed by 3 weeks tapering).

The multiple systemic manifestations in this case involving locomotor, skin, lymph node, parotid gland, epididymis and testes lead to think of multiple differentials including sarcoidosis, lymphoma, disseminated TB and systemic lupus erythematosus (SLE). Eventually, FNAC from lymph node and skin showed granulomatous inflammation suggesting TB. Repeated follow-up showed marked improvement of the skin lesion and arthralgia.

Disseminated TB is defined as tuberculous infection involving the blood stream, bone marrow, liver, or two or more noncontiguous sites, or miliary TB. Disseminated TB is a potentially lethal form of TB resulting from massive lymphohematogenous dissemination of *Mycobacterium tuberculosis* bacilli. It remains a diagnostic challenge for the physician all over the world. The symptoms are nonspecific and the duration of symptoms before diagnosis is variable. Therefore, it mimics a variety of diseases and requires a high index of suspicion.[1]

Although extrapulmonary TB has been observed for many centuries, the exact incidence of disseminated TB is still unclear. The emergence of the HIV/AIDS pandemic and widespread use of immunosuppressive drugs has changed the epidemiology of disseminated tuberculosis.[2] Definitive diagnosis of disseminated TB can be very difficult. Sometimes, clinical diagnosis is only confirmed after complete recovery with specific treatment. Disseminated TB lacks typical clinical symptoms and imaging diagnosis, so can easily be misdiagnosed resulting in delayed treatment. Since prognosis is worse in patients with delayed treatment, a high index of suspicion is required.

REFERENCES

1. World Health Organization. WHO Report: Global Tuberculosis Control. Geneva: World Health Organization; 2011.
2. Murray CJ, Lopez AD. Global mortality, disability, and the contribution of risk factors: Global Burden of Disease Study. Lancet. 1997;349:1436-42.

CASE 20

MIDDLE-AGED LADY WITH PROGRESSIVE DYSPHAGIA

CASE SUMMARY

A 48-year-old female presented with progressive dysphagia with regurgitation for last 2 years. Dysphagia was initially for solid food, and later she also developed dysphagia for liquid. She mentioned significant weight loss during the course of illness. She had history of whitening and bluish discoloration of her hands on exposure to cold. Later she developed burning and ulceration of her finger tips leading to amputation of fingers of both hands about 14 years back. Due to fall on fire at her 3 years of age, she progressively developed Marjolin's ulcer on her right leg for which she underwent amputation of her right leg up to mid-thigh about 12 years back. There was no history of fever, skin rash or pigmentation, oral ulcer, arthralgia, chest pain or cough.

On examination, she was ill-looking, afebrile, nasogastric (N-G) tube was in situ. Her body-built was below average. Skin tightening was present over her face and hands. Fingers of both hands were amputed and right leg was amputed up to mid-thigh, there was no joint swelling, deformity or restricted movement. Pulse was absent in radial, brachial, and femoral arteries bilaterally; and popliteal and arteria dorsalis pedis arteries in the left lower limb. Her BP was 100/70 mm Hg. Chest and abdominal examination was normal.

Investigation showed Hb—10.2 g/dL, white blood cell (WBC)—8,340/mm^3 (DC: N-65%, L-30%); platelet—2,50,000/mm^3; erythrocyte sedimentation rate (ESR)—78 mm in first hour; urine routine examination—albumin trace, pus cells were 2-4/ high-power field of microscope (HPF); red blood cell (RBC)—1-2/HPF. ECG, chest X-ray, serum creatinine and electrolyte were normal.

QUESTIONS

1. What is the most likely diagnosis?
2. What three abnormal findings may have been discovered on examination of hands?

3. What further investigations would you perform?
4. How would you manage her dysphagia?

DISCUSSION

Patient's history of color change of hands on exposure to cold indicates Raynaud's phenomenon. Her coexistence of Raynaud's phenomenon, skin tightening and dysphagia strongly suggests systemic sclerosis (SSc) as the most likely diagnosis here. In addition to the signs of Reynauds's phenomenon in the hands, skin thickening, subcutaneous calcification and telangiectasia should be looked for during examination and a history of breathlessness sought.

Further investigations performed in this patient are: Antinuclear antibodies (ANA) was positive (pattern: centromere). Anti-dsDNA and extractable nuclear antigen (ENA) antibodies profile—negative.

As there was esophageal involvement, barium swallow of esophagus was done which showed—stricture of mid-thoracic part of esophagus suggestive of: growth.

Endoscopy of upper gastrointestinal tract (GIT) revealed—luminal narrowing with circumferential ulcer.

So endoscopic biopsy from the esophagus was done, no malignancy was seen. Diagnosis—ulcer.

Then for histological evidence, skin biopsy was done which was compatible with scleroderma.

Final Diagnosis: Systemic Sclerosis

For management of dysphagia, esophageal stenting was done. After that there was significant relief of her dysphagia and she was able to swallow. So later on the N-G tube was removed.

Systemic sclerosis is an autoimmune disorder of connective tissue, which results in fibrosis of the skin, internal organs and vasculature. It is characterised typically by Raynaud's phenomenon, digital ischemia, sclerodactyly and cardiac, lung, gut and renal involvement.[1]

The peak age of onset is the fourth and fifth decades and overall prevalence is 10–20 per 100000, with a 4:1 female : male. It is subdivided into diffuse cutaneous systemic sclerosis (dcSSc: 30% of cases) and limited cutaneous systemic sclerosis (lcSSc: 70% of cases).[1]

Systemic sclerosis should be considered in patients with Raynaud's phenomenon, typical musculoskeletal or skin manifestations or unexplained dysphagia, malabsorption, pulmonary fibrosis, pulmonary hypertension, cardiomyopathies or conduction disturbances. Diagnosis can be obvious in patients with combinations of classic manifestations, such as Raynaud's phenomenon.

Diagnosis is clinical, but laboratory tests help with confirmation. Usually antinuclear antibodies (ANA), Scl-70 (topoisomerase I) and anticentromere antibodies are positive. ANA are present in >90% cases often with an antinuclear pattern.

Specific treatment is difficult and depends on symptoms. To date with the possible exception of hematopoietic stem cell therapy (HSCT), no therapy has been shown to significantly alter the natural history of SSc. Immunosuppressive agents used in other autoimmune diseases have generally shown modest or no benefit in SSc. Glucocorticoids alleviate stiffness and aching in early inflammatory-stage dcSSc, but do not influence the progression of skin or internal organ involvement. Since their use is associated with an increased risk of scleroderma renal crisis, glucocorticoids should be given only when absolutely necessary, at the lowest dose possible, and for brief period only.[2]

The prognosis in dcSSc is poor (5-year survival about 70%). Poor prognostic factors include older age, diffuse skin disease, proteinuria, high ESR, a low gas transfer factor for carbon monoxide (TLCO) and pulmonary hypertension.[1]

REFERENCES

1. Ralston SH, Penman ID, Strachan MWJ, Hobson RP. Davidson's principles and practice of medicine. 23rd ed. Edinburgh: Churchill Livingstone/Elsevier; 2018. p. 1037.
2. Jameson JL, Kasper DL, Longo DL, Fauci AS, Hauser SL, Loscalzo J. Harrison's Principles of Internal Medicine. 20th ed. NewYork: McGraw Hill Education; 2018.

CASE 21

DELIRIOUS YOUNG MAN WITH FEVER AND HEPATOMEGALY

CASE SUMMARY

A 32-year-old male, school teacher, resident of Faridpur (southern part of Bangladesh) was brought to hospital with the complaints of vomiting for 4 times and abnormal behavior with confusion for last 2 days. According to the statement of his relatives, he was quite well about 2 years back, then he developed high grade fever with chills and rigor. He had anorexia and gradually he noticed 3 kg weight loss. He consulted different physicians and took several courses of antibiotics and antipyretic, but his symptoms persisted. Then they took him abroad and there splenectomy was done after making a diagnosis of autoimmune hemolytic anemia with pancytopenia. Before the operation, he was given several courses of steroid but there was lack of preoperative vaccination. He was quite well after the operation up to last 2 days- when he was treated as a case of meningoencephalitis in a local clinic in Faridpur before coming to Dhaka Medical College and Hospital (DMCH). He was nondiabetic, normotensive, nonsmoker, nonalcoholic. On repeated query, no definitive history of jaundice was perceived. There was no history of abdominal distension, hematemesis or melena, chest pain, arthralgia, respiratory distress or hemoptysis.

On examination, he was ill-looking with average body build, anemic. His blood pressure was 100/60 mm Hg, pulse was 72 beats/min, temperature was slightly raised. There was no jaundice, cyanosis or edema. Bilateral gynecomastia and palmar erythema on both hands were found (Fig. 1), two spider nevi were found in the trunk. There was a scar mark in upper abdomen (Fig. 1). On admission, Glasgow Coma Scale (GCS) score was 10/15. Plantar response was equivocal on both sides and signs of meningism were absent. Abdominal examination revealed 6 cm firm, nontender hepatomegaly, no ascites. Chest examination was normal.

Investigations showed, complete blood count: Hb—9.89 g/dL, erythrocyte sedimentation rate (ESR)—82 mm in first hour, white blood

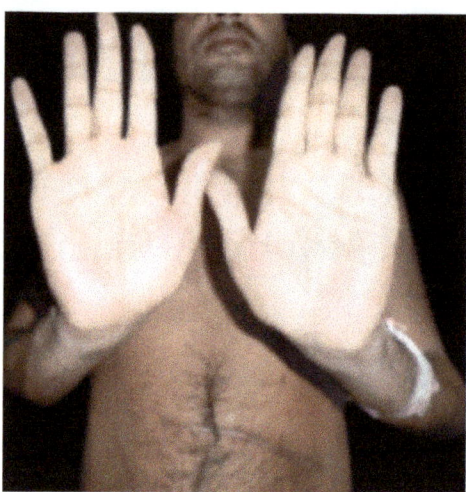

Fig. 1: Palmar erythema and splenectomy scar.

cell (WBC) count—13,500/cumm, neutrophils—75%, lymphocytes—21%]; platelet count—1,40,000/cumm, peripheral blood film (PBF) showed normal cell count and morphology; alanine aminotransferase (ALT)—101 U/L, aspartate aminotransferase (AST)—82 U/L, total protein—114 g/L, serum albumin—33 g/L, serum globulin—81 g/L, albumin to globulin (A:G) ratio was 1:2.5, prothombin time—12.2 seconds, serum ammonia—44 µmol/L, serum lactate dehydrogenase (LDH)—295 U/L; viral markers including HBsAg, anti-hepatitis C virus (HCV) antibody, anti-hepatitis B core (HBc) (total), HIV 1 and 2 were negative. Serum creatinine, serum electrolytes, blood glucose and serum Vitamin B12 and folate were within normal limit. Chest X-ray posteroanterior (P/A) view, ECG, upper gastrointestinal (GI) endoscopy and CT scan of brain were normal. Ultrasonography (USG) of whole abdomen showed hepatomegaly with status post-splenectomy; fibroscan of liver showed liver stiffness 6 kPa. Antinuclear antibodies (ANA) and anti-smooth muscle antibodies (ASMA) were negative.

QUESTIONS

1. What further investigation would you undertake to find out the cause?
2. How would you treat the patient?

DISCUSSION

The patient had spider angioma, palmar erythema and gynecomastia; all of which favored the *diagnosis of chronic liver disease (CLD)*. Initial presentation during admission was in favor of suspected hepatic encephalopathy. It was also confused with *overwhelming sepsis due to status post-splenectomy*.

After exclusion of all the possible causes of chronic liver disease and on the background of endemicity of the patient's residential area, previous history of pancytopenia, and significantly raised serum globulin level, *visceral leishmaniasis (kala-azar)* was also an important consideration here. Under strong clinical suspicion, blood for rK39 test was sent as its sensitivity is 100% and specificity is 95%[1,2] and the result came positive. For further confirmation, the test was repeated in a national centre [Institute of Epidemiology Disease Control and Research (IEDCR)] and found to be positive again.

It was not possible to take splenic aspirate due to previous splenectomy. So, *bone marrow examination* was done which revealed reactive marrow with 8–10% plasma cells. No malignant cell or granuloma, or any Leishman-Donovan (LD) body was found.

Finally *liver biopsy* was done as it is the gold standard and ultimate diagnostic tool for the detection of liver pathology in spite of normal fibroscan of liver.[3] Liver biopsy showed *periportal fibrosis and moderate infiltrate of chronic inflammatory cells. The histology activity index (HAI - Knodell score) was 11/22 (periportal +/-, bridging necrosis = 4, intralobular degeneration and focal necrosis = 3, portal inflammation = 3, fibrosis = 1)* (Fig. 2). *Further section revealed a few LD bodies within histiocytes in the portal areas. Kupffer cells were prominent* (Fig. 3).

So liver biopsy and rk39 test both showed result in favor of *CLD with visceral leishmaniasis (VL)*.

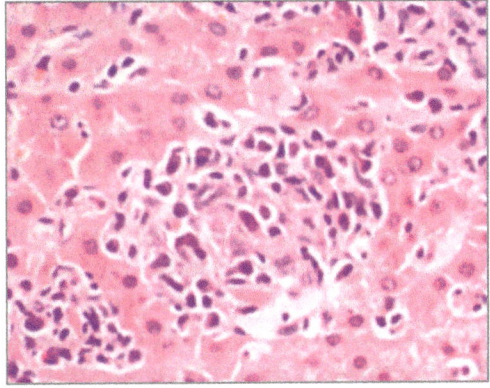

Fig. 2: Photomicrograph showing nodularity in the liver.

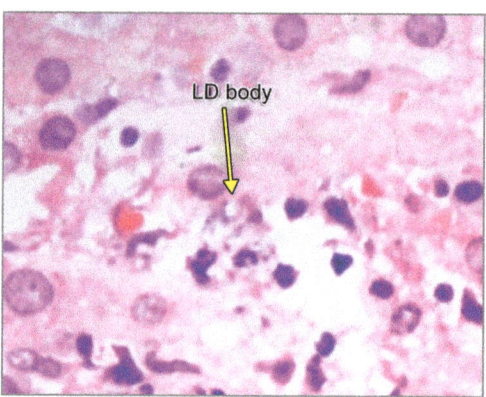

Fig. 3: Photomicrograph (H&E staining, x1200) showing single LD body.

Final Diagnosis: Chronic Liver Disease (CLD) due to Visceral Leishmaniasis (VL)

After confirmation of CLD and visceral leishmaniasis, the patient was treated with *single dose of liposomal amphotericin B*. Gut sterilizer and lactulose was also started.

The patient responded very well. Gradually he became conscious and well-oriented. He was vaccinated against all encapsulated organisms before discharge.

Kala-azar (VL) is a disease caused by parasites of genus *Leishmania*, which are transmitted by phlebotomine sandflies. The infection may be anthroponotic or zoonotic. An individual in an endemic area who has fever for more than 3 weeks, splenomegaly and positive rK-39 test should be diagnosed as a case of kala-azar.[4]

On the other hand, cirrhosis of liver is defined histopathologically. It includes decrease in hepatocellular mass, development of fibrosis to the point that there is architectural destruction with formation of regenerative nodule.

In our country, visceral leishmaniasis (VL) is a significant disease burden due to known endemicity, whereas chronic liver disease (CLD) due to various etiologies is also commonly encountered. In a recent Bangladesh study, it was found that initial diagnosis of CLD was made in 36% of the patients with VL; and that 9% of kala-azar patients were initially thought to have congenital hemolytic anemia.[5] But the simultaneous presence of both VL and CLD in the same person is very unlikely, and CLD due to VL is even rarer, but nonetheless, possible. Kala-azar often involves the liver due to effect of LD body itself or immunological response against it leading to altered biochemistry of liver.[5]

We investigated thoroughly pursuing both lines of diagnoses. Upper GI endoscopy and fibroscan of liver were normal. USG of abdomen showed hepatomegaly with normal echotexture of liver. So we could not find any evidence in favor of CLD. Moreover, we could not take splenic aspirate due to previous splenectomy and bone marrow examination revealed only elevated plasma cell count. In spite of all the negative features, under strong clinical suspicion, we sent blood for rK39 test and liver biopsy was taken, and the results were in favor of cirrhosis and VL. So, we ultimately concluded that our patient had both kala-azar and chronic liver disease. And in absence of any specific etiology for CLD, we came to believe that, these two conditions may have cause-effect relationship. So, when presented with such difficulty in distinguishing between CLD and VL, under strong clinical suspicion, gold standard investigations should be performed to confirm the diagnosis.

REFERENCES

1. Bern C, Jha SN, Joshi AB, Thakur GD, Bista MB. Use of the recombinant K39 dipstick test and the direct agglutination test in a setting endemic for visceral leishmaniasis in Nepal. Am J Trop Med Hyg. 2000;63(3-4):153-7.
2. Sundar S, Reed SG, Singh VP, Kumar PC, Murray HW. Rapid accurate field diagnosis of Indian visceral leishmaniasis. Lancet. 1998;351(9102):563-5.
3. Nudo CG, Jeffers LJ, Bejarano PA, Servin-Abad LA, Leibovici Z, De Medina M, et al. Correlation of laparoscopic liver biopsy to elasticity measurements (fibroscan) in patients with chronic liver disease. Gastroenterol Hepatol. 2008;4(12):862-70.
4. Sundar S, Rai M. Laboratory diagnosis of visceral leishmaniasis. Clin Diagn Lab Immunol. 2002;9(5):951-8.
5. Rashid A, Mamun A, Rasul C, Afrafuzzaman M, Hossain M, Rahman M. Jaundice in pediatric visceral leishmaniasis (Kala-azar) patients. J Medicine. 2008;8(1).

CASE 22

YOUNG LADY WITH SUDDEN UNCONSCIOUSNESS

CASE SUMMARY

A 40-year-old female presented with several episodes of sudden brief unconsciousness for a couple of months. Each episode lasted for a few minutes, after which she regained consciousness but remained disoriented. She had history of repeated vomiting and anorexia for same duration. This time after admission, immediate clinical evaluation revealed, her Glasgow Coma Scale (GCS) score was of 8/15, blood pressure was low (70/30 mm Hg), blood glucose was normal, but serum serum sodium level was low (104 mmol/L). After proper resuscitation, she regained her full consciousness within 24 hours. Her blood pressure was persistently low and postural drop was also present. Her obstetric history revealed, she was a mother of three children, all of them were born via normal vaginal delivery. About 6 years back, during her last child-birth, she had severe postpartum hemorrhage (PPH) due to retained placenta for which dilatation and curettage (D&C) was done. Afterwards, she faced difficulty in breastfeeding with her last child. On query, she also gave history of menstrual disturbance in the form of oligomenorrhea following her last delivery, and she had been amenorrheic for the last 2 years starting at the age of 38.

On examination, she was pale, lethargic, and body-built was below average. Skin was dry, coarse and wrinkled (Fig. 1A), breast started to atrophy and axillary hair was lost. Postural drop was found (on lying—90/50 and on standing—70/40). The rest of the examination was normal.

Investigations revealed: hemoglobin (Hb)—11 g/dL, white blood cells (WBCs)—11,000/cumm, platelet (PLT)—2,55,000/cumm, erythrocyte sedimentation rate (ESR) in first hour—60 mm, serial sodium level (104, 112 and 120 at different times), potassium (3.38, 3.45 and 3.5) and chloride levels were low (68, 78 and 83). Serum cortisol—0.75 ug/dL (low), serum cortisol (after short synacthen test)—1.14 ug/dL (low), adrenocorticotropic hormone (ACTH)—11.4 pg/dL (low), follicle-stimulating hormone (FSH)—13.27 IU/mL (lower limit of normal level), luteinizing hormone (LH)—4.67 IU/mL (lower

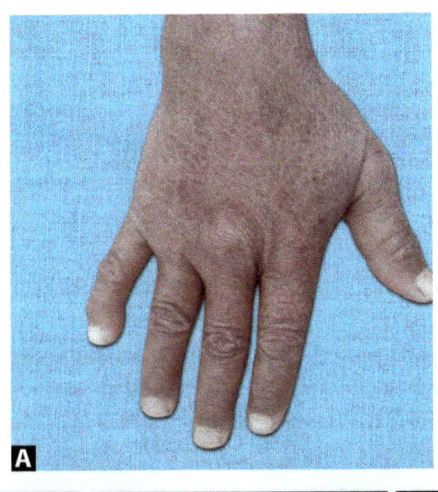
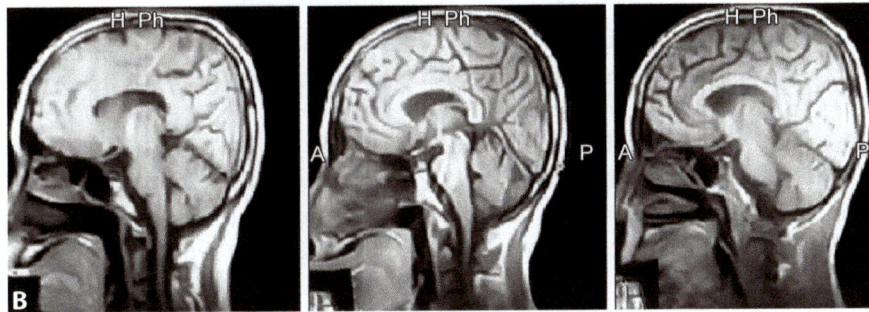

Figs. 1A and B: (A) Hand showing dry, coarse skin and fine wrinkling; (B) MRI of brain showing empty sella.

limit of normal level), growth hormone—0.072 ng/mL (low), thyroid-stimulating hormone (TSH)—6.70 IU/mL (raised), FT3—1.10 pg/mL (low), FT4—0.74 ng/dL (low) and serum aldosterone was in lower level of normal limit. Magnetic resonance imaging (MRI) of brain revealed partial empty sella (Fig. 1B).

QUESTIONS

1. What is the most probable diagnosis?
2. Would you suggest any further investigations for this patient?

DISCUSSION

Though all clinical features and biochemical findings were suggestive of partial Sheehan's syndrome, yet finding of raised TSH and low FT3, FT4 levels warranted further evaluation. Next, we did the following investigations: Antithyroperoxidase (TPO) antibody—1,400 IU/mL (very high); antithyroglobulin antibody—960 IU/mL (very high).

Final Diagnosis: **Partial Sheehan's Syndrome with Primary Hypothyroidism**

Ischemic damage to the pituitary has long been recognized as a cause of hypopituitarism. During pregnancy, the pituitary gland may be more sensitive to hypoxemia because of the hyperestrogenic state. Some degree of hypopituitarism has been reported in 32% of women with severe PPH.[1] The extent of pituitary damage determines the rapidity of onset as well as magnitude of pituitary hypofunction. The gland has a great secretory reserve and more than 75% must be destroyed before clinical manifestations are evident.

Presence of 50% of pituitary gland suffices for maintenance of normal functions. Partial or total hypopituitarism develops with necrosis of 70–90% of the gland.[1] It is believed that 32% of women with severe postpartum bleeding develop hypopituitarism.[1] However, the clinical features of hypopituitarism are often subtle and years may pass before pituitary insufficiency is recognized following an ischemic insult. Pituitary autoimmunity may play a role in the cause of hypopituitarism following PPH. However, slow clinical progression suggests factors other than ischemia in its pathogenesis.[1,2]

Even if PPH has been well managed, this complication cannot be excluded, and it can be life-threatening. It is necessary to consider this diagnosis in all patients presenting with a cardiovascular collapse during childbirth, whatever be the cause, and in the presence of the classic signs of pituitary insufficiency. In some cases, the pituitary necrosis is only partial and the syndrome can present in atypical and incomplete forms, further complicating the diagnostic procedure.

Our patient had PPH about 6 years back, and she presented in our hospital with severe hyponatremia associated with circulatory collapse. Gradually, over the course of 6 years, she developed lactational insufficiency, weakness, fatigue, lethargy, anorexia, oligomenorrhea and amenorrhea.

Both anti-TPO antibody and antithyroglobulin antibody were very high, which indicates "partial Sheehan's syndrome with primary hypothyroidism."

REFERENCES

1. Greenspan FS, Baxter JD. Endocrinological evaluation of the hypothalamic pituitary axis. Gardner DG, Shoback D, eds. In: Basic and Clinical Endocrinology, 4th edn. San Francisco/Appleton and Lange; 1994. pp. 91-3.
2. Goswami R, Kochupillai N, Crock PA, Jaleel A, Gupta N. Pituitary autoimmunity in patients with Sheehan's syndrome. J Clin Endocrinol Metab. 2002;87(9):4137-41.

CASE 23

YOUNG BOY WITH CHRONIC DIARRHEA AND FAILURE TO THRIVE

CASE SUMMARY

A 17-year-old boy presented with complaints of passage of loose stool for the last 3 years and gradual weight loss for the same duration. The stool frequency was 10–12 times per day and stool was pale, bulky, greasy, frothy, offensive, contained undigested food particles and sticky, which made it difficult to flush away. It was associated with nausea and abdominal fullness with no association with intake of wheat, burley or grains. For the last 3 months, he had a history of occasional blood-mixed stool which was not previously noticed. He had loss of appetite, and developed significant weight loss of about 15 kg over last three years. One-and-a-half-year back he had a history of poor vision at night and in dim light which persisted for a year. On query, he also complained of generalized body ache, difficulty in getting up from squatting position, tingling and numbness in both hands and feet for the last one year. He had no history of jaundice, cough, hemoptysis, oral ulceration, joint pain, tremor, palpitation, heat intolerance, itching, purpura or bruising. For these complaints, he got admitted to Dhaka Medical College Hospital (DMCH) several times and got empirical Category 1 anti-tuberculosis (TB) treatment for 2 months and then discontinued by himself, without any consultation. Four months later, he got readmitted and was given Category 2 anti-TB along with supplementation of vitamin A, vitamin D, calcium and minerals. Symptomatic improvement was observed during this period of taking anti-TB, but after a few months of completion, his bowel symptoms reappeared.

On physical examination, the patient was ill-looking, emaciated and mildly anemic (Fig. 1). His pulse was 84 beats/min, blood pressure was 110/70 mm Hg, respiratory rate was 20 breaths/min and temperature was normal. There was no lymphadenopathy, scar mark or pigmentation. All other parameters of general examinations were normal. Systemic examination

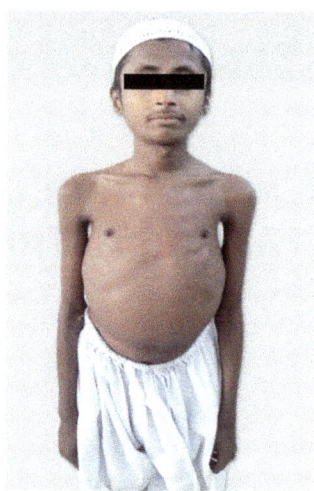

Fig. 1: Emaciated boy with distended abdomen.

revealed that abdomen was distended due to ascites, and no organomegaly was present. Pain and temperature sensation were diminished in gloves and stocking pattern. Joint position and vibration sensations were intact. Other systemic examinations revealed normal findings.

Investigations showed that hemoglobin level was variable. White blood cells (WBCs) showed neutrophilic leukocytosis. ESR was 70 mm in 1st hour. Peripheral blood film (PBF) showed normocytic normo—chromic anemia with neutrophilic leukocytosis. A chest X-ray showed normal findings. In stool and urine routine microscopic examination, no abnormality was found. Serum electrolytes and creatinine were normal, but serum albumin—2.5 g/dL, calcium—7.30 g/dL, and serum phosphate—1.4 mg/dL, levels were all low. Alkaline phosphatase level was high—342 U/L, vitamin D level was low—10.8 ng/dL, parathyroid hormone (PTH) level was high—218 pg/mg. Creatine kinase (CK) level was—70 U/L, serum vitamin B12 level was normal and iron profile showed serum iron—146 mg/dL, serum ferritin—117.35 mg/L and total iron-binding capacity (TIBC)—95 mg/dL. Anti-human immunodeficiency virus (HIV)[1,2] was negative, thyroid function test and serum cortisol were normal and ultrasonography (USG) showed: hepatomegaly with prominent intra-abdominal lymphadenopathy. USG-guided fine needle aspiration cytology (FNAC) from para-aortic lymph node showed: lymphocytes at various stages of maturation and histiocytes, and no granuloma or malignant cell was seen. Colonoscopy revealed normal findings. Upper gastrointestinal (GI) endoscopy showed flat folds in the duodenum with scattered tiny nodular swelling, and lumen was neither narrowed nor dilated. Histopathology from duodenal biopsy showed short and broad villi, and mildly elongated crypts. Lamina propria contained moderate number of chronic inflammatory cells including lymphocytes, plasma cells and a few eosinophils. Comment was chronic nonspecific duodenitis with partial villous atrophy. A few lymphoid follicles with germinal center were present. No granuloma was seen. Anti-tissue transglutaminase (tTG) was negative.

QUESTIONS

1. What differentials should be considered in this case?
2. What further investigations are needed to reach a final diagnosis?
3. How should this patient be managed?

DISCUSSION

Problem list for this young boy was such as: long history of malabsorption (bloody diarrhea), weight loss, stunted growth and features of various vitamin deficiencies such as night blindness, proximal myopathy and peripheral neuropathy. Based on these, our provisional diagnosis was inflammatory bowel disease (IBD). But colonoscopic finding was completely normal. Then considering clinical features and other investigations like high ESR (70 mm) with high Mantoux test (MT) (23 mm), anti-tubercular medication was also given. Initially, he responded well but his symptoms were not resolved completely. At this point besides intestinal TB, we also considered other differentials such as intestinal lymphoma, parasitic infestation and HIV infection. Negative HIV1 and HIV2 ruled out HIV infection. Stool routine microscopic examination also failed to reveal any ova or cyst. Though he had no gluten intolerance, biopsy from duodenum revealed villous atrophy, as a result anti-tissue transglutaminase (tTG) was also done but it was negative and celiac disease was excluded.

To reveal any obscure pathology of gastrointestinal tract, double balloon enteroscopy was done which showed scalloping of the mucosa with nodularity and reduced circular fold in jejunum (Fig. 2) with normal esophagus, duodenum and stomach; and jejunal biopsy report was suggestive of lymphoproliferative disorder (Fig. 3). Previously done ultrasonography also revealed intra-abdominal lymphadenopathy. So we did immunohistochemistry which revealed the following result: CD20 and CD5 were positive in most lesional lymphoid cells. CD3 and CD10 were negative. MUM1, CD138, kappa and lambda were all positive in many lesional cells and the final impression was: immunoproliferative small intestinal disease (IPSID) variety of extranodal marginal zone of lymphoma of mucosa-associated lymphoid tissue.

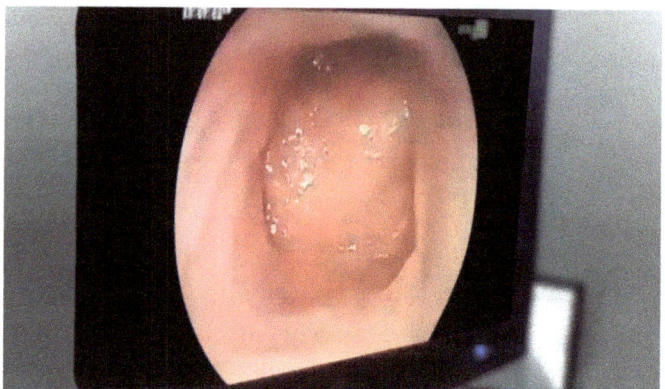

Fig. 2: Scalloping of mucosa with nodularity and reduced circular fold in jejunum.

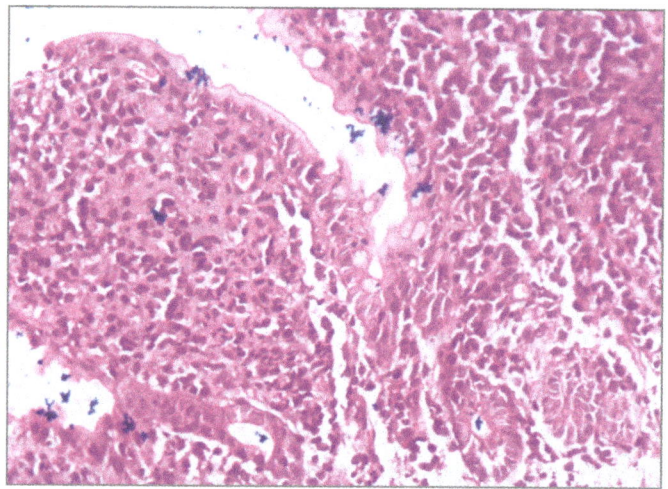

Fig. 3: Histopathology of tissue biopsy from jejunum showing dense infiltration of lymphoid cells in the mucosa, lamina propria and submucosa—suggestive of lymphoproliferative disorder.

Final Diagnosis: Malabsorption Syndrome due to Immunoproliferative Small Intestinal Disease

The patient was treated with tetracycline 250 mg four times daily for 3 months. With this, he was clinically improved and weight gain was about 10 kg.

Immunoproliferative small intestinal disease (IPSID) also known as alpha heavy chain disease, is a rare condition occurring mainly in Mediterranean countries, the Middle East, India, Pakistan and North America. It is a variant of B-cell lymphoma of MALT type and often associated with *Campylobacter jejuni* infection. The condition varies in severity from relatively benign to frankly malignant.[1]

It is postulated that IPSID occurs in patients with repeated intestinal infections.[2] Recent studies suggest association with *Campylobacter jejuni*.[3] It is postulated that this results in continuous chronic antigenic stimulation of IgA-secreting lymphoid tissue common in small intestine with a resultant clonal proliferation of IgA-secreting lymphoid cells. Subsequently, most cases lose the ability to synthesize light chain. In early stages it may be very difficult to differentiate IPSID from chronic inflammatory process by the reporting pathologists.[2]

The small intestinal mucosa is diffusely affected, especially proximally, by a dense lymphoplasmacytic infiltrate. Enlarged mesenteric lymph nodes are also common. Most patients are young adults who present with malabsorption, anorexia and fever. Serum electrophoresis confirms the presence of alpha heavy chains (from the Fc portion of IgA). Prolonged remissions can be obtained with long-term antibiotic therapy but chemotherapy [cyclophosphamide, vincristine, adriamycin, and prednisolone (CHOP)] is required for those who failed to respond or who have aggressive disease.[1]

REFERENCES

1. Ralston SH, Penman ID, Strachan MWJ, Hobson RP. Davidson's Principles and Practice of Medicine. 23rd ed. Edinburgh: Churchill Livingstone/Elsevier; 2018. p. 813.
2. Fine KD, Stone MJ. Alphaheavy chain disease, Mediterranean lymphoma, and immunoproliferative small intestinal disease: a review of clinicopathological features pathogenesis and differential diagnosis. Am J Gastroenterol. 1999; 94:1139-52. Comment in: Am J Gastroenterol. 2000;95:848.
3. Lankarani KB, Masoompour SM, Masoompour MB, Malekzadeh R, Tabei SZ, Haghshenas M. Changing epidemiology of IPSID in Southern Iran. Gut. 2005; 54:311-2.

CASE 24

MIDDLE-AGED MAN WITH FEVER, SPLENOMEGALY AND ARTHRITIS

CASE SUMMARY

A 52-year-old male, farmer by profession, known diabetic, was presented with the complaints of low-grade, irregular fever, anorexia for the last 3 months and right knee arthritis for the last 1 month. His fever mainly came around midnight, maximum recorded temperature was 101°F, subsided with paracetamol. He did not give any history of chills and rigor, night sweat, weight loss, cough, headache or seizure. He was treated as a case of diabetes mellitus with urinary tract infection (UTI) and received tablet nitrofurantoin and tablet domperidone without any improvement. Eventually, he developed right knee arthralgia followed by arthritis. Pain was persistent all through the day, having morning stiffness but no history of back pain or aggravating or relieving factors. Rest of his joints were normal. Along with these above-mentioned complaints, he was diagnosed as a case of disseminated TB and Category-1 anti-tubercular drugs were given empirically. Initially, he became afebrile for 2 weeks with improvement of his appetite and little improvement of his knee arthritis. However, his fever reappeared. During hospital stay, he developed right ankle arthritis, then left ankle arthritis, abscess under right knee joint, cellulitis on his right leg. He also developed hematuria, hematochezia and urinary incontinence, and was managed accordingly.

On examination, he was severely anemic and febrile (100°F). Examination of abdomen revealed nontender hepatomegaly of 2 cm, firm in consistency, smooth surfaced, regular-margined, no hepatic bruit, with nontender firm splenomegaly of 4 cm from the left costal margin toward right iliac fossa. There was no evidence of ascites. GALS (Gait, Arms, Legs, Spine) screening revealed he had difficulty in walking and needed assistance, right knee was found to be tender with raised temperature and patellar tap was present. All other findings were normal.

Investigations showed, hemoglobin (Hb%) was persistently low (ranging from 8.3 g/dL to 10.20 g/dL), persistently high erythrocyte sedimentation rate (ESR) in first hour (highest one was 120 mm), white blood cell (WBC) count was within normal limit though neutrophil counts were in higher ranges around 80% in multiple reports, persistently low platelet (PLT) count (ranging from 20,000/mm^3 to 65,000/mm^3), peripheral blood film (PBF)—microcytic hypochromic anemia and with thrombocytopenia, urine R/M/E—pus cell: plenty/HPF, albumin: trace, urine C/S—no growth, S. creatinine—1.62 mg/dL, 24 hours urinary total protein—1.54 g/24 hours, ANA and anti-ds DNA were negative, C3—1.09 g/L, C4—0.21 g/L, aspertate aminotransferase (AST)—34 U/L, AST—41 U/L, C-reactive protein (CRP)—174.03 mg/L, blood c/s—no growth, bone marrow study—normal, anti-HIV antibody-negative, ECG-normal, echocardiography—mild aortic sclerosis, CXR P/A view—normal, sputum for AFB and Gene Xpert—negative, synovial biopsy from right knee—acute and chronic synovitis. USG of whole abdomen—splenomegaly with multiple hypoechoic lesions in spleen suggesting TB, CT scan of W/A with contrast: hepatomegaly, splenomegaly with multiple hypodense lesions suggestive of microabscess, or infiltrative lesion, left-sided minimal subphrenic abscess. Pus from splenic abscess: microscopic features—total count: 160/mm^3 (polymorphs: 20%, mononuclear cell: 80%), no malignant cell identified; pus for AFB and Gram staining: AFB not found, pus cell: present, Gram negative coccobacilli: present, pus for culture: no growth, pus from abscess below right knee—*Acinetobacter* spp. (profuse growth), MRI of lumbosacral spine—normal, except some degenerative changes.

QUESTIONS

1. What are the differential diagnoses?
2. What should be the next diagnostic investigation?
3. How would you manage the case?

DISCUSSION

Considering the clinical findings, along with diabetes mellitus, our differential diagnoses for this patient were:
- Disseminated tuberculosis
- Lymphoma
- Systemic onset arthritis
- Disseminated melioidosis.

To reach the diagnosis, we targeted splenic lesion. Fine needle aspiration cytology (FNAC) from splenic lesion was done twice and findings were negative for malignant cell but reported as granulomatous inflammation,

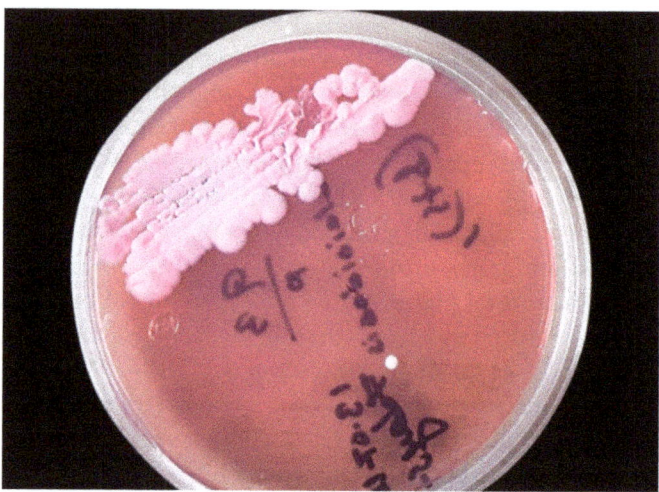

Fig. 1: Pus from splenic abscess was sent for culture: Growth of *Burkholderia pseudomallei* (profuse growth).

suggestive of tuberculosis. Since the patient did not adequately respond to previous anti-tubercular chemotherapy, we searched for an alternative diagnosis. As our clinical suspicion for melioidosis was high, we sent off the pus from splenic abscess for culture which revealed growth of *Burkholderia pseudomallei* (profuse growth) (Fig. 1).

Final Diagnosis: Disseminated Septicemic Melioidosis with DM

We treated the case with injection meropenem for 30 days, injection ciprofloxacin for 14 days and injection ceftazidime for 17 days and continued tablet co-amoxiclav (625 mg) TDS for 5 months. He had complete recovery after completion of the treatment.

Melioidosis (also called Whitmore's disease, Vietnamese tuberculosis) caused by *Burkholderia pseudomallei* is an infectious disease with a distinct geography, myriad clinical presentations and a complex pathogenesis. It is found in soil and fresh water more specifically in pooled surface water such as in paddy field. In Bangladesh, isolation of the organism from soil of Kapasia, Gazipur, in 2013, has already made this nation a definite country of melioidosis.[1]

Persons with certain medical condition like immunosuppressive states are strongly associated with severe infection and poor outcome. It is considered an opportunistic infection. But host compromise is not an essential prerequisite for the disease.

In our case, the patient was diabetic who presented with prolonged fever, arthritis, hepatosplenomegaly. Later on, he developed multiple abscess. In our country, tuberculosis is highly prevalent. So the physician thought of disseminated tuberculosis as a differential diagnosis initially. He was given Cat-1 anti-TB chemotherapy empirically but the response was not adequate. Reappearance of the symptoms and multiple abscess in different sites guided us to think of alternative diagnosis like melioidosis which also can show histological similarities with tuberculosis including caseation necrosis and granuloma. Clinical presentation can be acute (<2 months) or chronic debilitating form (>2 months). Pneumonia is the most common presentation and is involved in approximately half of all cases. Disseminated diseases can be presented as multiple abscesses in subcutaneous tissue and bones, internal organs (the spleen, prostate, kidney, liver), septic arthritis and osteomyelitis with or without septicemia.[2]

Confirmation of melioidosis is achieved with isolation of *B. pseudomallei* from clinical specimens (blood, urine, sputum, throat swab or pus from abscess or wound). Finally, in this case, pus from splenic abscess was sent for culture which revealed profuse growth of *Burkholderia*.

The treatment has two phases: an intensive phase followed by an eradication phase. The intensive phase involves intravenous antimicrobial therapy for minimum of 2-3 weeks with ceftazidime, imipenem or meropenem. The eradication phase consists of oral therapy with doxycycline plus co-trimoxazole for a minimum of 12 weeks.[3] In our case, due to extensive dissemination and severity, we continued prolonged intravenous antibiotics followed by prolonged maintenance phase.

A high index of suspicion is needed for confirmation of melioidosis. It requires awareness among the clinicians, training of microbiologist and laboratory technologist to identify suspect colonies in culture. Anti-TB chemotherapy should not be given hastily without any definite proof.

REFERENCES

1. News Medical. Melioidosis: deadly bacteria in Gazipur soil of Bangladesh. Bangladesh Med J. 2013;42(3):99.
2. Quan HB, Gao YY, Chen DX, et al. Observation on the clinical features of diabetes mellitus cases complicated with *Burkholderia pseudomallei* septicemia. China Tropical Medicine. 2006;6:1750-2.
3. Dance D. Treatment and prophylaxis of melioidosis. Int J Antimicrob Agents. 2014;43(4):310-8. doi:10.1016/j.ijantimicag.2014.01.005.

CASE 25

MIDDLE-AGED LADY WITH LUMPS AND LOW BACK PAIN

CASE SUMMARY

A 55-year-old lady presented with low-grade fever, multiple nodules in neck region, low back pain radiating to right lower limb and progressive weight loss for the last 2 months. The fever was not documented, intermittent with evening rise of temperature with night sweats and without any chills and rigor. She also noticed nontender multiple nodular swellings in the neck region, gradually increasing in number and size. Low back pain was moderate in intensity, more on movement and persisted throughout the day with radiation to the whole right lower limb and nonresponding to any pain killers. She also complained of significant weight loss in last 2 months. On query, she said that she had constipation, and denied any history of cough, hemoptysis, chest pain, other abdominal complaints, or tuberculosis exposure. She had been suffering from hemorrhoids for the last 7 years, and had history of cholecystectomy 5 years back. She was a postmenopausal woman for about last 10 years.

On general examination, the patient was vitally stable, severely anemic without jaundice, clubbing, koilonychia or leukonychia. Multiple lymph nodes were palpable in submandibular, cervical and right epitrochlear region. The largest one was in the submandibular region, about 2 cm in diameter, globular, nontender, firm to hard in consistency, mobile, discrete, free from underlying structure and overlying skin. Straight leg raise (SLR) test was positive on right side and gait was antalgic. On nervous system examination, jerks of right lower limb were exaggerated initially, later upper limb jerks were also affected with intact sensation, and plantar was extensor on right side. Spine was normal. Other system examination revealed no abnormalities.

Investigations revealed, complete blood count (CBC) with peripheral blood film (PBF): hemoglobin (Hb)—7.0 g/dL, erythrocyte sedimentation rate (ESR)—90 mm in first hour, white blood cell (WBC)—17,150/cumm, platelets—329,000/cumm, neutrophils—80.4%, lymphocytes—9.2%, monocytes—3.4%, basophils—6.7%, PBF—normocytic anemia with neutrophilic leukocytosis. Serum creatinine, electrolytes, uric acid, bilirubin, and alanine aminotransferase (ALT) were normal. Serum albumin—2.98 g/dL, calcium—13.25 mg/dL and lactate dehydrogenase (LDH)—847 U/L. Urine routine examination (RE): albumin—trace, pus cells—20-25/hpf, red blood cells (RBC)—2-4/hpf, culture and sensitivity (C/S)—growth of *Enterococcus faecalis* (10^5), anti-human immunodeficiency virus (HIV) 1 and 2—negative. Chest X-ray, posteroanterior (PA) view—consolidation in right middle lobe. Ultrasonography of the whole abdomen—multiple small simple right renal cortical cysts—Bosniak stage I with mild hydronephrosis (left kidney) and postcholecystectomy state.

QUESTIONS

1. What are the differentials?
2. What next investigations would you like to do to reach a confirmed an final diagnosis?
3. What would be the final diagnosis?

DISCUSSION

Clinically, disseminated tuberculosis was the provisional diagnosis as the lady presented with low-grade fever, multiple lymphadenopathy, low back pain and progressive weight loss. Differentials considered were lymphoma and distant metastasis of unknown primary tumor. Considering the provisional diagnosis and differentials, following investigations were done.

Magnetic resonance imaging (MRI) of dorsal spine with whole spine screening was done to find out the cause of low back pain with radiation to the right lower limb (Fig. 1). And it was suggestive of metastatic lesion in the vertebral column significantly involving sacral region causing cauda equinal compression resulting in spinal canal stenosis with infiltrative lesion (metastatic lesion) in the rest of the vertebral column.

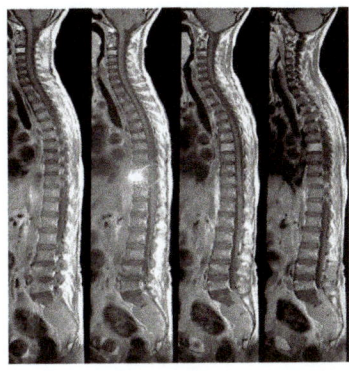

Fig. 1: Magnetic resonance imaging (MRI) of dorsal spine with whole spine screening.

Excisional biopsy and histopathology of lymph node revealed non-Hodgkin lymphoma (NHL), intermediate grade.

Bone marrow study was also done which showed active marrow with myeloid hyperplasia. In computed tomography (CT) scan of chest there was consolidation at medial segment of right middle lobe and lingular segment of left lung with left-sided mild pleural effusion and right paratracheal lymphadenopathy (7 mm × 6 mm). CT scan of abdomen was also done to see the extent of the disease. It showed mild hepatomegaly, bilateral hydronephrosis, right renal cortical cysts, moderate ascites and peripancreatic lymphadenopathy.

Final Diagnosis: Non-Hodgkin Lymphoma with Spinal Metastasis with Urinary Tract Infection

The most common presenting symptom of NHL is a painless swelling of the lymph nodes in the neck, axilla or groin. On the other hand, low back pain with concurrent radiculopathy in an otherwise healthy elderly patient is usually associated with degenerative disc disease, or lumbar disc herniation. Radiculopathy and back pain as first signs of NHL with spinal metastasis is rare, occurring in less than 5% of patients, and primary bone lymphoma is even rarer, accounting for only 3% of all primary bone malignancies. Spinal cord/cauda equina compression from NHL usually occurs due to an isolated primary or secondary deposit within the spinal canal or by extension from an adjacent nodal mass or collapsed vertebra.[1-3]

REFERENCES

1. McDonald AC, Nicoll JA, Rampling RP. Non-Hodgkin's lymphoma presenting with spinal cord compression; a clinicopathological review of 25 cases. Eur J Cancer. 2000;36(2):207-13.
2. Durr HR, Muller PE, Hiller E, Maier M, Bauer A, Jansson V. Malignant lymphoma of bone. Arch Orthop Trauma Surg. 2002;122(1):10-6.
3. Evans LS, Hancock BW. Non-Hodgkin lymphoma. Lancet. 2003;362:139-46.

CASE 26

YOUNG BOY WITH STROKE

CASE SUMMARY

A 12-year-old obese, right handed, normotensive, nondiabetic student presented with severe headache and vomiting for 15 days, weakness of right side of body for 4 days and sudden inability to talk for 2 days. He had no history of vertigo, blurring of vision, sensory disturbance, convulsion, urinary or stool incontinence, palpitation, chest pain, or any history of trauma. He never had similar episode before. He was nonsmoker and nonalcoholic and family history was unremarkable.

On examination, patient was conscious, but aphasia was present, and vital signs were completely normal. Nervous system examination revealed Glasgow coma scale (GCS) score was 9/15, no nystagmus, cranial nerves were intact, muscle power was 1/5 both in lower and upper limbs on right side. All reflexes were exaggerated in right side, with extensor plantar response. Coordination and sensory modalities were intact. Cardiovascular, respiratory and alimentary system examination revealed no abnormality.

Investigations showed Hb—15.1 g/dL; peripheral blood film—red blood cells are normocytic normochromic with matured white blood cells with normal distribution and normal platelet count. Serum electrolytes, creatinine, random plasma glucose and urinalysis were normal; lipid profile showed increased triglyceride level (277 mg/dL), others were within normal limit; electrocardiogram and chest X-ray were normal; echocardiography revealed a small patent foramen ovale with left to right shunt, no vegetation or thrombus was found; CT scan of brain showed acute moderately large left frontoparietal infarct, chronic small left parietal infarct and no evidence of intracerebral hemorrhage; MRI brain showed features of fibrolamellar cortical necrosis of left frontoparietal region suggestive of gliomatosis cerebri; immunology screening including antinuclear antibodies, hepatitis B surface antigen test, VDRL test, antihepatitis C virus, human immunodeficiency virus were all negative.

QUESTIONS

1. What could be the cause of stroke in this young boy?
2. What further investigation can lead to a final diagnosis at this stage?

DISCUSSION

Differential diagnoses or etiologies for young stroke are broad. Besides metabolic and hereditary causes three most common causes for stroke in young patient are:[1]
- Cardiac causes
- Hematological causes
- Vasculopathy in the form of aneurysm/malformation and vasculitis.

Here in our case a young boy with no apparent risk factors and having no obvious findings in clinical examination underwent several investigations to find out underlying cause of his stroke at this adolescent age. His hematological profile was completely normal. Though his echocardiography showed small patent foramen ovale but lack of vegetation and valvular disorders made it insufficient to explain the underlying etiology of his stroke. At this stage as CT scan showed multiple acute and chronic infarcts and MRI showed fibrolamellar cortical necrosis, we decided to go for digital subtraction angiogram (DSA).

Digital subtraction angiogram anteroposterior view revealed discontinuation of left internal carotid artery at supraclinoid level with multiple dural and meningeal vessels supplying the left middle cerebral artery and left anterior cerebral artery territory giving rise to the typical angiographic appearance of moyamoya disease (Fig. 1).

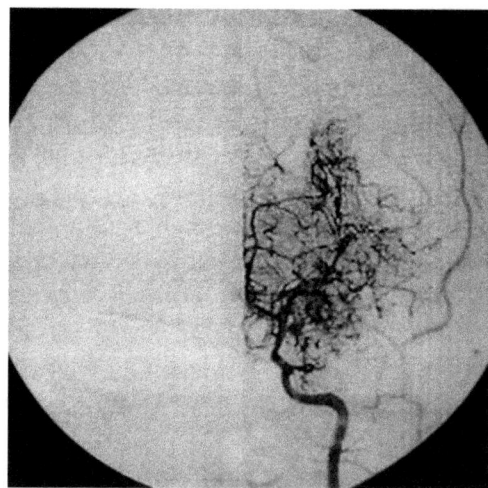

Fig. 1: Typical angiographic appearance (puff smoke) of moyamoya disease.

Final Diagnosis: Moyamoya Disease with Patent Foramen Ovale (Small)

Moyamoya disease is a rare, progressive cerebrovascular disorder caused by blocked arteries at the base of the brain at the basal ganglia. The name "moyamoya" means "puff of smoke" in Japanese and describes the look of the tangle of tiny vessels formed to compensate for the blockage. This disease was first described in Japan and is found in individuals around the world; its incidence is higher in Asian countries than in Europe or North America.[2]

The cause of moyamoya disease is not known. It is believed to be genetic. Familial moyamoya disease is autosomal dominant with incomplete penetrance that depends on age and genomic imprinting factors. Pathologically, moyamoya disease is characterized by intimal thickening in the walls of the terminal portions of the internal carotid vessels bilaterally. The proliferating intima may contain lipid deposits and causes varying degrees of stenosis or occlusion.[3,4]

The disease primarily affects children but it can also occur in adults. In children, the first symptom of moyamoya disease is often stroke, or recurrent transient ischemic attacks (TIA, commonly referred to as "mini-strokes"), frequently accompanied by muscular weakness or paralysis affecting one side of the body. Adults may also experience these symptoms that arise from blocked arteries, but more often experience a hemorrhagic stroke due to bleeding into the brain. Other symptoms may include headaches, seizures, disturbed consciousness, involuntary movements, vision problems, cognitive and/or sensory impairment.[2]

Treatment depends on type of the disease. In ischemic moyamoya, platelet antiaggregants, vasodilators, calcium channel blockers and corticosteroids can be tried. Anticoagulants are not useful. Surgical revascularization techniques like superficial temporal to middle cerebral artery anastomosis have produced good results and is considered the treatment of choice. Other important techniques include encephaloduroarteriosynangiosis (EDAS), encephalomyosynangiosis (EMS), and multiple burr hole.[2] In hemorrhagic moyamoya, there is no established therapy is available to prevent rebleeding.

There is a 4% risk of recurrent infarct or hemorrhage with the next 30 days after the surgical procedure but the 5 years survival rate after that is 96%.

REFERENCES

1. Beslow LA, Jordan LC. Pediatric stroke: the importance of cerebral arteriopathy and vascular malformations. Childs Nerv Syst. 2010;26(10):1263-73. doi:10.1007/s00381-010-1208-9.
2. Moyamoya disease information page, National Institute of Neurological disorders and stroke. Available from https://www.ninds.nih.gov/disorders/all-disorders/moyamoya-disease-information-page.
3. Roy Sucholeiki MD, Moyamoya Disease, Updated nov, 2018. Available from https://emedicine.medscape.com/article/1180952-overview.
4. Mineharu Y, Takenaka K, Yama Kawa H, et al. Inheritance Pattern of Familial Moyamoya Disease: autosomal dominant mode and genomic imprinting. J Neurol Neurosurg. Psychiatry. 2006;77(9):1025-9.

CASE 27

MIDDLE-AGED MAN WITH BACK PAIN

CASE SUMMARY

A 52-year-old gentleman, ex-smoker (5 pack-years), known diabetic and hypertensive presented with complaints of progressive upper and mid-back pain for 2 months. This insidious pain radiated to the front of the chest as a band-like sensation, aggravated by movements like bending, twisting and occasionally by taking deep breath or coughing, and relieved to some extent after taking rest. His pain was severe enough to hamper his night sleep. He consulted a physiatrist, followed by a rheumatologist and was diagnosed with spondylosis. He was treated with nonsteroidal anti-inflammatory drugs (NSAIDs) and physiotherapy but showed less significant improvement. After 3 days of admission, he developed sudden weakness of both lower limbs. Subsequently, he developed retention of urine and occasional overflow incontinence. He did not have any history of fever, weight loss, nausea, vomiting, hematemesis, melena, cough, hemoptysis, chest pain, or altered bowel habit.

The general examination findings were unremarkable apart from mild anemia and tenderness over dorsal spine as well as over few upper ribs and sternum. Nervous system examination revealed intact higher psychic function and cranial nerves. Motor examination showed muscle power 3/5 proximally and distally, knee jerks and ankle jerks were exaggerated bilaterally, and both plantar reflexes were extensor. All modalities of sensation were intact. The rest of the examination findings were unremarkable.

Investigation showed Hb level was—10.2 m/dL; white blood cells (WBC)—16,100/mm^3 (N: 75%, L: 15%, E: 2%, myelocyte: 5%); platelet (PLT)—470,000/mm^3; erythrocyte sedimentation rate (ESR) in first hour—31 mm; peripheral blood film (PBF)—normocytic anemia with leukocytosis; urine R/M/E—occasional red blood cells (RBCs) with trace albumin; serum electrolytes—normal; serum creatinine—0.99 mg/dL with serum calcium—11.1 mg/dL; serum albumin—40 g/L; serum inorganic phosphate—3.6 mg/dL; vitamin D—17.3 mg/mL; alkaline phosphatase (ALP)—388 U/L; C-reactive protein (CRP)—26 mg/L; hemoglobin A1C (HbA1C)—7%;

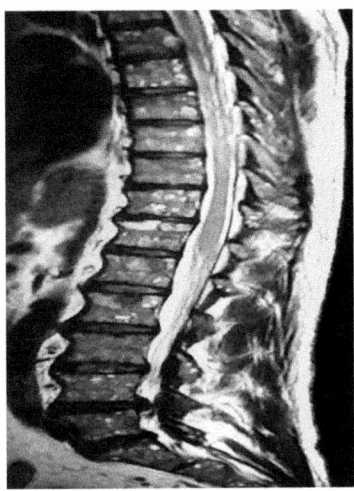

Fig. 1: Magnetic resonance imaging of spine showing gross osteoporosis.

thyroid function test—normal; chest X-ray posteroanterior view— suspected homogeneous opacity involving right apical region; computed tomography (CT) scan of the chest—normal; X-ray of the dorsal spine—suggestive of dorsal spondylosis with generalized osteopenia; X-ray of the lumbosacral spine—degenerative changes with generalized osteopenia. Ultrasonography (USG) of W/A—bilateral mild pleural effusion; 24 hours urinary electrolytes—sodium: 245.10 mmol, potassium: 48.16 mmol, chloride: 232.20 mmol, urinary calcium: 21.50 mg/dL; serum prostate-specific antigen (PSA)—normal; antinuclear antibody (ANA)—negative; human leukocyte antigen (HLA) B27—negative; serum protein electrophoresis—normal study; magnetic resonance imaging (MRI) of dorsal spine—features suggestive of osteoporotic changes; degenerative disk disease; MRI of lumbosacral spine—degenerative disk disease with osteoporosis (Fig. 1). CT scan of dorso-lumbar spine—osteoporotic change.

QUESTIONS

1. What should we do next?
2. What would be the diagnosis?

DISCUSSION

Our patient presented with back pain which was severe enough to disrupt his sleep, and pain was followed by paraparesis and urinary retention. It was obvious that he had spinal cord involvement. But the initial imaging studies did not give us a clue. At this point we did the following investigations:
- Bone mineral density (BMD)—osteopenia in lumbar vertebrae
- Bone marrow examination was suggestive of histiocytosis (foamy).

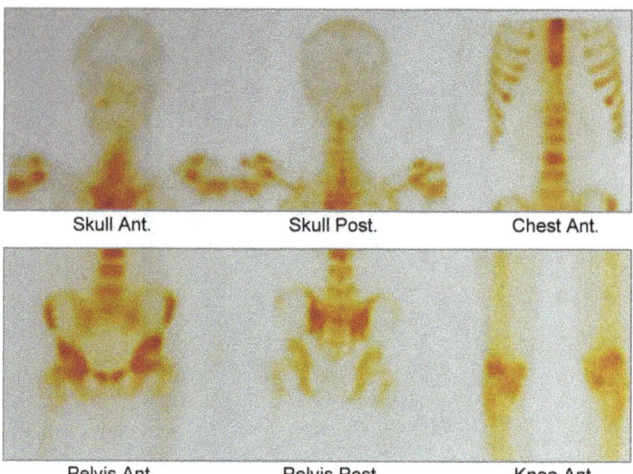

Fig. 2: Bone scan: Costovertebral and sacroiliac joint infiltration.

- Skeletal system scintigraphy—increased tracer uptake in T9 and T10 costovertebral junctions and left sacroiliac joint—suggestive of infiltrative bony lesion (Fig. 2).
- CT-guided fine needle aspiration cytology (FNAC) from vertebral lesion at sacrum—positive for malignant cell. Suggestive of metastatic adenocarcinoma.

So, after doing skeletal scintigraphy and CT-guided FNAC from suspected lesion, the diagnosis of metastatic adenocarcinoma came up. At this stage, we tried to find out the primary origin. But the patient did not have any specific symptoms suggesting site of origin. We planned to search some common sites.

- Upper gastrointestinal tract (GIT) endoscopy was done and biopsy was taken from an incidental ulcer at greater curvature. It revealed adenocarcinoma of the stomach.

Final Diagnosis: Adenocarcinoma of the Stomach with Bony Metastasis

Adenocarcinomas account for up to 60% of all cancers of unknown primary origin.[1] Adenocarcinomas are the most difficult metastatic tumor to accurately identify the primary site. Except few metastatic adenocarcinomas, which have distinctive histological features that allow for their site determination (e.g. colonic adenocarcinoma and bronchioloalveolar cell carcinoma), the majority of metastatic adenocarcinomas have histological features that are not distinctive enough to allow for a specific diagnosis of their origin.

Gastric adenocarcinoma is one of the most common malignancies worldwide.[2] It may be asymptomatic in earlier stages or cause only non-specific symptoms. In most of the symptomatic cases, the cancer has already metastasized by the time of diagnosis, which accounts for its poor prognosis. A 5-year survival rate for stomach cancer is less than 10%.

The most common sites of metastasis are liver (48%), peritoneum (32%), lung (15%) and bone (12%).[3] The spread of the disease to the bone is very rare. Our patient presented with this rare bony involvement without any GI symptoms.

Cancer of the stomach is difficult to cure unless it is found at an early stage. Surgery, radiotherapy and chemotherapy or combined approaches are the mainstay of the treatment.

REFERENCES

1. Hammar SP. Metastatic adenocarcinoma of unknown primary origin. Hum Pathol. 1998;29:1393–402.
2. Patru CL, Surlin V, Georgescu I, Patru E. Current issues in gastric cancer epidemiology. Rev Med Chir Soc Med Nat Iasi. 2013;117:199–204.
3. Ameur WB, Belghali S, Akkari I, Zaghouani H, Bouajina E, Jazia EB. Bone metastasis as the first sign of gastric cancer. Pan Afr Med J. 2017;28:95. doi:10.11604/pamj.2017.28.95.13787

CASE 28

MIDDLE-AGED FARMER WITH DIARRHEA AND GENERALIZED ITCHING

CASE SUMMARY

A 45-year-old male, farmer by profession, presented with the complaints of frequent passage of loose semisolid stool for last 6 months. Stool frequency was about 4–5 times/day, it was large in volume, contained undigested food materials and was associated with cramping mid-abdominal pain and bloating aggravated after taking fatty food and milk, but no relation with wheat made food. No blood or mucus was present in stool. He complained of intense itching of whole body associated with skin eruption and scaling for the last 6 months. He also had anorexia, weight loss of about 10 kg, generalized weakness and difficulty in standing from sitting position. On query, he mentioned having occasional low-grade fever which did not follow any diurnal pattern, not associated with chills and rigor subsided with sweating with or without taking antipyretic. He consulted a local physician and received some antibiotics, calcium, folic acid supplements, and some unknown over-the-counter drugs suggested by quacks. He was transfused three units of whole blood about 2 years back. He was nonsmoker, nonalcoholic and there was no history of contact with TB patient or any unprotected sexual exposure.

On examination, he was lethargic and cachexic, mildly anemic. Angular stomatitis, smooth tongue, generalized itchy, dry, hyperpigmented, scaly lesions and bilateral pitting edema were present (Figs. 1A to C). Pulse: 120/min, regular and blood pressure: 90/60 mm Hg (in lying) and 85/60 mm Hg (on standing). Abdominal examination revealed no abnormality. On digital rectal examination (D/R/E) Sentinel tag was present at 6 o'clock position, anal fissure at midline posteriorly. Anal tone was normal. Proctoscopy: Normal. Nervous system examination revealed bulk of muscle was reduced in all four limbs, power was normal but reflexes were absent in both upper and lower limbs, planters were bilaterally flexor, all sensations were diminished in gloves and stocking pattern except joint position and

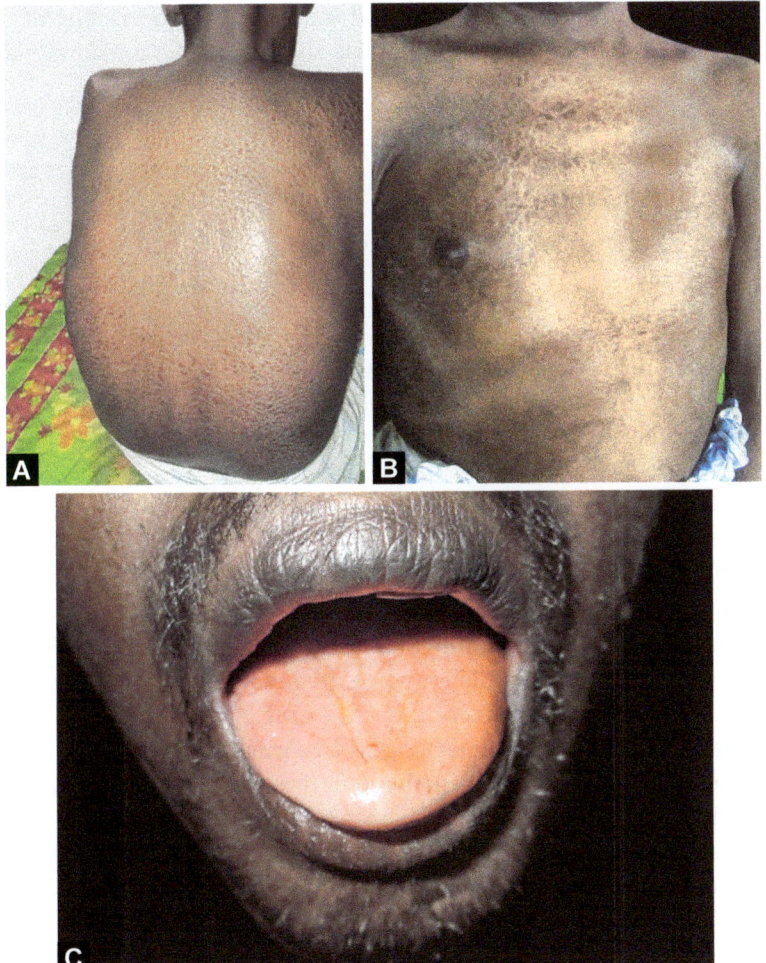

Figs. 1A to C: (A and B) Hyperpigmented scaly lesion over front and back of chest; (C) Smooth tongue.

vibration sense was intact. Features of proximal myopathy were present. The rest of the examination was normal.

Investigations showed, hemoglobin (Hb): 9.6 g/dL, WBC: 12,350/mm^3 (DC: N—71 %, L—17%, E—8%), Platelet: 656,000/mm^3, ESR: 6 mm in first hour. PBF showed normocytic normochromic anemia with eosinophilia with reactive thrombocytosis. Urine R/E showed albumin +, RBC: 4-6 HPF. S. albumin: 1.21 g/dL, S. ALP: 236 U/L. S. electrolytes: Na: 125 mmol/L, K: 2.77 mmol/L, Cl: 91 mmol/L, S. calcium: 6.87 mg/dL, corrected value: 9 mg/dL. S. magnesium: 1.89 mg/L. S. vitamin B12: 6.2 ng/mL, S. folic acid: 280 pg/mL. Serum creatinine, RBS, thyroid function test, CXR, USG of W/A, barium follow through of small intestine and endoscopy of upper GIT: normal. Sputum for AFB and MT test—negative. ANA and viral markers including HBs-Ag, anti-HCV, HIV 1 and 2—negative.

QUESTIONS

1. Suggest four possible diagnoses?
2. What further investigations would you like to do?

DISCUSSION

Our patient had malabsorption syndrome in the form of long standing frequent passage of semisolid stool, abdominal pain and weight loss, along with severe itching. Taking this history in account, following differentials were considered:
- Giardiasis/helminthiasis
- Intestinal tuberculosis
- Tropical sprue
- Coeliac disease.

In our case, clinical examination also revealed features of proximal myopathy and neuropathy which can be explained by nutritional deficiencies due to long standing malabsorption syndrome. To reveal the underlying cause, we did CT scan of abdomen which was normal, endoscopic biopsy from distal duodenum was taken which failed to reveal any significant pathology. Ileocolonoscopy and colonoscopic biopsy from rectal tissue revealed benign inflammatory rectal polyp. All these investigations ruled out possibilities of several pathologies of gastrointestinal tract.

Finally, stool routine microscopic examination revealed larvae of Strongyloides stercoralis (moderate), and stool culture showed no growth.

Final Diagnosis: Strongyloidiasis Leading to Malabsorption Syndrome

Strongyloides stercoralis is a very small nematode which parasites the mucosa of upper part of small intestine.[1]

Clinical features of strongyloidiasis depends on involvement of different systems.
- *Gastrointestinal manifestation*
  - Abdominal pain
  - Diarrhea
  - Steatorrhea
  - Weight loss.
- *Pulmonary manifestation*
  - Cough
  - Dyspnea
  - Wheeze.

- *Dermatological manifestation*
    - Urticaria
    - Larva currens: A highly characteristic pruritic, elevated, erythematous lesion advancing along the course of larval migration.
- *Neurological manifestation*
    - Seizure
    - Altered level of consciousness
    - Meningoencephalitis.
- *Besides strong clinical suspicion, diagnosis of Strongyloidiasis depends on several investigations:* CBC—eosinophilia
- *Diagnostic procedure*
    - String test
    - Doudenal aspiration
    - Immunodiagnostic tests (IFA, IHA, EIA, ELISA)
    - Repeated examination of stool.
- *Treatment for strongyloidiasis*: It is recommended for all persons found to be infected, whether symptomatic or not, due to the risk of developing hyperinfection syndrome and/or disseminated strongyloidiasis. Treatment options are as follows:[2]
    - Drug of choice: *Ivermectin,* single dose, 200 μm/kg orally for 1–2 days. Eradication rates are as high as 97%.
    - *Albendazole:* 400 mg orally twice daily for 7 days.

REFERENCES

1. Page W, Judd JA, Bradbury RS. The Unique Life Cycle of Strongyloides stercoralis and Implications for Public Health Action. Trop Med Infect Dis. 2018;3(2):53. doi:10.3390/tropicalmed3020053.
2. Centres for Disease Control and Prevention (CDC). Available from https://www.cdc.gov/parasites/strongyloides/health_professionals/index.html.

CASE 29

YOUNG MALE WITH NEUROPSYCHIATRIC ABNORMALITY

CASE SUMMARY

A 36-year-old, automobile driver was admitted with frequent episodes of irrelevant talk and agitation, recurrent attacks of left-sided hemiparesis and progressive dementia for last 3 years. All his episodes of hemiparesis were accompanied by generalized seizures, and resolved after a few days with conservative and supportive management. One month earlier, he had developed slurring of speech with echolalia and for the last 7 days before admission, he had become completely mute. There was no visual disturbance, fever or weight loss. He was nondiabetic, nonalcoholic, unmarried, and had no significant family history.

Examination revealed patient was depressed with intact consciousness. There were multiple hypopigmented macules on neck (Fig. 1A) and hyperpigmented macules on extensor surface of both lower limbs (Fig. 1B) with intact sensation. All tendon reflexes were exaggerated in left side with extensor planter response. Pupillary light reflexes were asymmetrical. Fundoscopy revealed no abnormality. Examination findings of the rest of the systems were normal.

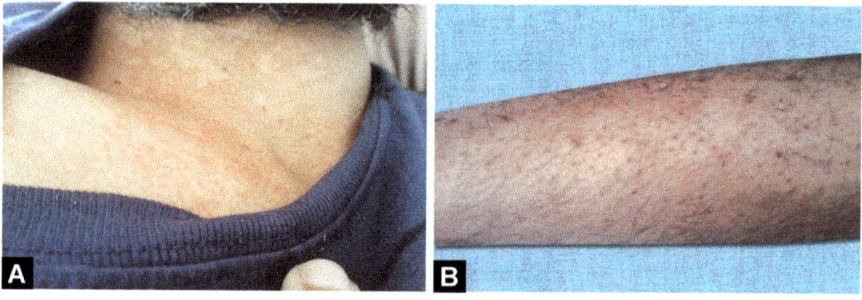

Figs. 1A and B: (A) Hypopigmented macules on neck region; (B) Hyperpigmented macules over extensor surface of lower limb.

Investigations revealed, CBC: mildly raised white blood cells (WBCs) count with high neutrophil. Liver, cardiac and renal function tests were normal. Vitamin B12 and folate levels were normal; MRI of brain showed hyperintensity of left posterior parietal lobe, tiny microvascular chronic ischemic changes involving the same area (Figs. 2 to 4). Anti-HIV 1 and 2 were negative; serum copper and ceruloplasmin levels were normal. Cerebrospinal fluid (CSF) study revealed—high WBC count with increased protein content.

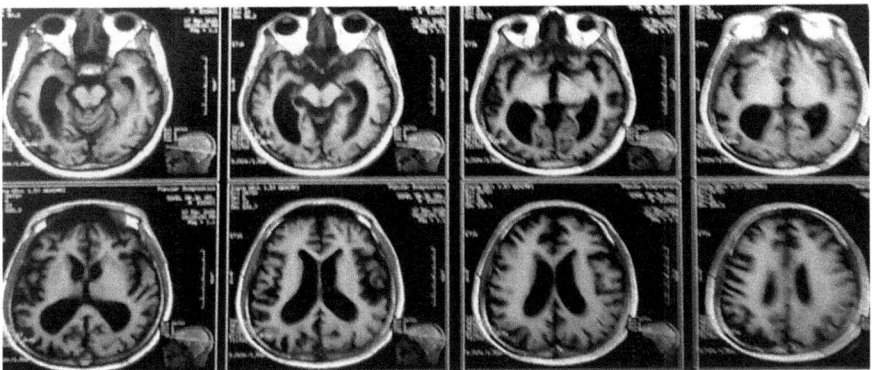

Fig. 2: MRI of brain, multiple axial cuts, T1 sequence.

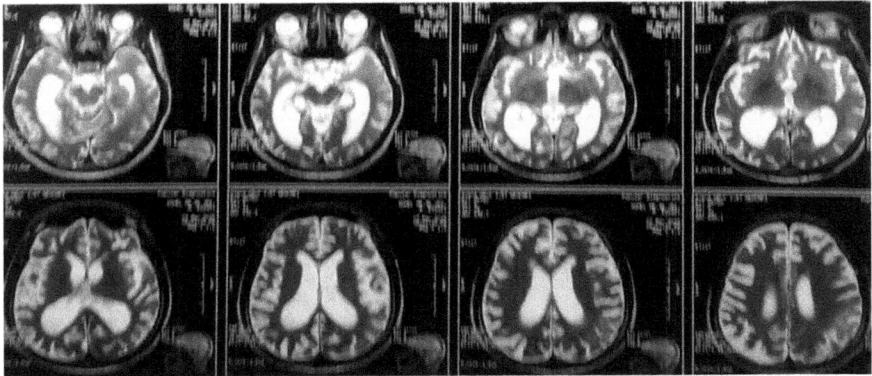

Fig. 3: MRI of brain, multiple axial cuts, T2 sequence.

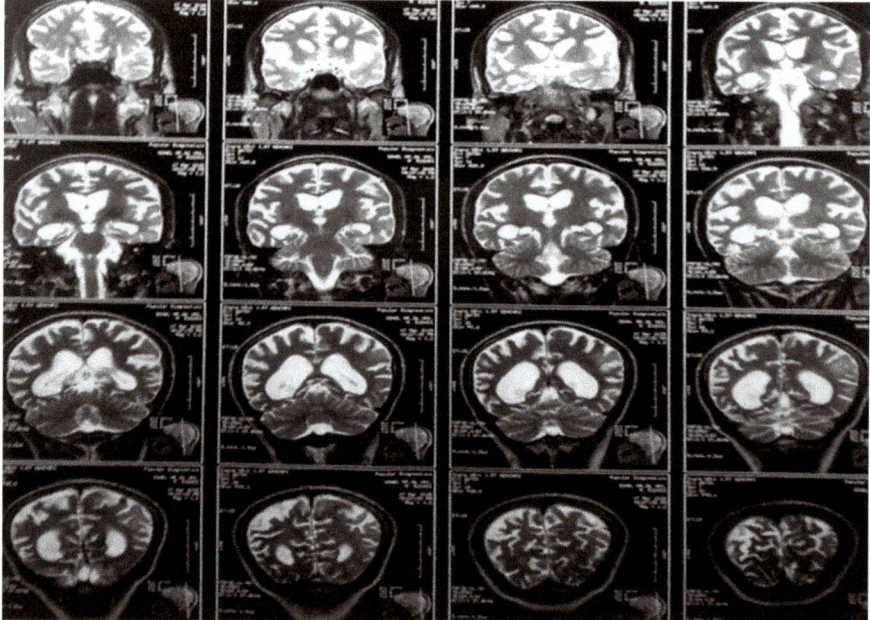

Fig. 4: MRI of brain, multiple coronal films, T2 sequence.

QUESTIONS

1. What are the possible differentials for this case?
2. What pertinent question should be asked in the history?
3. What investigations should be done next?

DISCUSSION

In this case the possible differentials were recurrent stroke, intracranial space-occupying lesions (ICSOL), multiple sclerosis and Wilson's disease. The findings in MRI of brain ruled out the possibilities of ICSOL and multiple sclerosis. There was no Kayser-Fleischer (K-F) ring, and serum copper and ceruloplasmin levels were normal—all of which disfavor Wilson's disease.

On repeated query, he admitted to have had previous casual sexual exposure and there was a history of genital (scrotal) ulcer with urethral discharge few months earlier to the onset of the symptoms.

Repeat CSF study findings were consistent with neurosyphilis, serology for Venereal Disease Research Laboratory (VDRL) test and *Treponema pallidum* hemaglutination assay (TPHA) were advised. VDRL was reactive and TPHA was positive.

Final Diagnosis: Neurosyphilis

The patient was treated with injection benzylpenicillin for 2 weeks. After treatment, he improved significantly. His behavioral abnormality was minimal and his spoken responses were better in comparison to that of the past.

Neurosyphilis is an infection of the nervous system caused by the spirochete *Treponema pallidum*. It usually occurs in people who have had chronic, untreated syphilis. It may take about 10-20 years after first infection and develops in about 25-40% of persons who are not treated.

The presentation of the disease may be in following ways:
- *Category 1—Neuropsychiatric disorders:* Including psychosis, delirium, and dementia.
- *Category 2—Cerebrovascular accident (CVA):* Acute, focal neurological deficit, compatible with a CVA or radiological evidence of stroke.
- *Category 3—Ocular:* Presentation with uveitis, visual loss, or optic nerve dysfunction.
- *Category 4—Myelopathy:* Acute, subacute, or chronic dysfunction of the spinal cord, including tabes dorsalis.
- *Category 5—Seizure:* Presentation with partial seizures, with or without secondary generalization, or myoclonus.
- *Category 6—Brain stem/cranial nerves:* Signs restricted to the brain stem and cranial nerves.[1]

CSF must be examined in all suspected cases of neurosyphilis. The diagnosis of neurosyphilis is made on a basis of CSF WBC count of 20 cells/μL or greater, CSF pleocytosis and/or a reactive CSF VDRL, and/or a positive CSF intrathecal *T. pallidum* antibody index.[2]

VDRL and treponomal antibody test is also sensitive except the chances of false positivity. The fluorescent treponemal antibody absorption (FTA-ABS) test is a reliable test with less chance of false positive result. Dark-field microscopy of the skin lesions is the most specific technique for diagnosis.

The treatment is injection benzathine penicillin for 2 weeks and olanzapine for psychosis and treatment of partner.

REFERENCES

1. Timmermans M, Carr J. Neurosyphilis in the modern era. J Neurol Neurosurg Psychiatry. 2004;75:1727-30.
2. Ahsan S, Burrascano J. Neurosyphilis: An Unresolved Case of Meningitis. Case Rep Infect Dis. 2015;2015:634259. https://doi.org/10.1155/2015/634259.

CASE 30

MIDDLE-AGED LADY WITH MASSIVE HEPATOMEGALY

CASE SUMMARY

A 46-year-old female, housewife came to hospital with the complaints of distension of the abdomen for 2.5 years which was gradual in onset and progressive in nature, it was not associated with any abdominal pain, vomiting, anorexia or weight loss. She also complained of occasional upper abdominal discomfort for the last 1 year. As her abdominal distension was increasing day by day along with persistent abdominal discomfort, she got herself admitted in a private clinic one month back. There she was investigated and was given three units of whole blood transfusion. On query, she mentioned that 2 years back she suddenly developed headache, dizziness, acute confusional state and generalized weakness and was admitted in a private clinic where MRI of brain findings were inconclusive, and she improved with symptomatic treatment. She was a known case of hypothyroidism with goiter for about 10 years and hypertensive for the last 2 years. She took tablet losartan (50 mg), tablet bisoprolol (2.5 mg) and tablet thyroxine (50 mg) regularly. Her menstrual cycle was regular with normal duration and flow with a history of using injectable contraceptives for several times 4–5 years back. Her bowel and bladder habits were normal. There was no history of fever, jaundice, oral ulcer, joint pain or leg swelling.

On examination, she was ill-looking, anemic. There was loss of lateral one-third of eyebrows. Palmar erythema was present. Thyroid gland was palpable, diffuse, size was about 5 cm × 10 cm, smooth surface, firm in consistency, nontender, and no bruit. Vitals were within normal limit. Abdominal examination revealed hugely distended abdomen, no tenderness. Liver was palpable, which was about 30 cm from the right costal margin and about 14 cm from the xiphoid process, smooth surface, firm, nontender, and no bruit. Liver span was 36 cm. Spleen was just palpable. Bedside urine for protein: (+++). The rest of the examination was normal.

Investigations showed: hemoglobin (Hb): 6.6 g/dL, WBC: 14,025/mm^3 (DC: N-70%, L-25%), platelet: 158,000/mm^3. ESR: 115 mm in first hour.

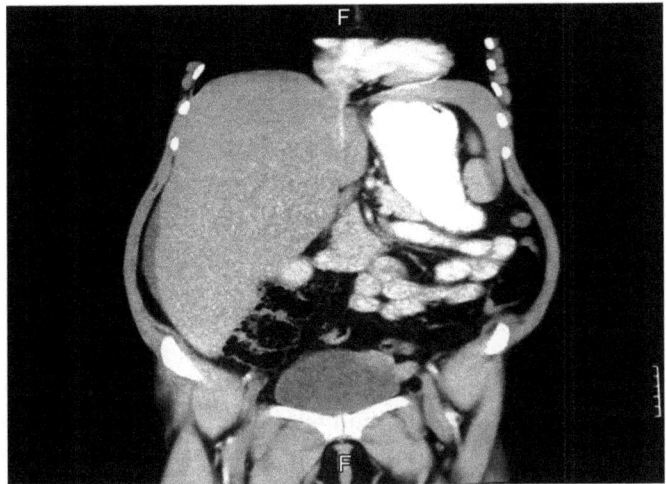

Fig. 1: CT scan of abdomen showing huge hepatomegaly, mild splenomegaly and ascites.

PBF—anisocytosis with anisochromia with fair number of macrocytes, microcytes and spherocytes, suggestive of hemolytic anemia. Reticulocyte count: 2.5%. Urine R/E: albumin present (+++). S. creatinine 1.7 mg/dL. Fasting lipid profile: normal except S. TG: 337 mg/dL and HDL: 26 mg/dL. TSH: 13.9 µIU/mL, free T4: 0.86 ng/dL, antithyroglobulin antibody: <20 IU/mL (negative), antithyroid peroxidase antibody: 238 IU/mL (positive). USG of thyroid: diffuse goiter. Liver function tests were normal except ALT: 68 U/L, alkaline phosphatase: 249 U/L. Viral markers HBs Ag, anti-HCV antibody, anti-HBc (total) antibody—negative. CXR, RBS, S. electrolyte, ECG, echocardiography: normal. Ultrasonography of whole abdomen showed liver was hugely enlarged in size occupying right hypochondrium, right lumber (right lobe), epigastric and left hypochondriac regions (left lobe). Hepatic parenchymal echogenicity was increased and echotexture was homogenous, spleen was mildly enlarged with minimal ascites. CT scan of abdomen also showed huge hepatomegaly, mild splenomegaly and ascites (Fig. 1). S. cortisol, S. ACTH, S. prolactin: normal. Coombs' test—direct and indirect: negative. Hb electrophoresis, barium follow through, barium enema of large gut, upper GIT endoscopy: normal. MT test: negative (2 mm). ICT for malaria and kala-azar: negative. Tumor markers: serum alpha-fetoprotein (AFP), CA-19.9, and CA-125 were negative.

QUESTIONS

1. Give four possible diagnoses.
2. What further investigations would you undertake?
3. How would you treat her?

DISCUSSION

For this case, along with hypertension with hypothyroidism, the additional possible diagnoses were:
- Storage disease (Gaucher's disease) with glomerulonephritis
- Nonalcoholic steatohepatitis with glomerulonephritis
- Amyloidosis
- Autoimmune hepatitis with glomerulonephritis.

Further investigations done in this patient:
- *Liver biopsy:* Stains performed: H & E, PAS and Congo red.
  - *Microscopic examination:* Sections correction-revealed liver tissue with mildly distorted hepatic lobular architecture. Many of the hepatocytes are swollen and some show vacuolated cytoplasm. Bridging fibrosis is present. The portal areas and the fibrous bands contain moderate number of chronic inflammatory cells. No foamy histiocytes are seen in the portal areas. Glycogen content of hepatocyte is reduced in the vacuolated cells. No amyloid deposit, granuloma or malignancy is seen. Definitive diagnosis could not be made.
- *Fibroscan of liver:* Fibrosis score: 42.2 kPa. Fibrosis stage: F4.
- *Bone marrow study:* Reactive marrow.

So, among all the confounding findings and laboratory evidences, yet with the diagnosis still illusive, we reflected that our patient had:
- History of neurological involvement (acute confusional state)
- Ascites
- Proteinuria (+++)
- Hemolytic anemia

Next, we did the following investigations:
- Serum ANA: Positive (value: 28.3), pattern: homogeneous.
- Anti-ds-DNA: Positive.
- ENA profile: Negative.
- 24 hours urinary total protein: 3 g/24 hours.
- Creatinine clearance rate: 82.5 mL/min (Range: 95–160 mL/min).

After establishing the diagnosis of systemic lupus erythematosus (SLE), we reviewed literatures[1,3] and case reports which solidified our conjecture that our patient's hepatomegaly was due to SLE.

Revised criteria for diagnosis of SLE according to 2015 American College of Rheumatology (ACR)/Systemic Lupus International Collaborating Clinics (SLICC) are given in Table 1.

Final Diagnosis: Systemic Lupus Erythematosus with Hypertension with Hypothyroidism

Patient was given tablet prednisolone (10 mg) 3 tablets once daily and was advised to come for follow-up after 2 weeks. In the next follow-up, there was improvement of her general well-being and significant relief of her abdominal

Table 1: 2015 ACR/SLICC revised criteria for diagnosis of SLE.[2]

Acute/subacute cutaneous lupus rash	Up to 2 points
• Malar rash	2 p
• Subacute cutaneous Lupus erythematosus (SCLE) rash	1 p
• Palpable purpura or urticarial vasculitis	1 p
• Photosensitivity	1 p
Discoid lupus erythematosus (DLE) rash or hypertrophic lupus rash	1 p
Non-scarring frank alopecia	1 p
Oral/nasal ulcers	1 p
Joint disease	1 p
Pleurisy and/or pericarditis	1 p
Psychosis and/or seizure and/or acute confusion	1 p
Kidney involvement	Up to 2 points
• proteinuria $\geq 3+$ or ≥ 500 mg/day or urinary casts	1 p
• Biopsy-proven nephritis compatible with SLE	2 p
Hematologic	Up to 3 points
• WBC count <4000/mm^3 or lymphocyte count <1500/mm^3 on ≥ 2 occasions or WBC count <4000/mm^3 along with lymphocyte count <1500/mm^3 in one occasion	1 p
• Thrombocytopenia <100,000/mm^3	1 p
• Hemolytic anemia	1 p
Serologic tests	Up to 3 points
• Low titer positive ANA	1 p
• High titer FANA= fluorescent antinuclear antibody test with homogeneous or rim pattern	2 p
• Positive anti-ds DNA	2 p
• Positive anti-Sm	2 p
• Antiphospholipid antibodies (aPLs)	1 p
• Low serum complement (C_3 and/or C_4 and/or CH_{50})	1 p

Note: The patients with 4 points out of 16, have definite diagnosis of SLE. With 3 points highly suggestive SLE, with 2 points probable SLE and with 1 point possible SLE are the diagnosis.

discomfort. On examination, there was no anemia and liver was palpable, about 22 cm from the right costal margin and about 12 cm from the xiphoid process, firm, nontender. Liver span was 30 cm. Spleen was not palpable. Follow-up investigations revealed:

- CBC: Hb 11.30 g/dL. ESR 30 mm in first hour
- Urine R/M/E: Albumin—trace
- 24 hours UTP: 1.1 g/24 hours
- LFT: S. Albumin: 43 g/L (previously: 36 g/L). S. SGPT: 42U/L (previously: 68 U/L). Alkaline phosphatase: 48 U/L (previously: 249 U/L).
- USG of W/A: Huge hepatomegaly with mild-to-moderate fatty change (right lobe 17.3 cm and left lobe 14 cm vertically) (previously 32 cm in CT scan of abdomen.) Prominent spleen (10.7 cm). (previously 14.2 cm in USG of W/A and 17cm in CT scan of abdomen.) No ascites (previously ascites in USG of W/A and CT scan of abdomen).

So, our patient was overall improved. Though rare, *hepatic involvement in SLE* may be in the form of fatty liver, portal inflammation and fibrosis, chronic active or chronic persistent hepatitis, cirrhosis, cholestasis, hepatic necrosis, granulomatous hepatitis, nonspecific reactive hepatitis, nodular regenerative hyperplasia, or hepatic infarction and arteritis.[3]

REFERENCES

1. Miller MH, Urowitz MB, Gladman DD, Blendis LM. The liver in systemic lupus erythematosus. Q J Med. 1984;53(211):401–9.
2. Revised criteria for diagnosis of SLE according to 2015 American College of Rheumatology (ACR)/Systemic Lupus International Collaborating Clinics (SLICC). Available from: https://sliccgroup.org/research/sle-criteria/
3. Grover S, Rastogi A, Singh J, Rajbongshi A, Bihari C. Spectrum of histomorphologic findings in liver in patients with SLE: a review. Hepat Res Treat. 2014;2014:562979.

CASE 31

YOUNG MALE WITH FEVER, RASH, JAUNDICE AND ANASARCA

CASE SUMMARY

A 27-year-old male, resident of Saudi Arabia, got admitted in Dhaka Medical College and Hospital, with high-grade fever, generalized pruritic maculopapular rash, progressively increasing jaundice and anasarca for the last 4 weeks. Two weeks prior to this illness, he experienced nonspecific body ache for which he was prescribed nonsteroidal anti-inflammatory drug (NSAID). Before this admission, he was admitted in a tertiary care hospital and was diagnosed as a case of expanded dengue syndrome with acute hepatic failure on the basis of positive dengue antibody. His medical documents revealed that during his illness he received a number of broad-spectrum antibiotics, including meropenem, tazobactam, and tigecycline. With time, his condition did not improve rather he developed maculopapular rash all over the body.

On examination, he was anemic, deeply icteric, febrile and hemodynamically stable. Multiple painless oral ulcers were present and both conjunctivas were congested. Desquamated maculopapular rash was present in trunk and limbs (Fig. 1A). He had firm, nontender hepatosplenomegaly. Ascites and bilateral pleural effusions were present.

Investigations showed anemia and persistent eosinophilia (highest 19.9%) with high erythrocyte sedimentation rate (ESR) and C-reactive protein (CRP). The liver enzymes were very high with normal alkaline phosphatase. Lactate dehydrogenase (LDH) was high with positive direct Coombs test. Both prothrombin time (PT) and activated partial thromboplastin time (APTT) were high. D-dimer and fibrinogen degradation product (FDP) were also high. Blood and urine culture did not show any growth. His dengue immunoglobulin M (IgM) and immunoglobulin G (IgG) as well as herpes simplex virus (HSV) IgM and IgG were positive. ANA and leptospira and human immunodeficiency virus (HIV) screen were negative. Chest X-ray

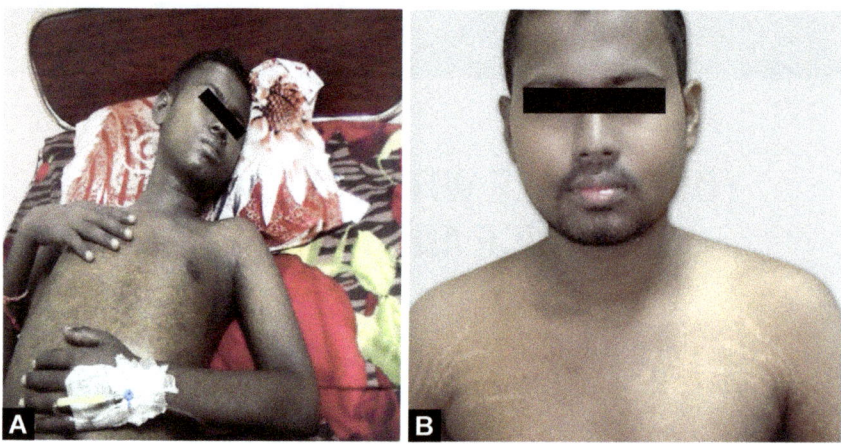

Figs. 1A and B: Photographs of the patient. (A) Desquamated maculopapular rash in trunk and limbs (before treatment); (B) After treatment.

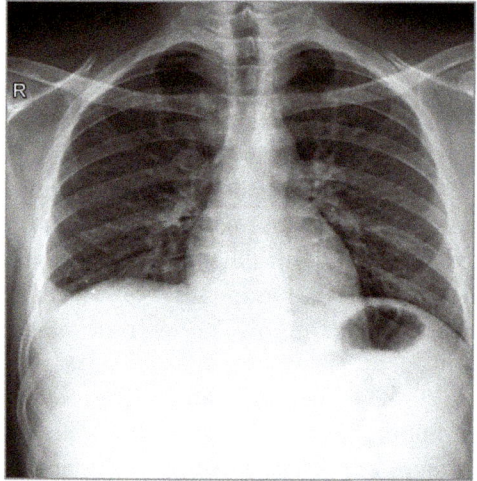

Fig. 2: Chest X-ray showing right-sided pleural effusion.

showed right-sided pleural effusion (Fig. 2). Ultrasonography of whole abdomen evidenced mild hepatosplenomegaly, ascites and prominent abdominal lymphadenopathy. Endoscopy of upper gastrointestinal (GI) tract was normal.

QUESTIONS

1. What are the differentials?
2. Which investigations would you like to do to reach the diagnosis?
3. What treatment will you commence?

DISCUSSION

Our patient was diagnosed as a case of expanded dengue syndrome evidenced by positive anti-dengue antibody and systemic involvement. Since this febrile patient presented with rapid development of anemia, jaundice, lymphadenopathy and hepatosplenomegaly- leptospirosis, SLE, leukemia, and lymphoma were probable considerations. But negative ANA, negative serology for leptospira and presence of generalized maculopapular rash following a viral illness guided us to think differently. Drug reaction was a strong possibility, especially because of history of receiving several broad-spectrum antibiotics and NSAIDs. In our case, presence of skin rashes, fever, lymphadenopathy, hematological abnormalities, internal organ involvement and presence of eosinophilia made the diagnosis of DRESS (Drug Reaction, Rash with Eosinophilia and Systemic Symptoms) syndrome evident.

DRESS syndrome is a delayed type IV hypersensitivity reaction thought to be mediated by antiviral T cells.[1] It is a severe, idiosyncratic multisystem reaction to drug. Medicines most commonly associated with DRESS syndrome are anticonvulsants, antibiotics (particularly beta-lactams), and allopurinol. Other medications that are known to be associated with DRESS include NSAIDs, captopril, mood stabilizers, and antiretrovirals.[2] In addition, a Japanese group consider human herpes virus 6 (HHV-6) reactivation to be diagnostic. However, as this syndrome is likely to occur 2–3 weeks after the onset of the rash, the diagnosis may be missed if reactivation is not measured at the correct time. Experts also debate whether reactivation is part of the syndrome or should be interpreted as a complication. In our case, herpes simplex virus types IgM and IgG were positive. To confirm the diagnosis, we decided to perform liver biopsy which showed diffuse hydropic change and feathery degeneration of the hepatocytes along with hepatocellular cholestasis. Portal tracts showed infiltration of acute and chronic inflammatory cells including few eosinophils which favored drug-induced hepatotoxicity.

Final Diagnosis: Drug Reaction with Eosinophilia and Systemic Symptoms Syndrome

He was treated with methylprednisolone and given supportive care. On discharge, his general condition improved, rash disappeared and anasarca resolved (Fig. 1B).

DRESS/drug-induced hypersensitivity syndrome (DIHS) is used to describe a severe drug hypersensitivity eruption associated with constitutional symptoms, such as fever, malaise, lymphadenopathy, hepatitis, myocarditis, interstitial nephritis, and pneumonitis. Long latency between symptoms and initiation of offending drug, and clinical worsening despite discontinuation of the culprit drug is considered as a characteristic feature. Out of the

Table 1: Diagnostic criteria of DRESS syndrome[3,4]

Criteria	No	Yes	Unknown
Fever	−1	0	−1
Lymphadenopathy two sites >1 cm	0	1	0
Circulating atypical lymphocytes	0	1	0
Peripheral hypereosinophilia	0	1 (10–19.9%)	2 (>20%)
Skin involvement:			
Extent of cutaneous eruption > 50%	−1	1	0
Cutaneous eruption suggestive of DRESS	−1	0	0
Biopsy suggesting DRESS	−1	0	1
One internal organ involved	0	1	0
Two internal organs involved	0	2	0
Resolution in >15 days	−1	0	−1
Laboratory result negative for at least three of the following: (1) ANA; (2) Blood C/S; (3) HAV/HBV/HCV serology; (4) Chlamydia Mycoplasma serology	0	1	0

Note: Scoring: 2—no case; 2 to 3—possible case; 5—probable case; >5—definite case.

diagnostic criteria (Table 1), our patient had peripheral hypereosinophilia, skin involvement, internal organ involvement (renal and bone marrow), negative autoantibody and serology, and scored 6; hence he was a definite case of DRESS syndrome. Oral steroids and supportive care are mainstay of treatment.

REFERENCES

1. Velema MS, Voerman HJ. DRESS syndrome caused by nitrofurantoin. Neth J Med. 2009;67:147–9.
2. Tas S et al. Management of drug rash with eosinophilia and systemic symptoms (DRESS syndrome): an update. Dermatology. 2003;206:353-56
3. Pannu AK, Saroch A. Diagnostic criteria for drug rash and eosinophilia with systemic symptoms. J Family Med Prim Care. 2017;6(3):693–4. doi:10.4103/2249-4863.222050.
4. Cacoub P, Musette P, Descamps V, et al. The DRESS Syndrome: a Literature Review. Am J Med. 2011;124(7):588–97.

CASE 32

DIZZY GENTLEMAN WITH ABDOMINAL PAIN

CASE SUMMARY

A 43-year-old man came to the hospital with three episodes of vertigo and recurrent abdominal pain in last 3 months. Each episodes of vertigo lasted for around 15 minutes, which was accompanied by nausea, and was unrelated to posture. Abdominal pain was central, of moderate intensity, nonradiating and triggered by meal. It resolved spontaneously after around 2 hours. He also gave a history of occasional blurring of vision and spontaneous gum bleeding for several times in the past.

Examination was completely unremarkable, except for palmar erythema and enlarged retinal vein on fundoscopy. Blood pressure was 140/90 mm Hg.

Investigation revealed hemoglobin (Hb)—17.6 g/dL, red blood cell (RBC) count: 8.13 M/μL, white blood cell (WBC)—15.58/cmm (N:72%), platelet—535/mm^3, erythrocyte sedimentation rate (ESR)—3 mm in first hour, hematocrit (Hct)—58.11%. Other reports including C-reactive protein (CRP) titer were normal.

QUESTIONS

1. What is the clinical syndrome?
2. What other investigations should be done in this case to establish the diagnosis?
3. What other physical signs could be present in this case?

DISCUSSION

This man fulfills the classic triad of hyperviscosity syndrome: mucosal bleeding, visual changes and neurological symptoms.[1] Hyperviscosity can be confirmed by measuring serum viscosity. Common causes of hyperviscosity syndrome: Waldenström macroglobulinemia, multiple myeloma, leukemia, polycythemia, thrombocytosis, myeloproliferative disease, sickle cell disease, spherocytosis and others. Our patient was a case of polycythemia rubra vera (PRV), which was subsequently confirmed by presence of JAK2 V617F mutation and panmyelosis of bone marrow.

Final Diagnosis: Polycythemia Rubra Vera

Polycythemia rubra vera, is one of the chronic myeloproliferative neoplasms (MPNs), characterized by clonal proliferation of myeloid cells. It can be distinguished from the other MPNs by elevated red blood cell mass.[1]

Most patients present incidentally with elevated hemoglobin or hematocrit or with symptoms of hyperviscosity such as headache, lassitude, dizziness, pruritus, epistaxis. Some may present with complications like thrombosis, bleeding.[1,2] Physical signs that may be found in PRV: splenomegaly (75%), hepatomegaly, plethora, hypertension (HTN), sausage-shaped enlarged retinal vein and palmar erythema.

JAK-2 V617F mutation is positive in 95% of cases. If JAK-2 mutation is negative, raised red cell mass and exclusion of other causes of secondary erythrocytosis can establish the diagnosis. Neutrophil and platelet counts may be frequently raised.

Treatment includes venesection, hydroxycarbamide or interferon alfa and intravenous 32P which is reserved for older patients.[2]

REFERENCES

1. Tefferi A. Clinical manifestations and diagnosis of polycythemia vera. In Rosmarin AG (Ed).UpToDate. Retrieved April, 2019, from http://www.uptodate.com/contents/clinical-manifestations-and-diagnosis-of-polycythemia-vera.
2. Ralston SH, Penman ID, Strachan MWJ, Hobson RP. Davidson's Principles and Practice of Medicine. 23rd ed. Edinburgh: Churchill Livingstone/Elsevier; 2018. p. 970.

CASE 33

YOUNG LADY WITH RECURRENT MULTIPLE SUBCUTANEOUS NODULES

CASE SUMMARY

A 28-year-old lady presented with multiple subcutaneous nodules in different parts of her body for the last 3 years. At first, she developed itchy rash with erythematous border in her submammary folds which was diagnosed as fungal infection and was treated accordingly. After a few days, she developed blisters all over the body followed by a tumor-like swelling beside her rectum which was surgically excised. Two months later she again noticed subcutaneous nodules on both arms, upper part of the chest and back, and along her midaxillary lines. Nodules were variable in size, shape and were painful, gradually increased in size. There was no fever, headache, weight loss, joint pain, skin rash or alteration in bowel and bladder habit. She was a regularly menstruating woman and mother of two children. Family history was unremarkable.

On general examination she was mildly anemic, with moderate ankle edema. Vital signs were normal. On abdominal examination, it was soft, nontender, non-distended, without any organomegaly. Local examination revealed multiple subcutaneous nodules over dorsal spine, upper chest, both arms, and midaxillary area. Largest one was on left arm 10×7 cm, firm in consistency, tender, rounded, overlying skin was red and shiny, but few were mobile and the rest were fixed with underlying structures; no overlying ulcer, discharge or sinus was found. Some other itchy lesions with well-circumscribed hyperemic margin with central hypoemic area were present over submammary fold, waist, groin and thigh. Other systemic examinations revealed no abnormality.

Investigations showed: Hb—10.7 g/dL; erythrocyte sedimentation rate (ESR) in first hour—53 mm; peripheral blood film (PBF)—normocytic anemia with normal white blood count and platelet count; renal and liver function test was normal; random blood sugar (RBS) was 5.3 mmol/L; chest X-ray posteroanterior view showed mild cardiomegaly and segmental consolidation in upper lobe; ultrasonography (USG) of the whole abdomen revealed two hypoechoic areas in each lower quadrant of abdomen revealed variable size and shape; cytoplasmic antineutrophil cytoplasmic antibodies (c-ANCA), perinuclear antineutrophil cytoplasmic antibodies (p-ANCA), anti-hepatitis C virus (HCV) and human immunodeficiency virus (HIV 1 & 2) were negative; tuberculin test revealed a 3 mm induration; X-ray dorsolumbar spine showed no bony or joint lesion; biopsy was taken from left arm nodule and histopathology revealed the presence of a malignant small round cell tumor suggestive of Ewing sarcoma/primitive neuroectodermal tumor (PNET).

QUESTION

1. What differentials could be considered in this case and why?

DISCUSSION

Considering the history and physical examination in this case, we had some differentials for her subcutaneous nodules like: tubercular subcutaneous nodule, lymphoma, melioidosis, multiple abscess, vasculitis, etc. Though she denied any low-grade fever, weight loss and other systemic features of tuberculosis, but due to wide prevalence of TB in our country and its diverse presentation, we searched for it. Vasculitis was another possibility but absence of prodromes, no joint involvement, and negative markers of vasculitis excluded the possibilities. Sarcoidosis and lymphoma were other considerations. Keeping those in mind after getting hypoechoic areas in abdomen, we decided to take biopsy and sent for histopathological examination which revealed PNET.

Final Diagnosis: Primitive Neuroectodermal Tumor

Primitive neuroectodermal tumors are a group of highly malignant tumors composed of small round cells of neuroectodermal origin that affect soft tissue and bone. Since PNETs exhibit great diversity in clinical manifestations and share pathologic similarities with other small, round cell tumors; classification of this family of tumors is challenging and controversial.

The PNET was first recognized in 1918 in an ulnar nerve—was thought to arise directly from nerves. In 1996 Batsakis et al. divided the PNET family of tumors into the following three groups based on the tissue of origin:[1]
1. CNS primitive neuroectodermal tumors (PNETs)—tumors derived from the central nervous system, e.g. Medulloblastoma.
2. Neuroblastoma—tumors derived from the autonomic nervous system.
3. Peripheral primitive neuroectodermal tumors (pPNETs)—tumors derived from tissues outside the central and autonomic nervous system.

The pPNETs are also classified as part of the Ewing family of tumors (EFTs), because immunohistochemical and cytogenetic studies suggest that both tumors have a common origin, and share the same reciprocal translocations, most commonly between chromosomes 11 and 22. But, while Ewing sarcoma is more common in bone, pPNETs are more common in soft tissues; and the latter often exhibits more aggressive clinical behavior with worse outcomes. Patients may have metastatic disease (commonly in lung, bone, bone marrow) at presentation and the rate of metastasis ranges from 20 to 31%.

pPNETs are further classified into:[2]
- Ewing's sarcoma (osseous and extraosseous)
- Malignant pPNETs or peripheral neuroepithelioma of bone and soft tissues
- Askin tumor (peripheral neuroepithelioma of the thoracopulmonary origin)
- Others: neuroectodermal tumor, ectomesenchymoma, peripheral medulloepithelioma.

Clinical symptoms depend on the site of presentation (thoracopulmonary region, pelvis, abdomen, extremities, and rarely, head and neck region), but invariably include pain and swelling of the surrounding structures due to mass effect.[2] Based on the distribution of lesions, our patient most likely had pPNETs.

Tissue biopsy with cytogenetic and immunohistochemical studies is paramount in diagnosing pPNETs. Typical histopathological findings include: monotonous collection of small, round, darkly (blue) stained cells. Electron microscopy reveals neurosecretory granules with microtubules and microfilaments. Short dendritic processes lie between cells in pPNETs which are absent in Ewing's sarcomas. Computed tomography (CT) scanning and magnetic resonance imaging (MRI) are essential in determining the limits of tumor involvement and ruling out metastatic disease. Bone marrow biopsy, technetium 99m bone scan, positron emission tomography (PET) scan may be indicated.[2]

The treatment plans depend on whether the disease is localized or metastatic. Current recommendations advocate:
- Complete surgical resection whenever possible
- Adjuvant or neoadjuvant chemotherapy (with vincristine/ doxorubicin/ cyclophosphamide and ifosfamide and etoposide[3])
- Radiotherapy.

Patients with metastatic disease uniformly have poor outcome ranging from zero to 25%, 5-year survival rates as compared with 40–79% for patients with localized disease.[4]

REFERENCES

1. Batsakis JG, Mackay B, el-Naggar AK. Ewing's sarcoma and peripheral primitive neuroectodermal tumor: an interim report. Ann Otol Rhinol Laryngol. 1996; 105(10):838-43.
2. Honrado CP. Primitive Neuroectodermal Tumors. 2018. [online] Available from https://emedicine.medscape.com/article/855644-overview [Accessed April 2019].
3. Carvajal R, Meyers P. Ewing's sarcoma and primitive neuroectodermal family of tumors. Hematol Oncol Clin North Am. 2005;19(3):501-25, vi-vii.
4. Scurr M, Judson I. How to treat the Ewing's family of sarcomas in adult patients. Oncologist. 2006;11(1):65-72.

CASE 34

ADOLESCENT GIRL WITH UNEXPLAINED CHRONIC LIVER DISEASE WITH SHORT STATURE AND PRIMARY AMENORRHEA

CASE SUMMARY

A 16-year-old unmarried girl presented with recurrent episodes of convulsion for the last 7 years and frequent passages of stool with frequent vomiting since birth. At the age 8, she first developed generalized tonic-clonic convulsion with urinary incontinence, postictal confusion, excessive sleepiness and several episodes of vomiting. That time after admission in hospital, she was diagnosed as a case of hepatic encephalopathy due to chronic liver disease (on the basis of liver biopsy) with short stature. Since then, she experienced similar episodes of convulsion 5-6 times followed by postictal confusion, amnesia, headache and several episodes of vomiting. She denied aura, lightheadedness or palpitation prior to convulsion, no history of weakness or numbness or speech difficulty after convulsion; no hematemesis, melena or bleeding from any other site, except occasional gum bleeding. Her mother also stated that her daughter had frequent passage of stool about 10-12 times per day up to age 5 years, later reduced to 3-4 times per day but the stool color and consistency was normal and unmixed with blood. There was no history of fever, abdominal pain, swelling, shortness of breath (SOB), cough, jaundice, itching, joint pain, skin rash, pigmentation, oral ulceration or Raynaud's phenomenon but history of undocumented jaundice 10 years back. Family history was significant—there was consanguinity of marriage between her parents and one of her three brothers died of liver disease. Her menstruation never started. She was born at term by uncomplicated vaginal delivery. Her developmental milestones were age-appropriate, except delayed head control and walking.

On physical examination, she was short statured but trunk and limbs were proportionate. Her height was 4 feet 6 inch, weight was 28 kg and BMI was 15.36 kg/m². Pulse was 80 beats per minute, blood pressure was 100/60 mm Hg, temperature 98°F, respiratory rate was 18 breaths per min. She was moderately anemic, was normally pigmented but axillary and pubic hair were absent. No thyromegaly or lymphadenopathy was found and there was no stigmata of liver disease. Nervous system examination revealed that the patient was fully conscious, oriented to time, place and person. Her speech, memory and intelligence were normal. Cranial nerve examination including fundoscopy revealed normal findings. Slit-lamp exam showed no Kayser-Fleischer ring. Muscle power was 5/5 in all four limbs with normal deep tendon reflexes. On admission, plantar responses were extensor bilaterally but later became flexor. All modalities of sensation were intact and coordination and gait was also normal. Abdominal examinations revealed enlarged liver, about 2 cm from the right costal margin along the midclavicular line, nontender, firm, smooth surfaced with well-defined margin. Upper border of liver dullness was in right 5th intercostal space (ICS) without any hepatic bruit. No other organomegaly was found. Shifting dullness was absent. Reproductive system examination showed underdeveloped breasts, Tanner stage III and absent pubic hair. External genitalia appeared normal with intact hymen and normal distal part of vagina. Other systemic examination revealed no abnormality.

Investigations showed low Hb level—7.3 g/dL. Total platelet count was also low. Peripheral blood film (PBF) showed normocytic normochronic anemia with thrombocytopenia. Liver function test showed normal bilirubin, alanine aminotransferase (ALT), alkaline phosphatase, but prothrombin time was 17.40 sec and serum albumin 2.71 g/dL. Her fasting lipid profile was always abnormal. Her initial triglyceride level was 575 mg/dL and subsequent tests were done yearly which showed values of 377 mg/dL, 169 mg/dL, 147 mg/dL and 228 mg/dL while the patient was on lipid-lowering medication. To find out the cause of liver disease, we did viral markers which were all negative, antinuclear antibody (ANA) was negative; serum ferritin, blood copper level, ceruloplasmin level and urinary copper level all were within normal range. We also did penicillamine challenge test which was negative. Endoscopy of upper gastrointestinal tract (GIT) showed grade II esophageal varices; liver biopsy showed moderate chronic hepatitis, fibro scan of liver showed fibrosis score 63.9 and fibrosis stage: F4. Due to her short stature, we assessed her hormone profile [thyroid-stimulating hormone (TSH), triiodothyronine (T3), total thyroxine (T4), luteinizing hormone (LH), follicle-stimulating hormone (FSH), prolactin, parathyroid hormone (PTH), adrenocorticotropic hormone (ACTH)], which were all found to be normal. Ultrasonography (USG) of the whole abdomen showed liver was enlarged and parenchymal echotexture was coarse and nonhomogeneous and having multiple echogenic solid masses, spleen was mildly enlarged, uterus infantile, left ovary could not be visualized. Magnetic resonance imaging (MRI) of brain showed hyperintensity in the caudate nucleus. Electroencephalogram (EEG) showed generalized encephalopathy. Karyotyping showed 46 XX.

For her treatment purpose, we did X-ray to determine her radiological age which was about 11–12 years. We also did her MRI of whole abdomen showing multifocal dysplastic nodules in both lobes of liver, infantile uterus and bilateral smaller ovaries. To exclude Gaucher's disease, we sent blood to see beta-glucocerebrosidase enzyme activity, which was found to be normal.

QUESTIONS

1. What are the possible diagnoses for this young girl?
2. Is there any correlation between dyslipidemia and chronic liver disease?

DISCUSSION

Considering all the problem lists: repeated convulsion, repeated vomiting, frequent passage of stool, poor appetite, short stature/failure to thrive, features of chronic liver disease (evident in liver biopsy) and features of hepatic encephalopathy, underdeveloped breast, primary amenorrhea, absent axillary and pubic hair, anemia, hepatomegaly, infantile uterus, smaller ovaries and early onset of symptoms at the age of 8, consanguinity of marriage between parents, death of younger brother at the age of 6, due to liver disease; we had the following differentials.

Apart from short stature and primary amenorrhea, chronic liver disease (CLD) due to:
- Wilson's disease
- Lysosomal storage disease.

Though young patient with CLD with neuropsychiatric symptom, our first consideration was Wilson's disease, but absence of KF ring, normal serum copper level, ceruloplasmin level and normal 24 hours urinary copper virtually excluded Wilson's disease.

Then our next consideration was storage disease. Normal beta-cerebrosidase level ruled out Gaucher's disease. Among all other lysosomal storage diseases, cholesteryl ester storage disease (CESD) was most probable as her lipid profile was always abnormal since her childhood. Her recurrent passage of stool and vomiting can also be explained by CESD where deposition of lipid particle in gut mucosa can give rise to these symptoms.

Then we decided to measure enzyme activity of lysosomal acid lipase and it was found to be 12.1 nmol/hr/mg, which indicates lower activity level and goes in favor of CESD.

We also did her parents' fasting lipid profile to exclude familial causes and that was found within normal limit. Thus, we diagnose our case as CESD. For her short stature and amenorrhea, we did not find any other underlying cause except chronic disease (CLD), which by affecting hypothalamic pituitary gonadal axis might cause amenorrhea.

Final Diagnosis: Cholesteryl Ester Storage Disease[1]

We treated our patient symptomatically and with atorvastatin and fibrates. As her radiological age was about 11-12 years (whereas chronological age was 16 years), so with consultation of endocrine department, we treated our patient with biosynthetic human growth hormone—somatropin (injection Norditropin SimpleXx 1 mg/day s/c) and she was responsive very well. Her hight increased about 2.5 cm within 3 months period of growth hormone treatment. For her short stature estrogen priming could be an option but contraindicated due to CLD. So during discharge, the patient was advised to continue growth hormone therapy.

Cholesteryl ester storage disease is inherited as an autosomal recessive condition.[2] So parents who are close relatives (consanguineous) have a higher chance to have children with a recessive genetic disorder. CESD affects males and females in equal number.[3] The majority of patients with CESD present an exon 8 splice junction mutation (E8SJM), G to A transition at position 1 (E8SJM) as one of the defective alleles in the *LIPA* gene.[4]

The symptoms and severity of CESD are highly variable. Some individuals may develop symptoms during childhood; others may have extremely mild cases that cause few symptoms. Still some individuals may not have any noticeable symptoms and may go undiagnosed until adulthood. CESD is characterized by alterations of blood lipoprotein profile; patients present with hypercholesterolemia, hypertriglyceridemia, high-density lipoprotein (HDL) deficiency with abnormal lipid deposition in many organs. Hepatomegaly usually becomes progressively worse eventually causing scarring (fibrosis) of the liver. In approximately one third of patients, the spleen may also be enlarged (splenomegaly). Abnormal enlargement of the adrenal glands (adrenomegaly) may also occur in few individuals.[2]

Cholesteryl ester storage disease is a type of lysosomal storage disorder, another closely associated disease is Wolman disease. In CESD, there is mutation for *LAL* gene which retains some enzyme activity while Wolman disease produces an enzyme with no residual activity or no enzyme at all and it is often fatal within the first 6 months of life.

Diagnosis of CESD may be suspected based upon identification of characteristic symptoms such as abnormally enlarged liver. Thus a thorough clinical evaluation, a detailed patient history (including family history) and specialized test that reveals deficient activity of the LIPA enzyme in certain cells of the body. Molecular genetic testing for mutations in the *LIPA* gene is also available.[4]

In 2015, the Food and Drug Administration (FDA) approved Kanuma (sebelipase alfa) as first treatment for LAL deficiency.[5] A hypolipidemic diet and statins are other therapeutic tools used against CESD. The combination of diet and drug administration has led to dramatic reductions in the levels of lipids such as cholesterol and triglycerides in the blood of affected individuals. A few individuals with CESD who developed CLD have been treated with a liver transplant with positive results.[4] Genetic counseling is recommended for affected individuals and their families. Other treatment is symptomatic and supportive.

REFERENCES

1. Karmaker M, Akter S, Kabir A, Azad KAK, Mollah AH. Cholesteryl ester storage disease – a rare presentation. J of Med. 2018;19(2):130-2.
2. Reiner Ž, Guardamagna O, Nair D, Soran H, Hovingh K, Bertolini S, Jones S, Ćorić M, et al. Lysosoml acid Lipase deficiency – an under-recognized cause of dyslipidaemia and liver dysfunction. Atherosclerosis. 2014;235(1):21-30.
3. Muntoni S, Wiebusch H, Jansen-Rust M, et al. Prevelence of cholesteryl ester storage disease. Arterioscler Thromb Vasc Biol. 2007;27(8):1866-8.
4. Cholesteryl ester storge disease. Available from: https://rarediseases.org/rare-disease/cholesteryl-ester-storage-disease/. Accessed on January 07,2018.
5. Burton BK, Balwani M, Feillet F, Bari I, Burrow TA, Grande CC, Coke M, Consuelo-sanchez A, et al. A phase-3 trial of sebelipase alfa in lysosomal acid lipase deficiency. N Engl J Med. 2015;373:1010-20. DOI: 10.1056/NEJMoa 1501365.

CASE 35

MIDDLE-AGED MALE WITH ATAXIA, DYSARTHRIA AND URINARY INCONTINENCE

CASE SUMMARY

A 55-year-old hypertensive male presented with progressive ataxia, dysarthria and urinary incontinence for the last 1.5 years. His family members also stated that he had gradual decline in mental ability and loss of memory severe enough to interfere with daily life for the last 6 months. The patient had no history of fever, trauma, convulsion or loss of consciousness. His bowel habit was normal. He was treated with antituberculosis medication 25 years back for his pulmonary tuberculosis (TB). No similar family history was present.

Examination revealed scanning speech and cerebellar signs were present including horizontal nystagmus, dysdiadochokinesia, dysmetria, and ataxic gait. Hypertonia was present in all four limbs. Reflexes were brisk with bilateral plantar extensor. Fundoscopy was normal.

All his routine blood tests, including complete blood count and urine routine examination, were normal. Ultrasound showed mild prostate enlargement. His calcium, vitamin B12 and folate levels were normal, and syphilis screening was negative. Computed tomography (CT) brain showed ventriculomegaly. Cerebrospinal fluid (CSF) pressure was normal, and fluid study was insignificant.

QUESTIONS

1. What are the differential diagnoses?
2. What is the next step of investigation?

DISCUSSION

In this patient, clinical features were suggestive of either lesion involving the cerebellum and spinal cord simultaneously, or demyelinating disease, or normal pressure hydrocephalus (NPH). The CT scan of brain showed ventriculomegaly which can be a presentation of NPH. However, it does not explain the cerebellar signs. Moreover, CSF pressure was normal. So we performed magnetic resonance imaging (MRI) of brain which showed cerebellar and brainstem atrophy and ventriculomegaly suggestive of olivopontocerebellar degeneration (Figs. 1 and 2).

In most individuals, spinocerebellar ataxia (SCA) presents at early age with ataxia and dysmetria. Later, they progress to dysarthria, diplopia and brainstem dysfunctions. As it is a dominantly inherited disease, suggestive family history is frequently present.[1] In this patient, the onset was late without any family history. That is why first we thought of few common possibilities and then performed the MRI of brain, and it showed a very rare

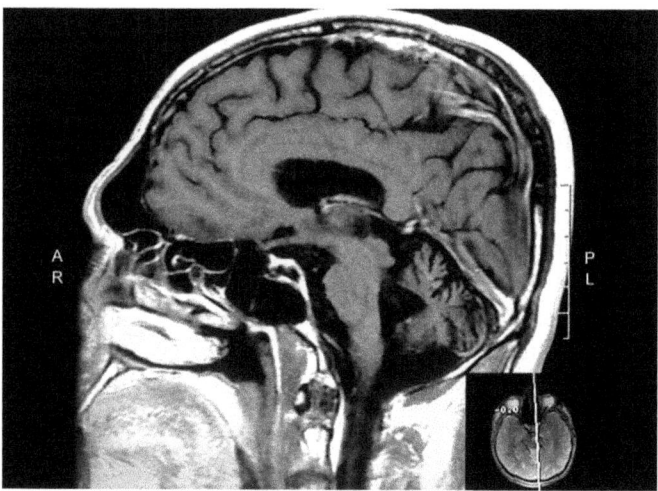

Fig. 1: Latest magnetic resonance imaging of brain olivopontocerebellar degeneration.

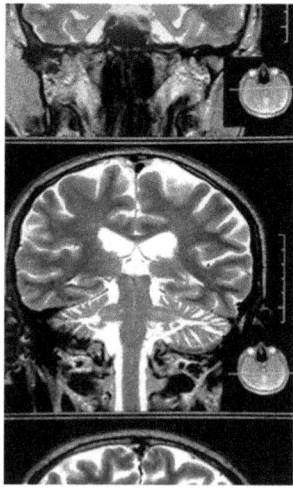

Fig. 2: Magnetic resonance imaging of brain showing ventriculomegaly.

disease with a rare presentation. The urinary incontinence was most likely due to involvement of lower spinal cord. Thus, we diagnosed him as a case of SCA (Figs. 1 and 2). Genetic testing and genetic counseling should have been performed.

Final Diagnosis: Spinocerebellar Ataxia

Spinocerebellar ataxia is a term referring to a group of hereditary progressive ataxias, those are characterized by slow degenerations in cerebellum, often accompanied with brainstem and other parts of central nervous system (less commonly the peripheral nervous system).[2] SCA is inherited in an autosomal dominant manner. There are many types of SCA. Around 30 types have been reported in the literature so far. Among them 1,2, 3, 5, 6, 7, 8, 10 and many more are dominant. The genetic testing is the confirmatory diagnosis and treatment is supportive. The learning of the case is that SCA can affect at any age and there might be denovo mutation which results in absence of suggestive family history.

It is a challenge for scientists and clinicians to identify which pathways are central to cerebellar integrity so that preventive and symptomatic therapies might be developed for individuals with SCA.

REFERENCES

1. Paulson HL. The spinocerebellar ataxias. J Neuroophthalmol. 2009;29(3): 227-37. doi:10.1097/WNO0b013e3181b416de.
2. Taroni F, DiDonato S. Pathways to motor incoordination: the inherited ataxias. Nat Rev Neurosci. 2004;5(8):641-55.

CASE 36

YOUNG LADY INFECTED WITH DUAL INTRACELLULAR PATHOGENS

CASE SUMMARY

A 30-year-old unmarried female garment worker, resident of Goffargaon, Mymensingh (northern part of Bangladesh) presented with double peak fever for 3 months and abdominal swelling for 1.5 months. Fever was intermittent, without chills and rigor, subsided with antipyretics but reappeared subsequently. Then she developed gradual distension of abdomen unassociated with pain, bowel-bladder complaints, or swelling of other parts of the body. She had no cough, neck swellings, bone or joint pain, rash or bleeding, headache, convulsion, or alteration of consciousness. She denied history of contact with tuberculosis (TB) patient, or of drug abuse or unprotected sexual exposure. Patient was immunized as per expanded program on immunization (EPI) schedule and gave no history of previous TB or jaundice. She lived in an earthen house with her family; none of her family members had similar illness.

On general examination, patient was moderately anemic, temperature was 99°F, other vitals were normal. Examination of abdomen revealed hepatosplenomegaly (liver: 7 cm and spleen: 8 cm). No abnormality was detected on examination of other systems.

Investigations revealed white blood cell (WBC) count of 2,200/ mm^3 (neutrophil: 880/mm^3, lymphocyte: 1,100/mm^3, monocyte: 150/mm^3, and eosinophil: 300/mm^3), red blood cell (RBC) count was 2.3 million/mm^3, hemoglobin (Hb): 7.8 g/dL, mean corpuscular volume (MCV): 108 fL, mean corpuscular hemoglobin (MCH): 33 pg, mean corpuscular hemoglobin concentration (MCHC): 31 g/dL. Platelet count was 185,000/mm^3 and erythrocyte sedimentation rate (ESR) was 125 mm in first hour. Peripheral blood film (PBF) showed macrocytic anemia with leukopenia (no malaria parasite seen); with normal serum vitamin B$_{12}$ and folate levels. Chest skiagram and electrocardiogram (ECG) were normal. Renal, hepatic and thyroid function tests were normal. HBsAg was negative. Ultrasonography of whole abdomen: suggestive of cystitis and hepatosplenomegaly. Upper gastrointestinal tract (GIT) endoscopy was normal. Immunochromatographic test (ICT) for kala-azar and rK39 were positive, but, *Leishmania donovani* (LD) bodies were not found in buffy coat. Amastigotes were found in splenic aspirate and that confirmed the diagnosis of visceral leishmaniasis (VL/kala-azar).

QUESTION

1. How would you manage this case?

DISCUSSION

Up to this point, there was no diagnostic dilemma, so we proceeded to start drug treatment for VL. During planning and initiation of management, the patient was explained her condition, treatment options with prognosis and related risks. At this point, under proper privacy and after understanding the gravity of the situation, she confessed that, due to social stigma and fear, she had concealed the history of being anti-HIV-1 positive for the last 4 years and that she had been taking HAART (with zidovudine, lamivudine, nevirapine) since the diagnosis of HIV infection had been made. She also provided relevant documents and reports- out of which, one report from a year back showed, the patient had CD4 count: 339/mm^3 of blood. We repeated CD4 count, which was 140/mm^3.

Final Diagnosis: HIV Infection with Visceral Leishmaniasis

Visceral leishmaniasis (VL) has emerged as an important infection associated with HIV, as it has significant clinical, diagnostic and epidemiological implications. The two infections are mutually reinforcing: HIV-infection imparts vulnerability to VL, while VL accelerates HIV replication and progression to AIDS. Further, coinfected patients serve as reservoirs of the parasite for the insect vector. As many as 35 countries throughout the world have reported cases of VL/HIV coinfection.[1] Notably, about half of coinfected patients develop full AIDS criteria within 2 months after the diagnosis of VL.[2]

Clinical manifestations of VL in HIV-infected people are almost the same as those in non-HIV-infected people. Usual features are fever, weight loss, hepatosplenomegaly and pancytopenia.

Indirect diagnostic methods such as serology for VL frequently fail; direct methods like aspirations (bone marrow, lymph node or splenic) are reliable but are invasive, require skilled microscopy, and have less value in treated and relapsing patients.[1] Peripheral blood analysis by polymerase chain reaction (PCR) has higher sensitivity and specificity to detect the parasite in coinfected patients. Recently, the use of real-time PCR has been shown to be a suitable tool for monitoring parasite load during the follow-up of coinfected patients, helping to predict the risk of relapses after treatment.[3] After confirmed diagnosis of VL, tratment should be started immediately, while continuing HAART. Liposomal amphotericin B is preferred for treatment of VL in HIV coinfected patients.

In contrast to the clinical manifestations, the course and prognosis of coinfected individuals differ importantly from those in non-HIV-infected individuals. It is characterized by significantly higher treatment failure rate regardless of the drug used and higher drug toxicity rates than those for VL in non-HIV-infected individuals. All coinfected patients will relapse—and eventually die—unless they are given antiretroviral therapy (ART).

During a 1-year follow-up in a comparative study, 53.7% of HIV-positive patients with kala-azar died compared with 7.5% of HIV-negative patients with kala-azar (p <0.001). Factors that predicted survival of HIV-positive patients were HAART, a high CD4+ cell count, and the use of secondary prophylaxis for VL.[2]

REFERENCES

1. Leishmaniasis and HIV coinfection. WHO. [online] Available from: https://www.who.int/leishmaniasis/burden/hiv_coinfection/burden_hiv_coinfection/en/
2. Alvar J, Aparicio P, Aseffa A, Den Boer M, Cañavate C, Dedet JP, Gradoni L, Ter Horst R, López-Vélez R, Moreno J. The relationship between leishmaniasis and AIDS: the second 10 years. Clin Microbiol Rev. 2008;21(2):334–59.
3. Monge-Maillo B, Norman FF, Cruz I, Alvar J, López-Vélez R. Visceral Leishmaniasis and HIV coinfection in the Mediterranean region. PLoS Negl Trop Dis. 2014;8(8):e3021. doi: 10.1371/journal.pntd.0003021.

CASE 37

YOUNG FEMALE WITH RECURRENT PAINFUL REDDISH SKIN NODULES WITH FEVER

CASE SUMMARY

A 19-year-old student presented with recurrent painful nodular reddish skin lesions for last 8 months and episodic fever for the same duration. She also developed malaise, anorexia, body ache, headache and extreme fatigability followed by painful red patches on the face, both arms and forearms, which turned into nodules on the same day. Skin lesions were associated with fever which was initially of low-grade, episodic, later became high-grade and more marked in the evening, sometimes associated with chills and rigor and subsided by sweating spontaneously or after taking antipyretic. The highest recorded temperature was 102°F. On subsequent attacks, she developed arthralgia of small joints of hands and feet without any morning stiffness. She also gave history of hair loss and significant weight loss of around 13 kg over the last 8 months but never had similar nodular swelling before. There was no similar illness in the family or contact with tuberculosis patient. She didnot give any history of oral ulceration, butterfly rash, purpuric rash, bone pain, photosensitivity, cough, chest pain, tingling or numbness and ocular disturbances or any bowel or bladder disturbance. With above complaints, she consulted several physicians and was diagnosed as a case of erythema nodosum and got treatment with corticosteroid and antituberculosis drugs but responses were inadequate.

On examination, she was depressed, mildly anemic with a body mass index (BMI) of 17.78 kg/m^2. Examination of skin revealed multiple ill-defined erythematous nodular lesions over the cheeks, flexor and extensor surfaces of both arms, forearms and both legs (Figs. 1A to C). The lesions were about 1–2 cm in diameter, reddish, and extremely tender. The interlesional areas were normal in color but tenderness was present. Old lesions were macular, bluish in color, had ill-defined margins with overlying desquamation. Sensation was intact on all lesions. There were no thickened peripheral nerves. All other systemic examination revealed no abnormality.

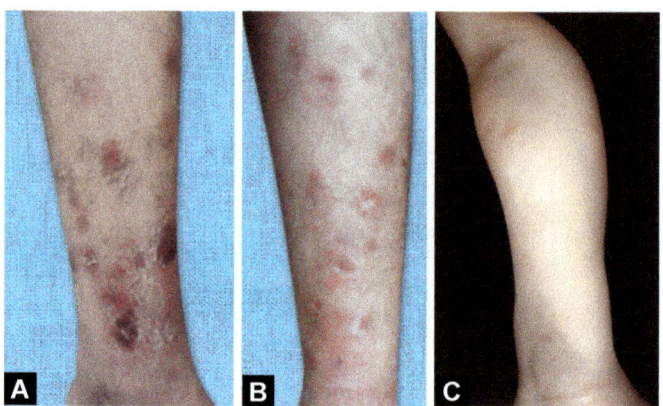

Figs. 1A to C: Multiple old and new lesions in both legs and right upper limb.

Investigations showed hemoglobin (Hb) level was 11 g/dL. Peripheral blood film (PBF) showed normocytic anemia with leukopenia. Erythrocyte sedimentation rate (ESR) was 40 mm for 1 hour. Serum creatinine, bilirubin and calcium were within normal limit but her urine showed trace albumin. Antistreptolysin O (ASO) titer and C-reactive protein (CRP), thyroid stimulating hormone (TSH) were all normal. Mantoux test (MT) was negative. Chest X-ray (CXR) posteroanterior (PA) view revealed normal study. Ultrasonography (USG) of whole abdomen showed mild pelvic collection in pouch of Douglas. Antinuclear antibodies (ANA) were positive but antidouble stranded deoxyribonucleic acid (anti-ds DNA) was negative. Extractable nuclear antigens (ENA) profile showed positive anti-Sjögren's syndrome-related antibody (anti-SSA Ab). Slit skin smear taken from earlobe, site of lesions and nasal septum was stained with modified Ziehl–Neelsen stain but Hansen's bacilli was not found. Then, skin biopsy showed infiltration of lymphocytes and histocytes in the subcutaneous adipose tissue, widening of the intervening septa along with fibrosis. No granuloma was seen and all the findings were compatible with erythema nodosum.

QUESTIONS

1. What is the most likely diagnosis?
2. What further investigations should be carried out to reach a final diagnosis?

DISCUSSION

Our initial differentials were erythema nodosum due to SLE, mycobacterial infection (including tuberculosis and leprosy), streptococcal infection, sarcoidosis, dermatomyositis and mixed connective-tissue disease (MCTD). After taking history, doing physical examination and even after doing initial investigations, causes of erythema nodosum were not borne out. Regarding mycobacterial infections, tuberculosis was our first consideration. But, there were no features of pulmonary tuberculosis, chest X-ray was normal, and MT was negative, disfavoring tuberculosis. Next, due to extensive presence of erythema nodosum, leprosy was a strong possibility, but initial negative slit skin smear was confusing. So, we decided to go for polymerase chain reaction (PCR) test for *Mycobacterium leprae*. PCR followed by gel electrophoresis done from skin tissue showed detection of *Mycobacterium leprae* DNA.

Final Diagnosis: Leprosy (Erythema Nodosum Leprosum)

DNA-based PCR assays can be 100% specific, while the sensitivity ranges from 34–80% in patients with paucibacillary (PB) forms to greater than 90% in patients with multibacillary (MB) forms of the disease.[1] Since finding *Mycobacterium leprae* is crucial in the confirmatory diagnosis of early leprosy, the use of PCR technique to enhance the ascertainment of difficult cases such as early PB and pure neural leprosy (PNL) is advisable and important in reaching a definitive diagnosis.

Treatment modalities given to the patient were nonpharmacological to provide education of the patient and party about the disease process and referral to a specialized leprosy center.

Pharmacological treatment includes antimicrobial treatment for 12–24 months with rifampicin, clofazimine, dapsone and corticosteroid, 40–80 mg daily with gradual reduction over 1–6 months.[2]

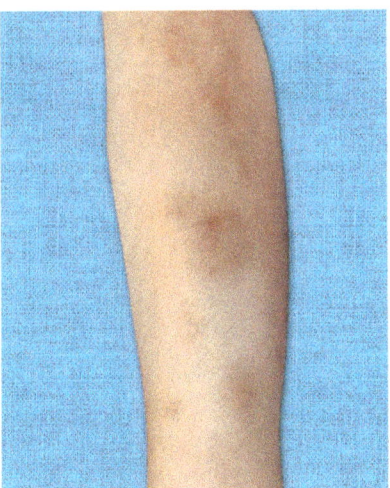

Fig. 2: Healed lesions in follow-up.

Our patient came in follow-up after 1 month and at that time fever was absent, skin lesions started to resolved (Fig. 2), pain subsided, weight gained up to 4 kg and her general well-being was also improved.

REFERENCES

1. Martinez AN, Talhari C, Moraes MO. PCR-Based Techniques for Leprosy Diagnosis: From the Laboratory to the Clinic. PLoS Negl Trop Dis. 2014;8(4):e2655.
2. Ralston SH, Penman ID, Strachan MWJ, Hobson RP. Davidson's Principles and Practice of Medicine. 23rd ed. Edinburgh: Churchill Livingstone/Elsevier; 2018;1037:268–70.

CASE 38

RELIGIOUS YOUNG BOY WITH FEVER DURING TRAVEL

CASE SUMMARY

A 16-year-old young boy from Republic of Chad, Africa came to Bangladesh for the Dawah activity of Tableeq-e-Jamaat (a religious movement of Sunni Muslims) and presented with the history of high-grade fever for 7 days, severe weakness leading to inability of walking or sitting without assistance for 1 day, drowsiness and disorientation for the last several hours. The boy was unable to give any history during admission. However, with the help of interpreter from Tableeq-e-Jamaat, history was taken with great difficulty from the attendant of the boy who only spoke in native language of Africa. According to them, they started their journey 14 days back. At first, they came to Egypt from Chad. On the fourth day, he developed high-grade, intermittent fever associated with chills and rigors, which subsided with profuse sweating. He became severely weak during febrile period, but felt better during afebrile period. He, along with his accompanied person, left Egypt with fever on the fifth day of their travel and came to Bangladesh. On the third day of arrival to Bangladesh, he consulted with a medicine specialist, and was diagnosed as a case of enteric fever and was treated with tab ofloxacin 400 mg twice daily, but there was no improvement. Moreover, he continued experiencing high-grade, intermittent fever (maximum temperature: 105°F). He again consulted with the previous physician. Immunochromatographic test (ICT) for malaria was done and came positive. He was prescribed oral quinine sulfate and doxycycline. After getting a single dose of medication, he became drowsy and nonresponsive. In that situation, he was admitted under our care. There was no significant history on systemic query. It was his first-time travel outside his country. One of his uncles recently suffered from malaria in Chad.

On examination, he was disoriented, Glasgow coma scale (GCS) score—11/15 (E4M5V1), moderately anemic, nonicteric, pyrexic (temperature: 104°F), dehydrated, blood pressure (BP)—80/60 mm Hg, p—110/m and features of meningism were absent. Complete evaluation of mental status could not be done as the patient was drowsy and there was language barrier. Cranial nerve examination could not be done due to his disorientation but fundoscopic examination revealed exudates and white central spots with hemorrhage on right eye (Fig. 1). Motor functions were intact. His plantar responses were extensor bilaterally. Gait could not be evaluated due to extreme weakness. On abdominal examination, there was splenomegaly. The rest of the systemic examination findings were normal. Bedside urine test for blood and protein was negative. Bedside capillary blood glucose (CBG) was 5.4 mmol/L. Rapid diagnostic test for malaria was positive (Fig. 2).

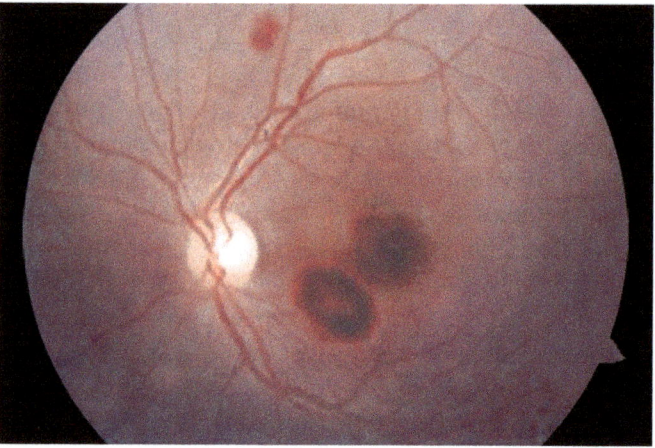

Fig. 1: Exudates with white central spots in hemorrhage found in fundal photograph.

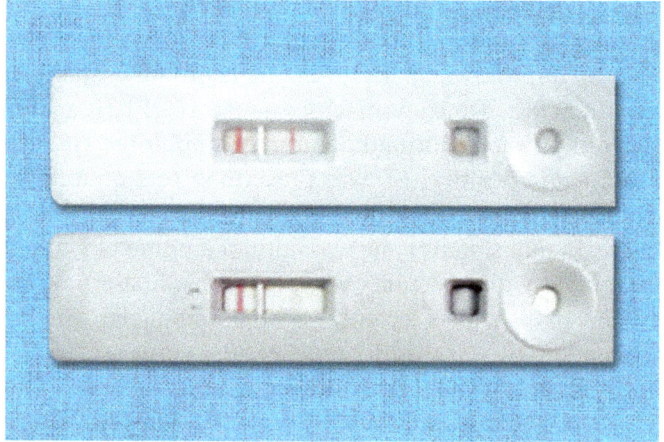

Fig. 2: Rapid diagnostic test positive in the case vignette

Investigation showed Hb%—7 g/dL, white blood cells (WBCs)—7,140/mm^3 (N: 65%, L: 25%), platelet (PLT)—101,000 mm^3, erythrocyte sedimentation rate (ESR) in first hour—35 mm, serum creatinine—1.02 mg/dL, alanine aminotransferase (ALT)—20 U/L, aspartate aminotransferase (AST)—54 U/L, malarial parasite (MP)—not found.

QUESTIONS

1. What is the single most likely diagnosis?
2. What further investigations can be done?
3. How would you manage this case?

DISCUSSION

Initially, the patient presented with flu-like symptoms such as headache, fever, shivering, arthralgia mimicking other conditions, such as sepsis, gastroenteritis and other viral diseases.

Our patient was initially treated as a case of enteric fever with antibiotics without any response. His deteriorating condition forced us to think alternatively. His residing area, pattern of fever, travel history, significant weakness leading to inability to walk and inability to eat, and gradually decreasing consciousness pointed us to make the diagnosis of cerebral malaria (CM). Then ICT for *Plasmodium falciparum* was done and the result came positive.

Final Diagnosis: Severe Malaria (Cerebral Malaria with Severe Prostration with Anemia)

After admission, the following treatments were given within 15 minutes:
- Intravenous (IV) artesunate 2.4 mg/kg (patient need 120 mg) body weight.
- IV fluid was given to prevent dehydration.
- Frequent monitoring of vital signs, blood glucose and urine output done.

After getting two more doses of artesunate at 12 and 24 hours, the patient became completely oriented and afebrile. Afterwards, he was treated with artemether and lumefantrine combination [atemisinin combination therapy (ACT)] for successive 3 days (total 6 doses). A single dose of primaquine was prescribed at the end of treatment.[1]

Cerebral malaria (CM) is a severe *Plasmodium falciparum*—malaria having case fatality around 20%. The tropical and subtropical regions are mostly affected.

Neurological symptoms which are predominantly found include unarousable coma (Glasgow coma scale score <11) or coma persisting >30 minutes after a seizure, focal or generalized convulsion, increased or decreased muscle tone, variable tendon reflexes, flexor or extensor plantar reflexes, abnormal posturing, nystagmus, conjugate gaze palsy, opisthotonus and drowsiness.[1]

Therefore, every patient of malaria with altered sensorium should be managed as severe malaria until proved otherwise.

There is a rapid proliferation of the parasites in the human body in relation to red cell invasion. Consequently, blood flow becomes stagnant in a large number of cerebral capillaries resulting in thrombotic occlusion of the capillaries. Hence, the peripheral blood film may initially be negative for malarial parasite. Repeated blood film may turn positive.

It has serious complications which include respiratory distress, acute kidney injury (AKI), hypoglycemia, acidosis, severe anemia, shock, hemoglobinuria, jaundice, bleeding tendency and extreme weakness.

Microscopic examination of blood films is a gold standard method. Antigen-based rapid diagnostic tests (RDT) are also used for early detection.

In CM, IV artesunate is preferable than IV quinine when available. ACT should be used which decreases resistance to any single drug component. Chloroquine drug resistant is high, so it should not be used in falciparum malaria. Multidrug resistance malaria is a public health threat. Prompt diagnosis is essential for timely initiation of appropriate therapy.

REFERENCE

1. Revised Malaria Treatment Regimen – 2017, 6th Version, National Malaria Elimination and Aedes Transmitted Disease Control Program, DGHS, Ministry of Health and Family Welfare, Bangladesh. Available from: http://www.dghs.gov.bd/index.php/en/publications/guideline.

CASE 39

MIDDLE-AGED MALE WITH RECURRENT OROGENITAL ULCERATIONS

CASE SUMMARY

A 60-year-old man presented with recurrent oral and genital ulcerations, frequent tiny vesicular eruptions all over the body which healed spontaneously, and intermittent fever for the last 1 year. He also had frequent attacks of sore throat, anorexia and significant weight loss. For the last 5–6 months, he had dry cough without hemoptysis. He gave no history of headache, visual disturbance, chest pain, abdominal pain or arthralgia. His bowel–bladder habit was normal. He had no history of thromboembolic manifestations. There was no known contact with infectious disease and no recent travel abroad. He was a nonsmoker, nonalcoholic and never used any intravenous (IV) recreational drugs.

On examination, he was ill-looking, emaciated, mildly anemic; and had nontender cervical and left supraclavicular lymphadenopathy. There was a small, almost healed ulcer on helix of right ear and also around glans penis. Multiple white patches were present on both sides of buccal mucosa. His pulse was 82/min, blood pressure (BP) 110/80 mm Hg, body temperature was normal and respiratory rate was 20 breaths/min. Examination of the chest revealed features of right-sided pleural effusion. The rest of the examination findings including fundoscopy were normal.

Investigations showed complete blood count (CBC) was normal except hemoglobin (Hb)—9.4 g/dL, erythrocyte sedimentation rate (ESR)—90 mm in the first hour. Peripheral blood film (PBF) showed features of microcytic hypochromic anemia. C-reactive protein (CRP)—94.3 mg/L. A chest X-ray (CXR) revealed encysted pleural effusion on right lower zone. The ultrasonography (USG) of W/A showed some enlarged lymph nodes (LN) in the peripancreatic and periportal region, a right-sided mild pleural effusion and trace ascites. Serum albumin was low. Urine routine examination and serum electrolytes were normal and blood culture and sensitivity test revealed no growth. Pathergy test was negative.

QUESTIONS

1. What important relevant history should be taken?
2. What further investigations would you like to do to reach final diagnosis?

DISCUSSION

The patient presented with history of recurrent orogenital ulceration, which initially lead us to think of Behçet's disease. But the absence of other essential diagnostic criteria[1] virtually excluded that diagnosis. The reference case also had repeated tiny vesicular eruptions all over the body, intermittent fever, frequent attacks of sore throat, dry cough and significant weight loss for the last 1 year. This history suggested immunodeficiency, hence, taking history regarding unsafe sexual exposure was important here, which on query, the patient admitted of having several years back.

After appropriate counseling, anti-human immunodeficiency virus (HIV) antibody test was carried out and anti-HIV 1 and 2 were positive. CD4 cell count was 130/mm^3 of blood.

To identify the cause of right-sided pleural effusion, pleural fluid study was done which revealed:
- Color: straw; appearance: hazy
- Cell count: 280/mm^3; N—10%, L—90%
- Biochemical: protein—41.5 g/L; glucose—1.8 mmol/L
- Adenosine deaminase (ADA): 89.7 U/L.

Next, we opted for pleural biopsy. Histopathology report stated: smear showed cellular debris and lymphocytes on the background of epithelioid histiocytes forming granuloma. Diagnosis: granulomatous inflammation, favoring tuberculosis.

Final Diagnosis: Acquired Immunodeficiency Syndrome (AIDS) with Right-sided Tubercular Pleural Effusion

TB is an opportunistic infection, and HIV weakens the immune system, increasing the risk of TB in people with HIV/AIDS. Worldwide, tuberculosis is one of the leading causes of death among people with HIV.[2] The presentation of pulmonary TB in HIV-infected patients is quite similar to that seen in HIV uninfected patients. Symptoms are usually present for several weeks to months. In the early stage of HIV disease, TB presents as a classic reactivation-type disease. But in advanced cases, patients are more likely to present with primary TB. There is increased prevalence of extrapulmonary TB, disseminated TB and sputum smear-negative, culture-positive TB in HIV-infected patients. For diagnosis, specimens should be collected and examined for acid-fast bacilli and culture should be done for mycobacteria. Diagnosis of TB in a HIV-infected individual is challenging. Fever, weight loss and malaise may be attributed to HIV itself. Therefore high index of suspicion is necessary to diagnose TB in an AIDS patient. These patients need simultaneous treatment for both AIDS and tuberculosis; however, when to start treatment and what medicines to prescribe requires individualizations since taking multiple drugs at the same time raises the risk of drug interactions and side effects.[2]

REFERENCES

1. Ralston SH, Penman ID, Strachan MWJ, Hobson RP. Davidson's Principles and Practice of Medicine. 23nd ed. Edinburgh: Churchill Livingstone/Elsevier; 2018. p. 1044.
2. [Internet] https://aidsinfo.nih.gov/understanding-hiv-aids/fact-sheets/26/90/hiv-and-tuberculosis--tb-[Accessed in April, 2019]

CASE 40

YOUNG MALE WITH RECURRENT ATTACKS OF FEVER AND JOINT PAIN

CASE SUMMARY

A 20-year-old nonsmoker, nonalcoholic farmer presented with recurrent high-grade intermittent fever and painful knee joints for three months. The joint pain was persistent, gradually progressive and this time was not associated with swelling, skin rash, oral ulcer or other systemic features. Two months earlier, he had similar episodes of high-grade fever which was accompanied by painful swelling in both knee joints (Fig. 1). He also mentioned to have occasional skin rash, neck swelling and discomfort in abdomen at that time. On the basis of clinical presentation and laboratory findings, he was diagnosed as adult-onset Still disease (AOSD) and was treated with injectable methylprednisolone and later prescribed oral prednisolone in tapering dose with azathioprine. He was symptom free for 2 weeks and

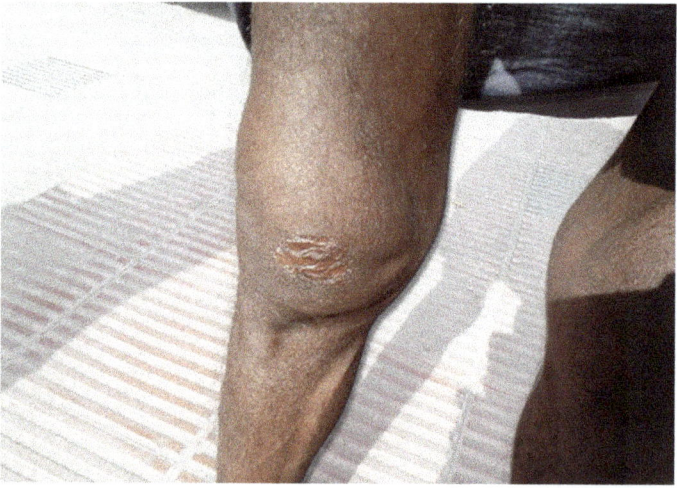

Fig. 1: Swollen left knee joint with traumatic scar mark found at the initial presentation.

then again developed same pattern of fever with joint pain. However, this time, there was no joint swelling. He was father of a 1-year-old baby. All of his family members were in good health.

General examination showed that he was ill-looking and emaciated, mildly anemic and febrile. All other systemic examination revealed no abnormality.

His investigation revealed anemia, leukopenia with high ESR. Peripheral blood film showed features of combined deficiency anemia. CRP and serum ferritin levels were high. Liver and renal function test reports were within normal limit. Ultrasonography of abdomen showed mild hepatosplenomegaly. Bone marrow examination revealed patchy areas of hypocellularity. Blood and urine culture did not grow any growth. Ultrasound of joint did not detect any fluid accumulation or any erosion. Autoantibody profile and serum ACE level were found normal.

QUESTIONS

1. What are the possibilities?
2. Should we stop azathioprine?

DISCUSSION

This male patient was successfully treated as a case of AOSD with immuno-suppressive earlier. Now the recent presentation can be explained by relapse of the AOSD, sepsis/septic arthritis, other connective tissue disease. Comparing him to his previous presentation, he was significantly improved except the fever. In this episode, fever was associated with arthralgia, but there was no arthritis. On query, he also admitted to use oral herbal medications for 2 weeks which he stopped after the onset of fever. His blood count was in favor of picture of sepsis with the background of using azathioprine and herbal medicine. All his autoantibody profile was negative which disfavors the possibility of connective issue disease. But both erythrocyte sedimentation rate and C-reactive protein were high with high ferritin level that points toward relapse of the primary disease.

We treated his sepsis with broad spectrum antibiotic. As the bone marrow was hypocellular, the question was: Should we stop azathioprine? But patient's AOSD was well controlled with it. Moreover, the herbal drug can also suppress the bone marrow. So, we continued the drug and prescribed him prednisolone to treat the relapse. Patient improved significantly. He was afebrile after 7 days and discharged. He came in follow-up 1 month later with improved well-being.

In this scenario, the decision was crucial if we should stop azathioprine or not. Had we have stopped it, then the relapse might have been more dangerous. So, we decided to continue azathioprine with proper support. We transfused him on several occasions. And later he improved.

Final Diagnosis: **Relapsed Still's Disease with Bone Marrow Suppression (Drug-induced)**

Adult-onset Still's disease is a systemic inflammatory disorder of unknown etiology that is a common cause of pyrexia of unknown origin and can also have serious musculoskeletal sequelae. The diagnosis is usually clinical. Yamaguchi criteria is one of the sensitive diagnostic clinical tools. According to these criteria, diagnosis requires at least five features, with at least two of these being major diagnostic criteria.

Major Criteria
- Fever of at least 39°C for at least 1 week
- Arthralgia or arthritis for at least 2 weeks
- Nonpruritic salmon-colored rash (usually over trunk or extremities while febrile)
- Leukocytosis (≥10,000/μL), with granulocyte predominance.

Minor Criteria
- Sore throat
- Lymphadenopathy
- Hepatomegaly or splenomegaly
- Abnormal liver function tests
- Negative tests for antinuclear antibody and rheumatoid factor.[1]

Adult-onset Still's disease is treated with immunosuppressive drugs. Steroids such as prednisolone are used to treat severe symptoms. Other commonly used medications include hydroxychloroquine, azathioprine, penicillamine, methotrexate, etanercept, anakinra, cyclophosphamide, adalimumab, rituximab and infliximab. The prognosis of AOSD is typically good, but the relapse rate is high. Literature review revealed that incidence happen in most of the cases during tapering prednisolone which is likely related to the speed of tapering and maintenance dose.[2] Clinicians must be aware of the possibilities of relapse and treat the presenting symptom accordingly.

REFERENCES

1. Yamaguchi M, Ohta A, Tsunemastu T, et al. Preliminary criteria for classification of adult Still's disease. J Rheumatol. 1992;19(3):424–30.
2. Liu Z, Lv X, Tang G. Clinical features and prognosis of adult-onset Still's disease: 75 cases from China. Int J Clin Exp Med. 2015;8(9):16634–9. Published 2015 Sep 15.

CASE 41

MIDDLE-AGED WOMAN WITH MULTIPLE LUMPS AND BUMPS

CASE SUMMARY

A 65-year-old hypertensive, diabetic housewife was admitted in hospital through outpatient department (OPD) with multiple nodular swelling on both upper limbs, and fatigue for the last 2 months. The woman was apparently well till she noticed few painless nodular subcutaneous swellings/lumps on the forearm, wrist and hands. These lumps developed on additive pattern within 1 week, and were enlarging slowly. She also complained of undue fatigue for the same duration with occasional shortness of breath on exertion.

Examination revealed multiple subcutaneous nodules on forearms and hands which were firm, nontender with smooth surface and indistinct margin with negative slip test. Nodules had no punctum, erythema, ulceration or dyspigmentation. The total number of nodules was 11 and the largest one measured 4 × 3 cm in size. The chest examination revealed bilateral scattered fine crackles.

Investigations showed that complete blood count (CBC) was normal except lymphopenia (17%). Erythrocyte sedimentation rate (ESR), C-reactive protein (CRP) titer, serum creatinine, serum electrolyte, serum calcium, alanine aminotransferase (ALT), and urine routine examination were normal. Electrocardiography (ECG) was within normal limit and chest X-ray (CXR) showed bilateral hilar lymphadenopathy. The Mantoux (MT) test was 0 mm at 72 hours.

QUESTIONS

1. What may be the diagnosis?
2. What should be the next course of action?

DISCUSSION

For this middle-aged lady with multiple subcutaneous nodules with exertional dyspnea, undue fatigue, and bilateral hilar lymphadenopathy—sarcoidosis was a strong possibility. If we only consider the multiple subcutaneous nodules, then neurofibromatosis, Dercum's disease, dermatofibroma and many other conditions come in mind. But since none of the aforementioned diseases could holistically explain all findings of our patient, we went for biopsy of the nodule, and histopathology showed many well-formed non-caseating granuloma made of epithelioid cell and giant cell, but lymphocyte counts were scanty, suggestive of sarcoidosis.

Along with clinical features, lymphopenia, anergy to MT test, bilateral hilar lymphadenopathy on CXR, and histological features of naked granuloma (scanty lymphocyte) all suggested Darier-Roussy syndrome, which is a variant of sarcoidosis.

Final Diagnosis: Darier-Roussy Syndrome (Subcutaneous Sarcoidosis)

Darier-Roussy syndrome (also known as subcutaneous sarcoidosis) is a cutaneous condition characterized by numerous deep-seated nodules on the trunk and extremities.[1] It affects 1-2% of patients with sarcoidosis. It has bimodal age distribution, with one peak at the third decade and another after fifth decade of life.

Patients often have less severe systemic disease. This syndrome is commonly associated with hilar adenopathy (extracutaneous systemic disease involvement).[2]

Diagnosis can be made by *subcutaneous sarcoidal or epithelioid granulomas with minimal lymphocytic inflammation.*[3,4]

Recommended treatment is oral glucocorticoids, response is noted usually within 4-8 weeks. Intralesional glucocorticoids may be used. Steroid-sparing drugs that have a role in subcutaneous sarcoidosis are hydroxychloroquine, methotrexate, clofazimine, thalidomide, dapsone, and allopurinol.[4,5]

REFERENCES

1. James WD, Berger TG. Andrews' Diseases of the Skin: Clinical Dermatology. Saunders Elsevier; 2006.
2. Deepak CL, Panchagnula R, Swetha J, Kori D. A case of Darier-Roussy sarcoidosis. IJCR. 2016;1(1):CS2.
3. Yanardağ H, Pamuk ON, Karayel T. Cutaneous involvement in sarcoidosis: analysis of the features in 170 patients. Respir Med. 2003;97(8):978-82.
4. Ahmed I, Harshad SR. Subcutaneous sarcoidosis: is it a specific subset of cutaneous sarcoidosis frequently associated with systemic disease? J Am Acad Dermatol. 2006;54(1):55-60.
5. Heller M, Soldano AC. Sarcoidosis with subcutaneous lesions. Dermatol Online J. 2008;14(5):1.

CASE 42

MIDDLE-AGED MALE WITH FEVER, BACK PAIN AND CHEST WALL PAIN

CASE SUMMARY

A 60-year-old farmer presented with a 3-month history of low-grade fever, loin pain on both sides associated with occasional vomiting. He also had constipation and fresh per rectal bleeding for the last 2.5 months. In addition, he suffered from generalized weakness and substantial weight loss and also complained of low back pain and chest wall pain. He gave a history of passage of dark colored urine which was painless. With these complaints, he got admitted to a hospital about 1 month back and was diagnosed as a case of acute pyelonephritis with benign enlargement of prostate (BEP) with hemorrhoids with hypertension and was treated conservatively. He felt better for some days but again he faced the same problems. He had lost 6 kg of weight during this course of illness.

On examination, he was afebrile and severely anemic. He had no lymphadenopathy and vitals were within normal. Abdominal examination revealed 6 cm firm, nontender hepatomegaly. Renal angle tenderness was present bilaterally. Rest of the examination was unremarkable.

On investigation, hemoglobin (Hb): 3.5 g/dL, WBC: 8,340/mm^3 (DC: N—65%, L—30%), platelet—38,000/mm^3. ESR—140 mm in first hour. PBF—normocytic normochromic anemia with thrombocytopenia. Urine R/E—albumin present (+), pus cells—8–10/HPF, RBC—plenty. Urine C/S showed growth of *Staphylococcus* spp. Urinary total protein—3.70 g/24 hr, S. creatinine—2.3 mg/dL. S. urea—58 mg/dL. CXR revealed multiple osteolytic lesions in left clavicle and multiple ribs. USG of W/A showed hepatomegaly, bilateral early renal parenchymal disease and enlarged prostate. PSA—0.79 ng/mL.

QUESTIONS

1. What is the most likely diagnosis?
2. Suggest some investigations to confirm the diagnosis?

DISCUSSION

This middle-aged man presented with history of low-grade fever, generalized weakness, weight loss, low back pain and chest wall pain. Investigations showed severe anemia, thrombocytopenia with very high ESR. There was also evidence of renal impairment and CXR revealed multiple osteolytic lesions in left clavicle and multiple ribs.

Multiple myeloma was the most likely diagnosis.
For confirmation, following investigations were done:
- X-ray skull lateral view—showed multiple punched out lesions.
- Urinary Bence Jones protein—absent.
- Plasma protein electrophoresis—showed monoclonal gammopathy.
- Bone marrow study: The marrow was diffusely infiltrated by sheets of both mature and immature plasma cells (about 70%), consistent with multiple myeloma.

Final Diagnosis: Multiple Myeloma with Recurrent Pyelonephritis with Hypertension and BEP with Hemorrhoids

Multiple myeloma is a debilitating malignancy characterized by a proliferation of malignant plasma cells in the bone marrow and a subsequent overabundance of monoclonal paraprotein (M protein).

Most patients present with sign/symptoms related to the infiltration of plasma cells into the bone or other organs and also due to kidney damage from excess light chains. Presenting symptoms include anemia, bone pain, fatigue, generalized weakness, hypercalcemia, weight loss, renal insufficiency and neurological disease like peripheral neuropathy, radiculopathy, cord compression and CNS involvement.

Due to immune dysfunction, there is increased chance of infection as well.[1]
According to international working group criteria for diagnosis:
- Clonal bone marrow plasma cells ≥10% or biopsy-proven bony or soft tissue plasmacytoma.

Plus one of the following:
- Presence of related organ or tissue impairment—anemia (hemoglobin <10 g/dL), renal insufficiency (creatinine >2 mg/dL), increased plasma calcium level (serum calcium >11 mg/dL), and bone lesions (one or more osteolytic lesions ≥5 mm in size on skeletal radiography).
- Presence of a biomarker associated with near inevitable progression to end-organ damage ≥60 percent clonal plasma cells in the bone marrow. Also not all patients will have an M-protein in serum and/or urine.[1]

Although multiple myeloma remains incurable, several drug therapies, autologous stem cell transplantation, radiation, and in certain cases surgical care, are valuable in treatment of patients with multiple myeloma.

Asymptomatic patients without any end-organ damage should be monitored carefully. In symptomatic patient, supportive management should be started immediately.
- High fluid intake—to treat hypercalcemia and renal failure
- Bisphosphonates—to reduce bone pain and skeletal events
- Analgesia
- Allupurinol—to prevent urate nephropathy
- Plasmapheresis for hyperviscosity
- Antibiotic for infections.

Standard treatment options include chemotherapy with or without hematopoietic stem cell transplantation (HSCT) and radiotherapy for emergency treatment of spinal cord compression and pathological fracture.

In younger patients, standard treatments are combination chemotherapy such as CTD (cyclophosphamide, thalidomide, dexamethasone) or VTD (bortezomib, thalidomide, dexamethasone). After maximum response, autologous HSCT should be performed in fitter patient.

In older patients, common combinations is thalidomide with melphalan with prednisolone, or lenalidomide with melphalan with prednisolone.[2]

REFERENCES

1. Rajkumar SV. Clinical features, laboratory manifestations, and diagnosis of multiple myeloma. In: Basow DS (Ed). Waltham: UpToDate, 2011.
2. Ralston SH, Penman ID, Strachan MWJ, Hobson RP. Davidson's Principles and Practice of Medicine. 23rd ed. Edinburgh: Churchill Livingstone/Elsevier, 2018.

CASE 43

YOUNG LADY WITH MULTIPLE JOINT PAIN AND MUSCLE WEAKNESS

CASE SUMMARY

A 33-year-old woman presented with joint pain involving both knee joints, both wrist joints, small joints of hands and elbow which was associated with morning stiffness for the last 1 year, but there was no history of joint swelling. She also complained of muscle weakness that was more marked during standing and while climbing up the stairs. She noticed pallor of fingers on exposure to cold temperatures for the last 3 months and developed hoarseness of voice for the last 15 days. She mentioned unusual fatigability and significant weight loss during this course of illness. Her menstrual flow and cycle was normal. She had no history of fever, headache, skin rash, photosensitivity, oral ulceration, or respiratory distress. Her bowel and bladder habit was normal.

On examination, her face was pigmented with beaked nose with generalized hyperpigmentation of skin involving face, upper limbs and lower limbs up to the ankle joint. There was skin tightening on the face and upper limbs. Her pulse—82/min, blood pressure (BP)—100/70 mm Hg and temperature—normal. Tenderness of small joints of hand was present without joint swelling, telangiectasia or dactylitis. Nervous system examination revealed muscle power 4/5 with predominant weakness of proximal muscle group, normal deep tendon reflexes and plantar was bilaterally flexor. The rest of the systemic examinations were normal.

Investigations showed complete blood count (CBC)—normal hemoglobin (Hb) and cell counts, except erythrocyte sedimentation rate (ESR)—30 mm in the first hour. C-reactive protein (CRP)—19.6 mg/L. Creatine phosphokinase (CPK)—258 U/L. Chest X-ray (CXR), ultrasonography (USG) of W/A, thyroid profile, serum cortisol, serum ACTH, urine R/E, serum creatinine and serum electrolytes were normal.

QUESTIONS

1. Suggest three possible diagnoses.
2. What may be the further query pertinent in this case?
3. What further investigations would you like to do?

DISCUSSION

The patient had arthralgia with morning stiffness, proximal myopathy and history of Raynaud's phenomenon. She had tightening of skin with generalized hyperpigmentation over the face and body.

Possible diagnoses in this context are systemic sclerosis, systemic lupus erythematosus (SLE) and overlap syndrome.

Asking questions about *dysphagia and pregnancy loss* is important in this case.

On query, this patient mentioned about difficulty in deglutition associated with vomiting for the last 8 months. She had history of three pregnancy loss in the form of intrauterine death (IUD), each occurred at 6–7 months of pregnancy, last incidence occurred 3 years back. All this information led us to search for antiphospholipid antibody because antiphospholipid syndrome (APS) occurs in association with SLE or another rheumatic or autoimmune diseases.

Further investigations done in this patient:
- Antinuclear antibody (ANA): Negative
- Anti-double-stranded deoxyribonucleic acid (anti-ds DNA): Negative
- Extractable nuclear antigen (ENA) profile: Negative
- Antiphospholipid antibody immunoglobulin M (IgM): Negative
- Antiphospholipid antibody immunoglobulin G (IgG): 17.5 U/mL (positive)
- Skin biopsy: Epidermis—unremarkable. Dermis showed dense collagen fiber, paucity of fatty tissue around the adnexal structure and infiltration of chronic inflammatory cells. Comment: compatible with systemic sclerosis.

Final Diagnosis: Secondary Anti-phospholipid Syndrome due to Systemic Sclerosis

This patient should be managed symptomatically. Treatment of antiphospholipid syndrome depends on patient's clinical features and the presence or absence of thrombotic events. Asymptomatic individuals in whom blood test findings are positive for antibody, do not require specific treatment. Prophylaxis for thromboembolism is needed during surgery or hospitalization, along with management of associated autoimmune disease. Low-dose aspirin is used widely in this setting.[1,2]

REFERENCES

1. Del Papa N, Vaso N. Management of antiphospholipid syndrome. Ther Adv Musculoskelet Dis. 2010;2(4):221–7. doi:10.1177/1759720X10365969.
2. Ralston SH, Penman ID, Strachan MWJ, Hobson RP. Davidson's Principles and Practice of Medicine. 23rd ed. Edinburgh: Churchill Livingstone/Elsevier; 2018. pp. 977–8.

CASE 44

MIDDLE-AGED MALE WITH HYPERPIGMENTATION AND WEIGHT LOSS

CASE SUMMARY

A 57-year-old male, smoker, alcoholic, presented with hyperpigmentation for last two years and weight loss for 6 months. His hyperpigmentation was generalized, nonpruritic, gradually progressive in nature and without any skin lesion (Figs. 1A and B). It also involved palms and soles along with hard palate. Previously, he was diagnosed with hepatitis B virus infection with bilateral adrenal mass in a tertiary care hospital. He was treated conservatively with oral antiviral medication and, despite treatment, all his symptoms persisted. The evaluation of adrenal mass was incomplete. Then he developed occasional episodes of vomiting without any other gastrointestinal symptoms.

On examination, he was emaciated; leukonychia was present, and hyperpigmentation was more marked over face as well as lips, gums, cheek, hard palate, trunk and all four limbs including palms and soles. Blood pressure

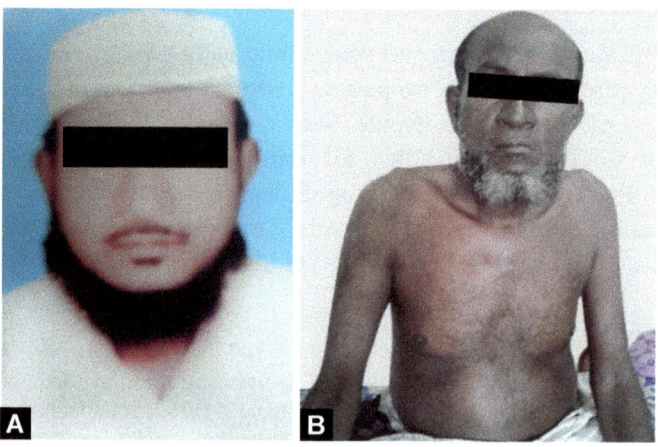

Figs. 1A and B: (A) Patient's photograph taken several years before disease-onset; (B) Patient's photograph taken after hospitalization, showing generalized hyperpigmentation.

was 90/60 mm Hg in supine and 90/50 mm Hg in standing position. Non-tender, firm hepatosplenomegaly was found in abdominal examination.

Investigations showed: complete blood count, erythrocyte sedimentation rate, renal function and liver enzymes were within normal limit; Mantoux test and chest X-ray were insignificant, prothrombin time was mildly raised; serum album was low; albumin: globulin ratio was altered, serum LDH and iron profile was normal. His early morning serum ACTH was 66.8 pg/mL; serum cortisol was 95.5 nmol/L; serum sodium was 130 mEq/L; potassium was 5.1 mEq/L. HIV screening was negative. Short Synacthen test was positive. Ultrasound of abdomen showed hepatosplenomegaly which was heterogeneous in texture. Both adrenal glands were enlarged.[1] Later CT of abdomen was performed which showed mild heterogeneously enhancing soft tissue density mass measuring 7×4.5 cm on left and 5.5×4.7 cm on right adrenal region.

QUESTIONS

1. What are the most likely differentials?
2. What should be the next step of investigation?

DISCUSSION

This patient had clinically and biochemically proven Addison's disease. To find out the underlying cause, we considered few differentials, which were: disseminated tuberculosis, hereditary hemochromatosis, histoplasmosis and lymphoma. Serum iron profile was normal which excluded hemochromatosis. Peripheral blood film showed no abnormality.

Then we performed ultrasound-guided aspiration from the suprarenal mass and cytology revealed necrotic debris containing a few histiocytes and lymphocytes. There were tiny round to oval bodies in macrophages, which were consistent with histoplasmosis. Then Gomori methenamine-silver (GMS) staining was performed which confirmed histoplasmosis.

Final Diagnosis: Disseminated Histoplasmosis with Addison's Disease

Histoplasmosis is a fungal infection caused by a fungus called *Histoplasma capsulatum*. Individuals affected with histoplasmosis are predominantly asymptomatic, those who develop clinical manifestations are usually immunocompromised or are exposed to a high quantity of inoculum. Clinical presentations include:
- Acute pulmonary histoplasmosis
- Chronic cavitary pulmonary histoplasmosis
- Progressive disseminated histoplasmosis
- Mediastinal lymphadenitis

- Broncholithiasis, mediastinal granuloma, fibrosing mediastinitis
- Lung nodules
- Inflammatory syndrome (pericarditis, arthritis, erythema nodosum).[2]

Few skin manifestations are common, e.g. erythema nodosum, papulonodular or ulcerating nodules. Radiological investigation may show inhomogeneous soft shadows (in acute infection) to calcifications (in long-standing cases) in lung, liver, spleen, etc. For which reason, it is always confusing with pulmonary tuberculosis. Laboratory detection is done by antigen detection, serology or culture. Combined urine and serum antigen testing have a high sensitivity of 90%. Culture is definitive but takes a long time of 12 weeks. However, another way to diagnosis is to determine the histopathological characteristics of the intracellular yeasts. Histoplasmosis is diagnosed by visualizing intracellular microorganisms in biopsy and/or culture. Periodic acid-Schiff (PAS) and GMS staining methods are routinely used for identification.[3]

Acute histoplasmosis may not need treatment. If severely symptomatic, may need 3 months of treatment (itraconazole 200 mg twice daily for 3 months). In chronic cases, the treatment may be prolonged up to 12-24 months. In severe pulmonary disease, the treatment of choice is amphotericin B followed by itraconazole along with methylprednisolone.[4]

REFERENCES

1. Drenthen LCA, Roerink SHPP, Mattijssen V, de Boer H. Bilaterally enlarged adrenal glands without obvious cause: need for a multidisciplinary diagnostic work-up. Clin Case Rep. 2018;6(4):729-34. Published 2018 Mar 3. doi:10.1002/ccr3.1340.
2. Knox KS, Hage CA. Histoplasmosis. Proc Am Thorac Soc. 2010;7:169-72. doi: 10.1513/pats.200907-069AL.
3. Rajeshwari M, Xess I, Sharma MC, Jain D. Acid-fastness of histoplasma in surgical pathology practice. J Pathol Transl Med. 2017;51(5):482-7. doi:10.4132/jptm.2017.07.11
4. Ralston SH, Penman ID, Strachan MWJ, Hobson RP. Davidson's Principles and Practice of Medicine. 23rd ed. Edinburgh: Churchill Livingstone/Elsevier; 2018. pp. 303-4.

CASE 45

YOUNG MALE WITH PROLONGED FEVER AND WEIGHT LOSS

CASE SUMMARY

A 24-year-old male presented with the complaints of low-grade fever with evening rise of temperature for the last 5 months. Fever was associated with anorexia, nausea and occasional vomiting. He gave history of about 13 kg weight loss within last 5 months. He was treated by a local physician and was given several antibiotics without any significant improvement. For the last 5 days, he had upper abdominal pain, dull in nature which was resolved after conservative treatment. He had no history of contact with known tuberculosis (TB) patient, any history of travel or I/V drug abuse. All systemic enquiries revealed nothing significant. His bladder and bowel habit was normal.

On examination, he was ill-looking, malnourished and mildly anemic. Pulse—90 beats/min, blood pressure—100/60 mm Hg, temperature: 100°F. Abdominal examination revealed tenderness over the left upper abdomen and mild splenomegaly. The rest of the examination was normal.

Complete blood count (CBC) showed Hb—10.2 g/dL; erythrocyte sedimentation rate (ESR)—84 mm in first hour with normal cell counts; peripheral blood film (PBF)—normocytic normochromic anemia. Urine routine examination (R/E), serum creatinine, liver function test (LFT), chest X-ray (CXR), barium follow through were normal; blood and urine culture test showed no growth; Mantoux test (MT) was 20 mm; sputum for acid-fast bacillus (AFB)—no AFB found; anti-HIV 1 and 2—negative.

QUESTIONS

1. Suggest two possible diagnoses for this case.
2. What further investigations would you like to do?

DISCUSSION

From the above scenario of a young male with low-grade fever, weight loss, abdominal pain, having low Hb (10.2 g/dL), high ESR (84 mm in 1st hour), MT-20 mm and mild splenomegaly; two possible diagnoses were: disseminated tuberculosis and lymphoma. Clinically, the man had no lymphadenopathy but had splenomegaly. So, ultrasonography of the whole abdomen was done which revealed splenomegaly with a hypoechoic area (34 mm × 28 mm) in lower part of the spleen suggestive of *splenic abscess*.

- *CT scan of whole abdomen with contrast was done which revealed*: Multiple non-enhancing hypodense areas are noted in splenic parenchyma. Multiple benign space-occupying lesion (SOL) in spleen.
- *Then USG-guided fine needle aspiration cytology (FNAC) from splenic lesion was done which showed*: Acute and chronic inflammatory cells with degenerated material. Epithelioid microgranuloma was noted. Inflammatory giant cells present. Negative for malignant cell. *Suggestive of splenic tubercular abscess*.
- *Gram staining of splenic material*: no microorganism found.
- *AFB staining of splenic material*: AFB present.
- *Colonoscopy* was also done and terminal ileum and whole colon were found to be normal.

Final Diagnosis: Tubercular Splenic Abscess

Spleen is one of the unusual sites for TB and isolated tubercular splenic abscess is a rare presentation in immunocompetent host. In general, fever of unknown origin, abdominal pain and enlarged spleen is common in various infections, splenic infarction and lymphoma. Tubercular splenic abscess may also have underlying HIV infection, so it should be ruled out.[1] In preantibiotic era, splenectomy was performed as the treatment of choice for splenic TB. Now treatment of splenic TB is same as that of pulmonary TB except it should last longer than 6 months.[2]

Splenic TB can be missed because of its rarity and nonspecific symptoms. So, high index of suspicion is necessary in patients with fever and splenomegaly residing in TB endemic areas.

REFERENCES

1. Gupta PP, Fotedar S, Agarwal D, Sansanwal P. Tuberculosis of spleen presenting with pyrexia of unknown origin in a non-immunocompromised woman. Lung India : official organ of Indian Chest Society. 2008;25(1):22-4. doi:10.4103/0970-2113.44134.
2. Divyashree S, Gupta N. Splenic Abscess in Immunocompetent Patients Managed Primarily without Splenectomy: A Series of 7 Cases. Perm J. 2017;21:16-139. doi:10.7812/TPP/16-139.

CASE 46

YOUNG BOY WITH DIARRHEA AND GENERALIZED SWELLING

CASE SUMMARY

A 16-year-old boy presented to us with a history of diarrhea for 1 year. He had loose stools 5–6 times/day, not related with any food intake, and stool was watery, bulky, frothy, foul smelling and pale in color. Subsequently, he developed progressive generalized swelling, which first appeared on his face and then expanded to the whole body. Six months later, he developed blurring of vision which was associated with occasional frontal headache, dull in nature but not associated with eye pain, nausea or vomiting. During this disease period, he occasionally noticed cramping type of muscle pain and a nonspecific pain in his whole body without any feature of arthritis. He also complained of poor appetite and he lost about 10 kg weight during this course of illness.

On physical examination, the patient's face was puffy and was mildly anemic. His nail was brittle and koilonychia was present (Fig. 1). There was

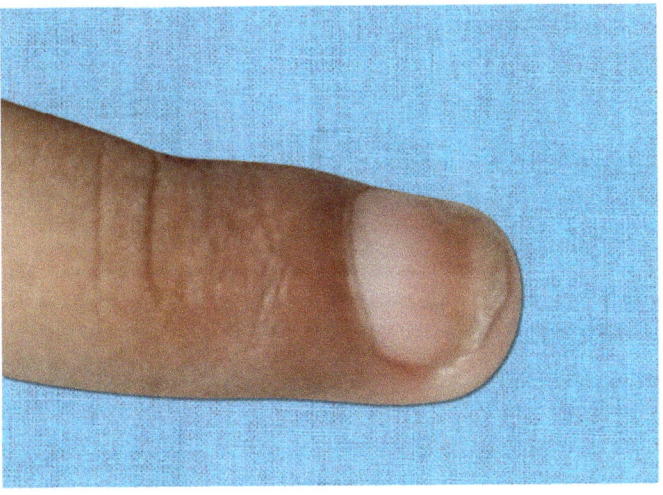

Fig. 1: Brittle nail.

glossitis. Bilateral leg edema was present and ascites was evident by positive shifting dullness. Jaundice and other signs of liver disease were absent. Vital signs were within normal limit. Bedside urine albumin test was negative. On fundoscopy, there was bilateral frank papilledema. Signs of meningeal irritation were absent.

On investigations, hemoglobin (Hb) was 10 g/dL and white blood cells (WBCs) count was 8,500/mm^3, where neutrophil count was 79.1% and lymphocyte count was low (14.6%) and peripheral blood film (PBF) was normal. Serum albumin was very low (1.30 g/dL). Corrected calcium level was also low (5.19 mg/dL). Routine urine examination was normal including nil urinary protein. All liver function tests and renal function tests including serum creatinine and serum electrolytes were normal. Thyroid function test and parathyroid hormone level were normal. Serum iron profile revealed iron deficiency evidenced by serum iron level of 26 µg/dL, serum ferritin level was 16 µg/dL and serum total iron binding capacity was 600 µg/dL. Stool routine examination revealed features of malabsorption, where fat globules and starch granules were present. Stool for the occult blood test (OBT) was negative. Antibodies for human immunodeficiency virus (HIV) I and II were non-reactive. Chest X-ray was normal. Ultrasonography (USG) of whole abdomen showed prominent fluid filled bowel loops in the abdomen and mild ascites. Computed tomography (CT) scan of head was normal. Cerebrospinal fluid (CSF) study and CSF pressure were also normal. On endoscopy, in duodenum, there was irregular whitish nodule with some mucosal elevations in the background of whitish mucosa (Figs. 2A and B). Colonoscopy was normal.

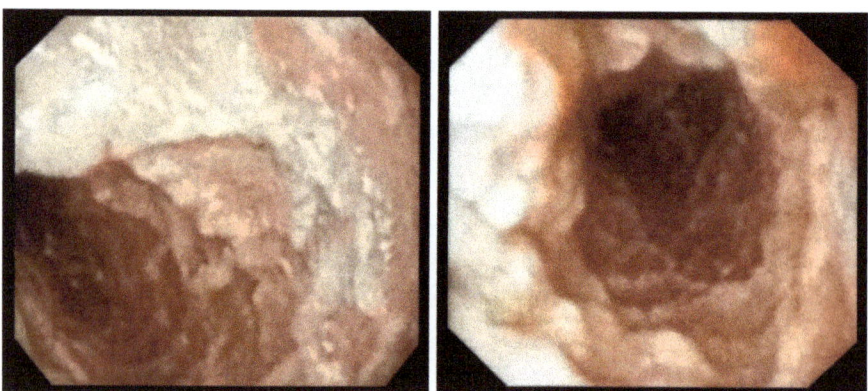

Figs. 2A and B: Endoscopic image showing irregular whitish nodule with some mucosal elevations in the background of whitish mucosa in duodenum.

QUESTIONS

1. Give some differential diagnoses.
2. What investigation you want to do next to reach the diagnosis?
3. What is the cause of his unexplained papilledema?

DISCUSSION

Our initial diagnosis was protein-losing enteropathy due to coeliac disease or tropical sprue which may have caused malabsorption. Stool for OBT was negative and also colonoscopy disfavored inflammatory bowel disease.

We did a duodenal biopsy which revealed:
- Edematous lamina propria
- Intraepithelial lymphocytes are mildly increased (15–20/100 enterocyte).
- The lamina propria also revealed congestion and increased number of chronic inflammatory cell.
- No granuloma or malignancy was seen.

We sent for antitissue transglutaminase (tTG) level which came out negative.

After that we tried to correlate all the things again and found that the patient's blood count showed lymphopenia; USG showed dilated intestinal loops and endoscopy revealed whitish nodule on the background of whitish mucosa, which may have been due to lymph leakage, and a similar picture can be found in primary intestinal lymphangiectasia which is the rarest cause of protein losing-enteropathy which can also cause malabsorption.

Though our biopsy report was not suggestive, we did not find any dilated lymphatic vessels, but to find out the actual picture, multi-dot biopsy or video-capsule endoscopy was required as intestinal lesions were segmental and localized.

Final Diagnosis: Primary Intestinal Lymphangiectasia (Waldmann's Disease)

While searching for the cause of papilledema in our patient, we reflected on his low corrected calcium level and found that, one of the rarest causes of papilledema is hypocalcemia. Hypocalcemia and papilledema leading to blurring of vision were first reported in 1903, and since then, approximately 50 cases had been recorded.[1] After correction of calcium level, his fundoscopic findings became normal and vision was improved.

Primary intestinal lymphangiectasia (PIL) is a rare cause of protein losing enteropathy characterized by dilated intestinal lacteals resulting in loss of lymph fluid in small bowel lumen.[2]

Usually PIL is diagnosed before 3 years of age but can be manifested and diagnosed in older age.[3]

Typical clinical presentations are edema that includes bipedal edema, pleural effusion, ascites (also may be chylous ascites) with abdominal pain, diarrhea and features of malabsorption.[4]

Laboratory findings of protein losing enteropathy include reduced level of serum albumin, gamma globulin, cholesterol, transferrin but diagnosis can be confirmed by an increase in alpha-1 antitrypsin clearance. Diagnosis of PIL as a cause of protein losing enteropathy can be established by endoscopy and histopathology from intestinal biopsy specimen. Typical endoscopic findings are scattered white spots, white villi, and chyle-like substances covering the mucosa. Histopathological examination can confirm the presence of dilated lymphatic vessels.[5,6]

The main management of PIL is dietary modification. Diet with low-fat and supplementary medium-chain triglycerides are widely prescribed as effective management. Octreotide (somatostatin analog) has shown beneficial improvement in PIL patients.[3,5]

REFERENCES

1. Vukovic DR, Pajic SMP. Hypocalcemia Induced Severe Heart Insufficiency and Visual Acuity Impairment– Will Calcium Supplementation Improve Heart and Eye Function? Blood Lymph. 2014;4:130. doi: 10.4172/2165-7831.1000130
2. Alshikho MJ, Talas JM, Noureldine SI, et al. Intestinal lymphangiectasia: Insights on management and literature review. Am J Case Rep. 2016;17:512–22.
3. Vignes S, Bellanger J. Primary intestinal lymphangiectasia (Waldmann's disease). Orphanet J Rare Dis. 2008;3:5. doi:10.1186/1750-1172-3-5
4. IIsa HM, Al-Arayedh GG, Mohamed AM. Intestinal lymphangiectasia in children. A favorable response to dietary modifications. Saudi Med J. 2016;37(3):199–204. doi:10.15537/smj.2016.2.13232
5. Grand RJ (2019). Protein-losing gastro enteropathy. In Grover S (Ed.), *UpToDate*. Retrieved January 17, 2019 from https://www.uptodate.com/contents/protein-losing-gastroenteropathy.
6. Asakura H, Miura S, Morishita T, Aiso S, Tanaka T, Kitahora T, Tsuchiya M, Enomoto Y, Watanabe Y. Endoscopic and histopathological study on primary and secondary intestinal lymphangiectasia. Dig Dis Sci. 1981;26:312–20.

CASE 47

UNMASKING OF THE CAUSE OF LYMPHADENOPATHY IN A YOUNG GIRL

CASE SUMMARY

A 20-year-old girl presented with a swelling on her right side of neck for the last 2 months. At first, it was small and nontender, but gradually it increased in size and became tender. She also mentioned, about 1 month back, she developed high grade, intermittent fever, and highest recorded temperature was 103°F. Fever was associated with pain in multiple small and large joints on both upper and lower limbs, but the joints were not swollen. She also noticed rash on her face which was exacerbated by exposure to sunlight. During the period of her hospital admission, her rashes become more extensive and appeared over both upper and lower limbs. She also developed periorbital swelling with puffiness of face. She had noticed an increased loss of hair. She denied history of night sweats and oral ulcer. She had tubercular lymphadenitis about 3 years back and she completed regimen of anti-tuberculosis (TB) drugs.

On examination, she was ill-looking, moderately anemic with facial puffiness and periorbital edema. Scaring alopecia was present on the scalp. Butterfly rash was present on her face, and multiple erythematous, raised rashes were present on all four limbs. A lymph node was enlarged on right posterior auricular region which was about 3 × 3 × 1 cm, firm in consistency, tender, not fixed to overlying skin and underlying structure. Vital signs were within normal limit. Other systemic examinations were unremarkable.

Investigations showed hemoglobin (Hb) was 8.5 g/dL, white blood cell (WBC) was 1,340/mm^3, platelet was 120,000/mm^3, erythrocyte sedimentation rate (ESR) was 65 mm in the first hour. Peripheral blood film revealed normochromic normocytic anemia with thrombocytopenia. Urinalysis revealed +++ proteinuria and red blood cells (RBCs): 0–2 (5% dysmorphic)/HPF. Urinary total protein (UTP) was: 3.45 g/24 hours. Serum creatinine and serum electrolytes were normal. Chest X-ray was normal. Fine needle aspiration cytology (FNAC) from submandibular lymph node showed inflammatory changes. Antinuclear antibody (ANA) and anti-double stranded deoxyribonucleic acid (anti-dsDNA) were negative repeatedly. P-ANCA and C-ANCA were also negative. Skin biopsy report was noncontributory.

QUESTIONS

1. What is the most likely diagnosis?
2. What further investigation is needed to solve the case?

DISCUSSION

All the clinical features were consistent with SLE but two important diagnostic markers, antinuclear antibody (ANA) and anti-double stranded DNA (anti-dsDNA) were negative repeatedly.

Our next investigation was extractable nuclear antigen (ENA) profile. It revealed anti-Ro/SSA and anti-ribosomal P protein (RPP) were positive. Renal biopsy was consistent with mesengial proliferative lupus nephritis (ISN/RPS class II).

Final Diagnosis: Systemic Lupus Erythematosus (Lupus Nephritis)

Antinuclear antibody negative systemic lupus erythematosus (SLE) is extremely rare. ANA is an important diagnostic marker for diagnosis of SLE and also recognized by its inclusion in the both American College of Rheumatology (ACR) and Systemic Lupus International Collaborating Clinics (SLICC) criteria for the classification of SLE.[1,2]

In 1976, Koller et al. 1st reported ANA-negative lupus of five patients, who were ANA-negative but clinical features were consistent with SLE.[3]

ANA-negative SLE patients are known to have a higher prevalence of anti-Ro (anti-SSA) antibody and cutaneous manifestations. Anti-RPP antibody is highly specific for SLE, though present in a minority of patients.[4,5]

The two most commonly used tests to detect ANA are indirect immunofluorescence ANA test (IF-ANA: gold-standard test) and enzyme immunoassay (EIA)/enzyme linked immunosorbent assay (ELISA). For ANA-negativity in SLE-patients, several reasons have been demonstrated in case studies. Technical factors, or prozone effects may be responsible. Other explanations include binding of ANA with immune complexes (found in lupus nephritis) which are undetectable by IF-ANA, or due to loss of ANA through profuse proteinuria. In case of renal involvement, ANA may become positive later, upon clinical recovery.[6-8]

REFERENCES

1. Hochberg MC. Updating the American College of Rheumatology revised criteria for the classification of systemic lupus erythematosus. Arthritis Rheum. 1997; 40:1725.

2. Petri M, Orbai AM, Alarcón GS, et al. Derivation and validation of the Systemic Lupus International Collaborating Clinics classification criteria for systemic lupus erythematosus. Arthritis Rheum. 2012;64:2677.
3. Koller SR, Johnston CL Jr, Moncure CW. Lupus erythematosus cell preparation-antinuclear factor incongruity. A review of diagnostic tests for systemic lupus erythematosus. Am J Clin Pathol. 1976;66:495–505.
4. Maddison PJ, Provost TT, Reichlin M. Serological findings in patients with "ANA-negative" systemic lupus erythematosus. Medicine. 1981;60:87–94.
5. Bloch DB. Antiribosomal P protein antibodies. In Curtis MR (Ed), UpToDate. 2018. Retrieved 2019 from https://www.uptodate.com/contents/antiribosomal-p-protein-antibobies
6. Linder E, Miettinen A. Prozone effects in indirect immuno-fluorescence. Scand J Immunol. 1976;5:513–9.
7. Blomjous FJ, Feltkamp-Vroom TM. Hidden anti-nuclear antibodies in seronegative systemic lupus erythematosus patients and in NZB and (NZB XN2 W) F1 mice. Eur J Immunol. 1971;1:396–8.
8. Persellin RH, Takeuchi A. Antinuclear antibody-negative systemic lupus erythematosus: loss in body fluids. J Rheumatol. 1980;7:547–50.

CASE 48

YOUNG BOY WITH A HIDDEN, DEADLY AND RARE COMPLICATION

CASE SUMMARY

A 15-year-old boy presented to us with 2 months' history of behavioral abnormality mainly manifested by repetition of same work, forgetfulness, lack of concentration and emotional lability in the form of smiling without any reason. He had to leave his school because of this illness. Subsequently, he developed recurrent jerky movements of the whole body and incurred repeated falls. Gradually, it became more severe and occurred more frequently and patient became bedridden. It was not associated with any tongue bite or bowel bladder incontinence. He came from a low socioeconomic family and was an issue of nonconsanguinity. His birth and development history was uneventful and his vaccination status was incomplete. Patient visited several physicians for this condition and was treated as a case of psychosis, without any improvement. His past medical and surgical history was uneventful, except his mother mentioned that at the age of 8, he suffered from fever with maculopapular rash.

On examination, patient was bedridden but conscious. His vital parameters were normal. He was disoriented, emotionally labile, and smiled inappropriately during conversation. His speech was incoherent and memory could not be evaluated. Pupils were bilaterally equal and reacting to light. All cranial nerves were intact and there was no Kayser-Fleischer (KF) ring on slit lamp examination. There was frequent myoclonic jerky movement involving whole body, more predominant on the left side. Motor examination revealed generalized rigidity, muscle power was normal. All deep reflexes were diminished. Plantar response was bilaterally flexor. Gait, and sensory functions could not be evaluated, and signs of meningism were absent. Examination of other systems revealed no abnormality.

Routine blood examinations revealed no abnormality. Urinary copper, serum copper level was normal. Magnetic resonance imaging (MRI) of brain and cerebrospinal fluid (CSF) study was normal. Electroencephalography (EEG) showed: In both hemispheres, there was high voltage sharp and slow waves (repeated bouts); more on provocation. Final suggestion was generalized epileptiform discharge.

QUESTIONS

1. What is the most likely diagnosis?
2. What investigations are needed to diagnose this case?
3. What are the treatment options and prognosis of this disease?

DISCUSSION

Patient presented with behavioral abnormality and inappropriate smiling, was mistakenly suspected as a case of psychosis initially and treated without any improvement.

Suspicion for Wilson's disease was there as patient presented with neuropsychiatric symptoms at this young age. Investigations were negative along with absent history of jaundice and Kayser-Fleischer ring.

Another possibility was postencephalitic syndrome.

At 8 years of age, history of fever associated with maculopapular rash with typical symptoms suggested measles infection. Myoclonic jerky movement and incomplete vaccination status and repeated positive EEG findings pointed toward a rare diagnosis, subacute sclerosing panencephalitis (SSPE), which also can present with neuropsychiatric symptoms.

So, our next step of investigation was to do measles antibody in blood and CSF. Measles antibody IgG was positive in both blood and CSF.

Final Diagnosis: Subacute Sclerosing Panencephalitis

The SSPE is a rare, fatal and progressive complication of infection with measles virus. It occurs after many years of measles infection, on average (7–10 years). Early age infection (<2 years) with measles virus has shown some association with this complication. Prognosis is poor; usually death can occurs within 1–3 years.[1]

Usual early symptoms are behavioral changes, deterioration in cognitive function, psychiatric manifestations. Later, with disease progression, myoclonic jerks can develop.

Diagnosis can be made by clinical suspicion, characteristics EEG findings (periodic repeated complexes), measles infection evidence (immunological), measles antibody in CSF, ribonucleic acid (RNA) of measles virus in brain sample [real-time polymerase chain reaction (RT-PCR)].[1,2]

Measles vaccination status has an association with the disease and showed that vaccination can prevent SSPE.[3]

SSPE is not curable, but isoprinosine (oral), alpha interferon (intrathecal) can be given to improve survival.[4]

REFERENCES

1. William JB, Jennifer SR, Luis E. et al. Subacute sclerosing panencephalitis: more cases of this fatal disease are prevented by measles immunization than was previously recognized. J Infect Dis. 2005;192(10):1686-93.
2. Gutierrez J, Issacson RS, Koppel BS. Subacute sclerosing panencephalitis: an update. Dev Med Child Neurol. 2010;52(10):901-7.
3. Campbell H, Andrews N, Brown KE, et al. Review of the effect of measles vaccination on the epidemiology of SSPE. Int J Epidemiol. 2007;36(6):1334-48.
4. Garg RK. Subacute sclerosing panencephalitis. J Neurol. 2008;255(12):1861-71.

CASE 49

MIDDLE-AGED FARMER WITH A BAGGY ABDOMEN

CASE SUMMARY

A 55-year-old farmer was admitted in hospital with swelling of the abdomen for 6 months. He first noticed that the girth of his abdomen was increasing and the abdomen felt heavier than before. The swelling was generalized and was slowly progressive. It was not associated with pain or bowel disturbance. He also complained of shortness of breath while lying on his back, but it was not associated with cough. There was no history of fever, joint pain and jaundice or weight loss.

Examination revealed a well-oriented man with normal vital signs, and symmetrical distended abdomen with full flank and everted umbilicus. Fluid thrill was positive. There were no features of chronic liver disease and heart failure.

Investigation revealed hemoglobin (Hb)—9.5 g/dL, mean corpuscular volume (MCV) 98 fL and erythrocyte sedimentation rate (ESR)—25 mm in first hour. White blood cells (WBCs), platelet, liver function test (LFT), renal function test (RFT), serum electrolyte, urine routine and microscopic examination prothrombin time (PT) and chest X-ray (CXR) all were normal, except alanine aminotransferase (ALT)—67 IU/L. Ascitic fluid study revealed total WBC—30/mm^3, lymphocyte—95%, and protein—4.8 g/dL. Serum ascites albumin gradient (SAAG)—1.0 g/dL, adenosine deaminase (ADA) was normal, and acid-fast bacilli (AFB) and Gram's stain were negative. Ultrasonography (USG) of W/A showed huge ascites. An endoscopy of the upper gastrointestinal tract (GIT), echocardiography and urinary total protein were unyielding.

QUESTIONS

1. What are the causes of high protein ascites?
2. What should be the next course of action?

DISCUSSION

Common causes of high protein (>2.5 g/L) and low SAAG ascites are peritoneal malignancy, tubercular peritonitis, pyogenic peritonitis and pancreatic ascites. To find out peritoneal pathology in such cases accurately, the best test is peritoneal biopsy and histopathology. In our case, before jumping to this, we did thyroid function test which revealed primary hypothyroidism. Subsequently, the patient was placed on thyroxine replacement therapy with complete resolution of symptoms.

This was an exceptionally rare presentation of hypothyroidism with only ascites.

Final Diagnosis: Primary Hypothyroidism

Incidence of ascites in hypothyroidism has been reported as <4%. Also, as a presenting complaint, it is very uncommon.[1] The exact cause is not established, but possible hypotheses include increased capillary permeability leading to extravasation of plasma protein; obstruction to lymphatic flow caused by hyaluronic acid; and diminished water diuresis due to excess antidiuretic hormone (ADH).

Proper identification of myxedema ascites prevents inappropriate diuretic use, repeated paracentesis, liver biopsy and peritoneal biopsy. Though ascites due to hypothyroidism is rare, yet, it is easy to treat. Treatment with thyroid hormone replacement therapy leads to regression of the ascites. High index of suspicion is required to establish the etilogy, especially if the ascitic fluid has a high protein content.[2]

REFERENCES

1. Khalid S, Asad-Ur-Rahman F, Abbass A, et al. Myxedema Ascites: A Rare Presentation of Uncontrolled Hypothyroidism. Cureus. 2016;8(12):e912. doi:10.7759/cureus.912
2. Ji JS, Chae HS, Cho YS, Kim HK, Kim SS, Kim CW, Choi KY. Myxedema ascites: case report and literature review. J Korean Med Sci. 2006;21(4):761–4. doi:10.3346/jkms.2006.21.4.761

CASE 50

MIDDLE-AGED LADY WITH RECURRENT ODYNOPHAGIA AND MULTIPLE ULCERS

CASE SUMMARY

A 60-year-old housewife, nondiabetic, hypertensive, nonsmoker and betel-leaf chewer, presented with a long history of difficulty in swallowing for 7 years and bilateral neck swellings with overlying ulcerations in right side of the neck for last 2 months. Her problems started with dysphagia and globus sensation and progressed to odynophagia, more marked at the base of the tongue and mainly associated with solid food intake. She consulted ear, nose and throat (ENT) specialists and underwent surgery for removal of soft tissue mass from the base of the tongue, which relieved her symptoms for the next 2 years, after which, odynophagia recurred and she underwent second similar surgery. Two years later, she developed a painless swelling near the right angle of mandible, with ulceration of the overlying skin; which subsided after antibiotic therapy. Two years after that, her dysphagia recurred, for which a biopsy was taken, but surgery was not repeated. Then she developed multiple painless neck swellings bilaterally. A couple of days later, one swelling from the right side discharged pus and became ulcerated, followed by another ulceration on the same side. For these painful ulcers, an ENT specialist prescribed her prednisolone for 2 months, which she took irregularly, but her symptoms worsened. Then she got admitted in the Department of ENT and was transferred to the Department of Medicine, Dhaka Medical College Hospital (DMCH). There was no history of contact with tuberculosis (TB) patient. She denied history of fever, cough, anorexia, significant weight loss, jaundice, bleeding or unsafe sexual exposure. She gave no history of convulsion, headache, visual disturbance, skin rash, oral ulcer or joint involvement. There was no family history of similar type of illness or any malignancy. Her allergic history and travel history were unremarkable.

On general examination, the patient was ill-looking, obese and mildly anemic. Her vitals were normal. Lymph node examination revealed bilateral supraclavicular and submandibular lymphadenopathy and palpable jugular

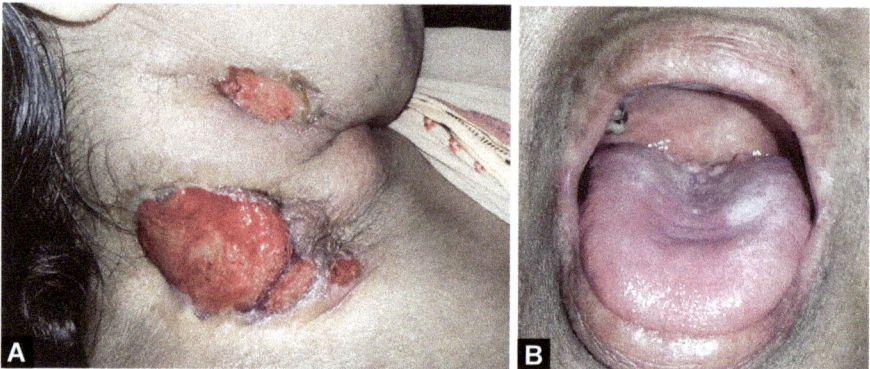

Figs. 1A and B: (A) Multiple ulcers over right cervical and right submandibular regions; (B) Nodules over the posterior part of the tongue.

group in right side; the largest one measuring 8 cm × 5 cm. Some nodes were tender, others were nontender, some were matted and others were discrete, firm, mobile, and free from underlying structure and overlying skin. There was no discharging sinus. There were multiple tender and mobile ulcers over right supraclavicular and submandibular regions (Fig. 1A), largest one being 8 cm × 6 cm, with undermined edge, floor was covered with slough, pus and red granulation tissue, bleeding on touch and base was free. Local temperature was raised and adjacent skin was blackish. On gastrointestinal system examination, some nodules were seen over the posterior part of the tongue (Fig. 1B). No other abnormality was detected. Other systemic examinations revealed normal findings.

The patient had mild anemia with hemoglobin (Hb): 10.5 g/dL, hematocrit (HCT): 36.5%, neutrophilic leukocytosis with white blood cell (WBC) count: 13,500/mm^3, platelet count: 550,000/mm^3, erythrocyte sedimentation rate (ESR): 92 mm in first hour. C-reactive protein (CRP) was normal and Montoux test (MT) was negative. X-ray chest posteroanterior (PA) view revealed no abnormality. Several histopathology reports were available, done each time a surgery was performed, at an interval of at least a year, all of which commented *malakoplakia* (Table 1). Subsequent ultrasonography (USG)-guided fine-needle aspiration cytology (FNAC) from right and left supraclavicular lymph node revealed *sinus histiocytosis with massive lymphadenopathy*.

QUESTIONS

1. What differential diagnoses should be considered in this case of recurrent lesions?
2. What are the management options?

Table 1: Several previous histopathology reports.		
Specimen	**Histopathological findings**	**Comment**
Soft tissue from base of the tongue and lingual surface of epiglottis	Polypoid pieces of tissue, lined by squamous epithelium. The underlying stroma shows dense infiltration of foamy histiocytes, admixed with polymorphs, lymphocytes. The foamy histiocytes contain **Michaelis–Gutmann bodies**, which have laminated as well as targeted appearance. These are periodic acid-Schiff (PAS) positive and positive for iron. No malignant cell seen	Malakoplakia
Swelling and ulceration near right angle of mandible	Similar findings	Malakoplakia
Polypoid growth on suprahyoid supraglottis (right and left side)	Similar findings	Malakoplakia
Tissue from base of tongue (right side)	Similar findings	Malakoplakia

DISCUSSION

Initially, in this case, apart from hypertension, our differentials for the rest of the scenario were:
- Low-grade lymphoma
- Disseminated tuberculosis
- Actinomycosis
- Malakoplakia.

The absence of systemic features and other clinical clues as well as nonsupportive complete blood count (CBC) and other investigations virtually excluded these differentials, except malakoplakia.

To see the extent of the disease, 3D reconstructive computed tomography (CT) scan of head and neck region was done, revealing *mass lesion involving base of the tongue and parapharyngeal space, bilateral cervical, and mediastinal lymphadenopathy* (Fig. 2), more marked on right, and left-sided maxillary sinusitis.

Almost all of the previous histopathology reports pointed unidirectionally toward malakoplakia, but this lady did not receive adequate treatment for the condition previously. So, for confirmation of the diagnosis, we went for biopsy and histopathology of left cervical lymph node which revealed dense

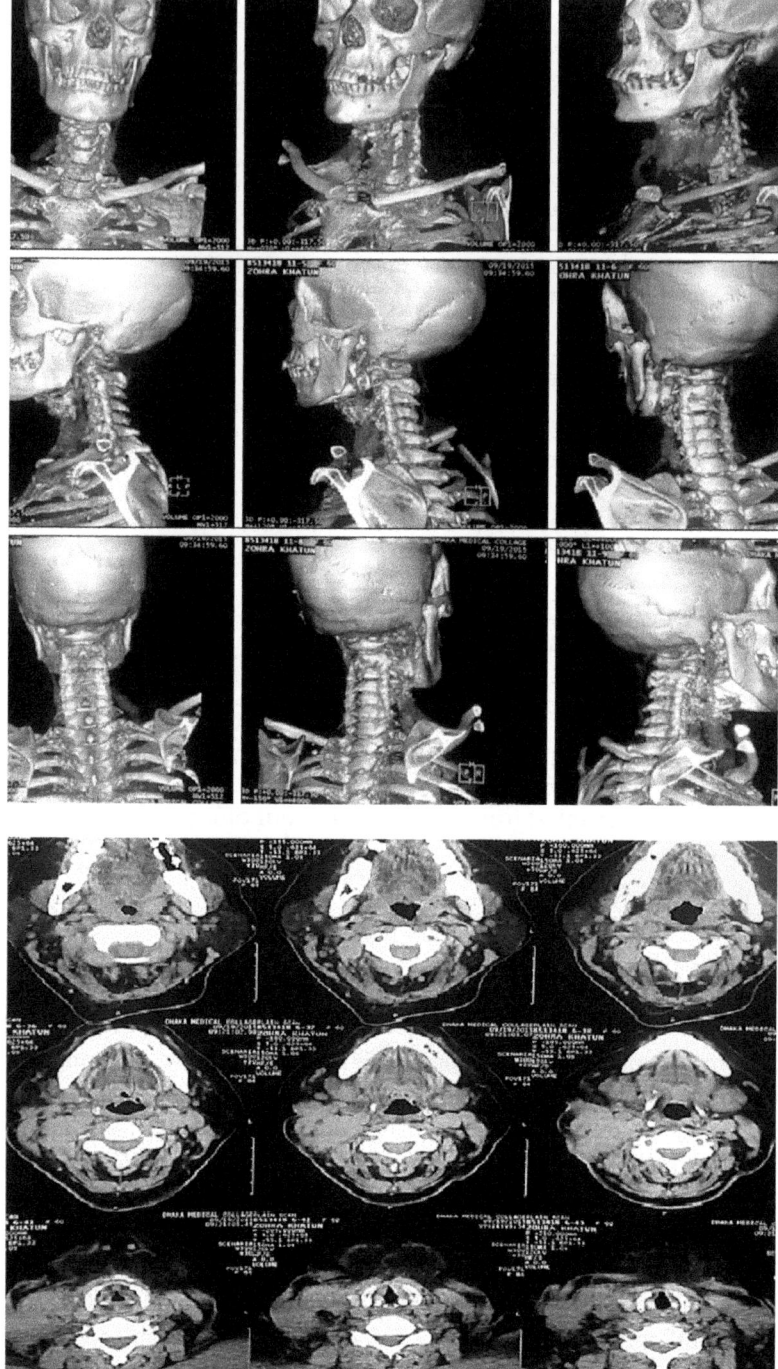

Fig. 2: 3D reconstructive CT scan of head and neck showing mass lesion involving base of the tongue and parapharyngeal space; bilateral cervical, and mediastinal lymphadenopathy- more marked on right.

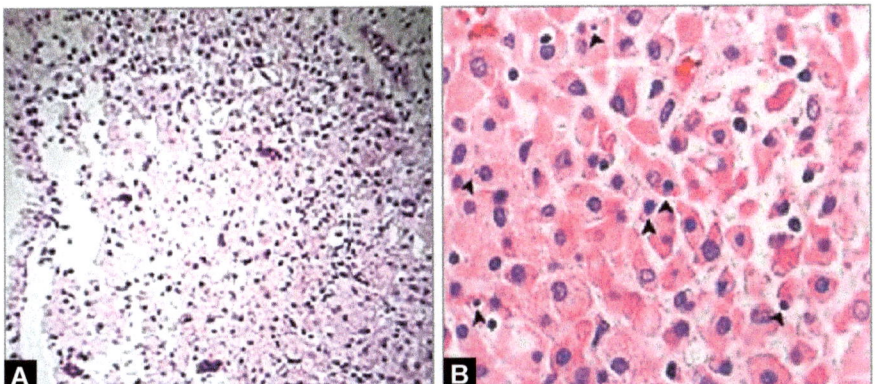

Figs. 3A and B: Histopathology smear showing histiocytes mixed with acute and chronic inflammatory cells. Some histiocytes contain Michaelis–Gutmann bodies (arrowheads).

collection of foamy histiocytes mixed with a good number of polymorphs and lymphocytes. No malignancy was seen. Conclusion was *lipogranuloma*. Simultaneously, a wedge biopsy was taken from soft tissue neck (right side) which showed histiocytes mixed with acute and chronic inflammatory cells. Some of the histiocytes contained round inclusions, consistent with Michaelis–Gutmann bodies (Figs. 3A and B). A few other histiocytes contained bacteria within the cytoplasm. No malignant cell was seen. Conclusion was *Malakoplakia*.

Final Diagnosis: Malakoplakia of the Tongue and Skin with Hypertension

This lady was treated with antibiotics (ciprofloxacin and cotrimoxazole) for 6 months, with surgical intervention. She was cured with complete resolution of lymphadenopathy and ulcers.

"Malakoplakia" is derivative of Greek *malakos* (soft) and *plakos* (plaque). It is a rare chronic acquired granulomatous inflammatory disease. Very few cases have been reported worldwide, with involvement of genitourinary tract (mainly bladder), gastrointestinal tract, pancreas, retroperitoneum, thyroid gland, lymph nodes, lung, bone, joint and brain. Primary cutaneous malakoplakia is an even rarer entity. Females are more commonly affected than males with a 4:1 ratio. Patients usually present after 50 years of age, though it can occur in any age group. Risk factors include immunosuppressive therapy after organ transplantation, lymphoma on chemotherapy, postradiotherapy, carcinoma of the breast postmastectomy, myelodysplastic syndrome, diabetes mellitus, alcoholism, rheumatoid arthritis, dermatomyositis, lupus vulgaris, concomitant urinary tract infection and prolonged therapy with systemic corticosteroids.

The exact pathogenesis is unclear but is probably due to the defective phagolysosomal activity of macrophages/monocytes. Dystrophic calcification occurs on affected sites. The most common bacteria involved are

Escherichia coli, Klebsiella, Proteus, Pseudomonas aeruginosa, Mycobacterium avium, Mycobacterium tuberculosis, Shigella, Staphylococcus aureus and *Enterococcus. Rhodococcus equi* is the most commonly associated microbe in HIV-infected patients.[1]

No typical clinical presentation has been described. Cutaneous malakoplakia is very rare and may manifest as erythematous papules, plaques, subcutaneous nodules, abscesses with or without fluctuation,[1] fistula to ulcers and nonhealing surgical wounds, cystic and polypoid masses. Malakoplakia of the tongue is even rarer, and neither has obvious association with immunosuppression nor internal organs involvement. When occurs, it usually affects the base of the tongue. Patients commonly present with a globus sensation or, less frequently, odynophagia.

Microscopically, the presence of Michaelis–Gutmann bodies is pathognomonic for malakoplakia. Culture studies, magnetic resonance imaging (MRI) and positron-emission tomography (PET) scans can be used for diagnosis and follow-up.

Infections to consider include tuberculosis, Whipple's disease, lepromatous leprosy, fungus (*Cryptococcus*), and parasites[1] (*Leishmania*). Malakoplakia has associations with foreign-body granuloma, sarcoidosis, lymphoma, xanthoma, Langerhans cell histiocytosis, fibrous histiocytoma, granular cell tumor and hemophagocytic syndrome.

As malakoplakia is a least-thought-of differential diagnosis for tongue and skin lesions, patients initially undergo excision biopsy, but wide surgical excision alone is not usually recommended as recurrence can occur after surgery. Additional treatment is usually required with antibiotics (quinolones, trimethoprim-sulfamethoxazole). Antibiotic therapy directed against *E. coli* in combination with surgery provides the best chance of cure. Bethanechol and ascorbic acid can be used in combination with antibiotics and surgery. Discontinuation or dose reduction of immunosuppressive drug therapy is usually needed to effectively treat malakoplakia.[2,3]

Malakoplakia of the skin or tongue may heal spontaneously and usually has an excellent prognosis, if there is no internal organ involvement.[2]

REFERENCES

1. Anwar MB. A middle aged man with generalized swelling. In: Ahasan HAMN, ed. Interesting 50 cases: a compilation of case reports in medicine, 1st ed. Dhaka: Medicine Department of Dhaka Medical College Hospital; 2013. pp. 87–90.
2. Dyall-Smith D. Malakoplakia of the skin and tongue. Derm Net NZ. 2010. [Online] Available from: https://www.dermnetnz.org/topics/malakoplakia-of-the-skin-and-tongue
3. Gómez AG, Botero ML, Calle CA, Serna FL. Malacoplakia: case report in tongue and review of the literature. Med Oral Patol Oral Cir Bucal. 2008;13(6):E352–4.

CASE 51

MIDDLE-AGED MAN WITH WEIGHT GAIN AND BREATHLESSNESS

CASE SUMMARY

A 45-year-old ex-smoker, non-asthmatic construction worker was admitted with the complaints of unintended weight gain with swelling of whole body, and constipation for the last 5 years; breathlessness and productive cough for the last 3 months. He noticed gradual swelling of his body over the last 5 years, which started from the face and then involved all four limbs and abdomen. He had constipation with passage of hard stool 1-2 times per week, without any abdominal or rectal pain or per-rectal bleeding. He also suffered from exertional breathlessness for the last 3 months, which worsened after climbing stairs. It was not associated with orthopnea, chest pain or palpitation. He complained of cough with scanty whitish sputum production for the last 3 months. There was no hemoptysis, halitosis, fever or history of contact with patient of tuberculosis. He mentioned having hair loss, fatigue and repeated attacks of sinusitis for as long as he can remember, but had no anosmia or hearing-difficulty. He did not have anorexia, cold intolerance, increased somnolence, loss of libido and also had normal bladder habit. Several years back, he was diagnosed as a case of subfertility after semen analysis; and never had any child out of his two marriages which terminated in divorces.

On examination, he appeared depressed and overweight (Fig. 1). He had hoarseness of voice, slurred speech, macroglossia; puffy face, periorbital swelling, non-pitting edema; dry, coarse, thickened skin; and sparse body hair; without thyromegaly. His vitals were normal. Systemic examination revealed vesicular breath sound with bi-basal coarse crackles. His apex beat was situated in the right 5th intercostal space. On abdominal examination, a non-tender left hypochondriac mass was palpable, which was (6 × 5) cm, firm in consistency, ill-defined, round-margined, free from skin, non-ballotable and moved with respiration. This mass gave the impression of palpable left-sided liver, and upper border of liver dullness was in the left 5th intercostal

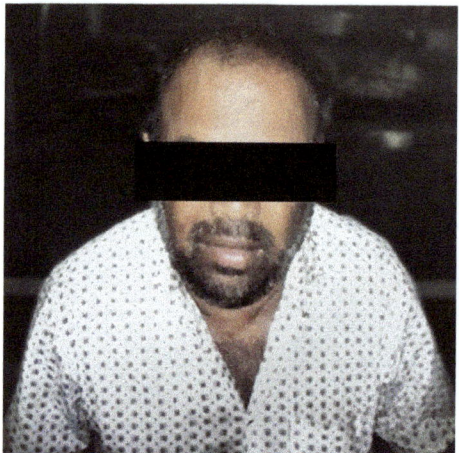

Fig. 1: Photograph of the patient.

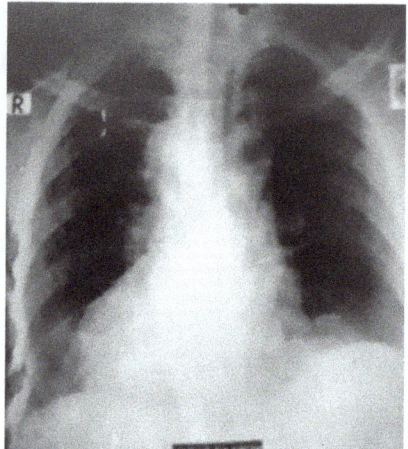

Fig. 2: X-ray chest P/A view showing dextrocardia.

space. There was no other organomegaly, lymphadenopathy or ascites. All of his deep reflexes were diminished, with delayed relaxation of ankle jerks. Rest of the examination findings seemed normal.

Investigations revealed: hemoglobin—68%, WBC—7,000/mm^3 (neutrophil 70%, lymphocyte 20%, eosinophil 3%, monocyte 7%), platelet count: 2,30,000/mm^3, ESR—50 mm in first hour. Urine R/M/E, serum creatinine, serum electrolytes, RBS—were normal. Liver function tests showed serum bilirubin—0.8 mg/dL, ALT—28 U/L, AST—32 U/L, serum total protein—7.5 g/dL, albumin—5.2 g/dL, A-G ratio was 2.3:1, prothrombin time—14 seconds, INR—1.17. X-ray chest P/A view demonstrated dextrocardia, increased transverse diameter of cardiac shadow with obtuse cardiac angle (Fig. 2). Sputum study: Gram staining—no organism, AFB—not found, C/S—no growth. ECG tracing was congruent with dextrocardia. Echocardiography—dextrocardia with no RWMA with good LV systolic function (EF 63%). X-ray PNS OM view—chronic pansinusitis. Serum TSH—62.5 mU/L (normal—0.2-4.5 mU/L), free T4—4.71 pmol/L (normal 9—21 pmol/L). Endoscopy of upper GIT—gastritis with situs inversus. Abdominal ultrasonography—situs inversus, hepatomegaly with fatty change; a large cyst in liver containing multiple daughter cysts.

QUESTIONS

1. Could you explain all of this patient's symptoms and signs with a single diagnosis?
2. What is your provisional diagnosis?
3. What further investigations would you perform to establish your diagnosis/diagnoses?

DISCUSSION

This gentleman presented with classic features of hypothyroidism, and investigations also demonstrated that. While performing physical examination, the discovery of dextrocardia on the background of history of chronic sinusitis and subfertility made this case very fascinating and put the provisional diagnosis of Kartagener syndrome (KS) on the table. We suspected bronchiectasis as the cause of his breathlessness, which was yet to be established. The suspicion that the left hypochondriac mass found during examination was hepatomegaly was proven correct, with possibly a hepatic hydatid cyst. So, we performed the following investigations.

- Ciliary function test (saccharin test): 30 minutes = prolonged (normal up to 20 minutes)
- Antibody against thyroid peroxidase (anti-TPOAb): 1,000 IU/L (normal up to 35 IU/L)
- Antithyroglobulin antibody: 15 IU/L (normal up to 40 IU/L)
- HRCT scan of chest: Dextrocardia with early bronchiectatic changes (Fig. 3)
- CT scan-guided aspiration and microscopic examination of aspirate from hepatic cyst: no scolices or hooklets found (Fig. 4)
- Indirect hemagglutination test (IHA) of aspirate for antibody against *Echinococcus granulosus*: positive.

Final Diagnosis: Kartagener Syndrome with Primary Hypothyroidism due to Autoimmune Atrophic Thyroiditis with Hepatic Hydatid Cyst[1]

Kartagener syndrome (KS) is also termed as sinusitis-bronchiectasis-situs inversus (triad) syndrome. It is a type of primary ciliary dyskinesia (PCD, also called immotile ciliary syndrome) in which there is presence of situs inversus totalis. Manes Kartagener first recognized this clinical triad as a distinct congenital syndrome in 1933. KS is a rare autosomal recessive genetic disorder

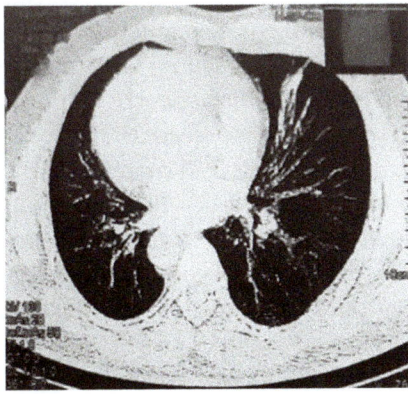

Fig. 3: HRCT scan of chest showing dextrocardia with early bronchiectatic changes.

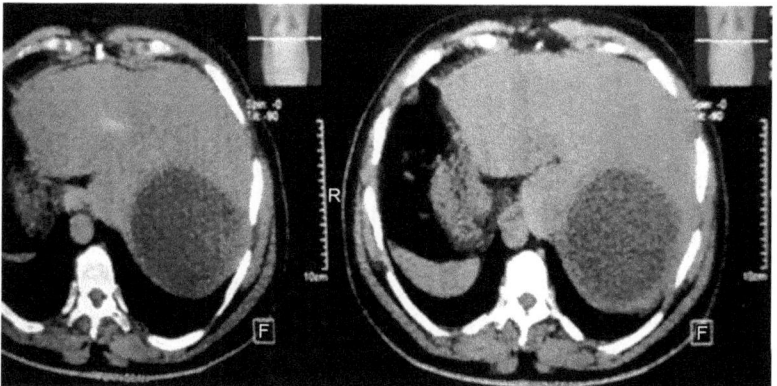

Fig. 4: CT scan of abdomen showing situs inversus, hepatomegaly with a large cyst in liver.

in which ciliary dyskinesia occurs due to dysfunction or lack of the dynein arms resulting in the disruption of the coordinated ciliary movement and the propulsion of the mucus. Defective function of cilia lining the respiratory tract (upper and lower, sinuses), Eustachian tube, middle ear, fallopian tube in female, and also of the flagella of sperm in male may present with neonatal respiratory distress; frequent lung, sinus and middle ear infections beginning in early childhood; and infertility. The situs inversus usually poses no clinical problem.[2-5]

Kartagener syndrome is typically suspected based on the presence of characteristic signs and symptoms. A diagnosis can be confirmed by biopsy and histopathology from an area covered with cilia—such as the sinuses or the airway. Genetic testing can also be used to confirm the diagnosis.[2,3]

Treatment should be according to manifestations: aggressive measures to enhance mucus clearance (chest percussion and postural drainage, oscillatory vest, breathing maneuvers) and prompt antibiotic therapy as directed by C/S for bacterial bronchitis, sinusitis and otitis media; consideration of lobectomy for localized bronchiectasis; lung transplantation for end-stage lung disease; sinus surgery for extensive sinus infections; consideration of grommet tube placement for chronic otitis media; speech therapy and hearing aids if needed. Surgical intervention may be necessary for congenital heart disease. Intracytoplasmic sperm injection (ICSI) or artificial insemination by donor sperm could be done for male infertility. Routine immunizations (including influenza and pneumococcal vaccine) should be ensured.[3]

Our patient had hepatic hydatid disease, also referred to as echinococcosis, caused by infection with the larval stage of the dog tapeworm *Echinococcus granulosus*.

Autoimmune atrophic thyroiditis may manifest with constipation, fatigue, inability to tolerate cold temperatures, weight gain, puffy face and joint stiffening.

We managed this patient with chest physiotherapy (postural drainage), antibiotics, oral thyroxine and albendazole, and discharged him with improving symptoms. He was advised for vaccination and regular follow-up.

Kartagener syndrome itself is a rare entity that entices researchers worldwide, and its simultaneous presence with autoimmune thyroiditis and echinococcosis in the same individual makes this case truly one of a kind.

REFERENCES

1. Anwar MB, Ahasan HAMN. Interesting 50 cases: a compilation of case reports in medicine. Department of Medicine; Dhaka Medical College Hospital. 2013. p. 24.
2. Primary Ciliary Dyskinesia. National Organization for Rare Disorders (NORD). Updated 2015; https://rarediseases.org/rare-diseases/primary-ciliary-dyskinesia/.
3. Zariwala MA, Knowles MR, Leigh MW. Primary Ciliary Dyskinesia. 2007 Jan 24 [Updated 2015 Sep 3]. In: Adam MP, Ardinger HH, Pagon RA, et al., (editors). GeneReviews® [Internet]. Seattle (WA): University of Washington, Seattle; 1993-2019. Available from: https://www.ncbi.nlm.nih.gov/books/NBK1122.
4. Primary ciliary dyskinesia. Genetics Home Reference. April 2014; http://ghr.nlm.nih.gov/condition/primary-ciliary-dyskinesia.
5. Primary ciliary dyskinesia. Orphanet. May 2014; http://www.orpha.net/consor/cgi-bin/OC_Exp.php?lng=en&Expert=244.

CASE 52

YOUNG LADY WITH LEG ULCER AND PSYCHOSIS

CASE SUMMARY

A 32-year-old woman, a school teacher by profession, presented with the complaints of multiple joints pain and swelling for the last 6 years, and generalized weakness for the last 3 months. Six years back, she first developed knee joint pain which was relapsing and remitting in nature and responded well to nonsteroidal anti-inflammatory drugs (NSAIDs). Over the next 2 years, she experienced pain in small joints of hands and feet and also in wrist, elbow and shoulder joints. Joint involvement was symmetrical and was associated with significant morning stiffness. At that time she was diagnosed as a case of rheumatoid arthritis (RA) on the basis of clinical criteria and laboratory findings. She was being treated with methotrexate and with this she was in remission. Meanwhile she noticed bluish discoloration of fingers on exposure to cold which tuned red on warming. About 1.5 months back, she noticed a blister on her left lower leg which turned into a rapidly spreading discharging ulcer which was initially very painful and itchy but improved after taking antibiotic without complete healing. For the last 20–25 days, the patient also experienced bizarre episodes of headache, blurring of vision associated with talking difficulty and mouth deviation which resolved spontaneously. She also gave history of alopecia and weight loss of about 2 kg over 2 months and low-grade fever and malaise. After admission, she developed some psychiatric symptoms and was diagnosed as a case of organic psychosis and had three episodes of melena though bowel habit was normal previously. On query, she gave no history of mouth ulcer or dryness, photosensitivity, skin rash, muscle pain or weakness. There was no history of dysphagia, dyspnea, hemoptysis, hematemesis or hematuria. No similar illness was found in the family.

On examination, she was anxious but well oriented with average body built. The patient was moderately anemic with objective evidence of hair fall with pulse 90 beats/min, blood pressure (BP) 100/60 mm Hg, temperature 100°F, respiratory rate (RR) 16 breaths/min. Local examination revealed a

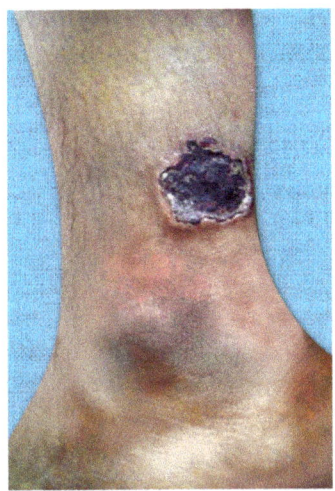

Fig. 1: Round ulcer covered with a blackish crust on lateral aspects of left lower leg.

round ulcer about 2–2.5 cm in size on lateral aspects of left lower leg above the lateral malleolus. Floor of the ulcer was covered with a blackish crust with a regular margin without any discharge (Fig. 1). On musculoskeletal examination, there was mild tenderness on metacarpophalangeal (MCP) and proximal interphalangeal (PIP) joints of both hands and wrist joints on squeezing but there was no bony deformity or periarticular swelling of any joint. Opthalmoscopic examination revealed a flame-shaped hemorrhage on right fundus in 10 o'clock position. Other systemic examination revealed no abnormality.

Investigations showed complete blood count (CBC): neutrophilic leukocytosis with reduced hemoglobin (Hb), with raised mean corpuscular volume (MCV) and with reduced platelet count. Peripheral blood film (PBF) showed features suggestive of hemolytic anemia with thrombocytopenia. Serum total bilirubin was 1.05 mg/dL and serum lactate dehydrogenase (LDH) was 1827 U/L. Both direct and indirect Coombs' tests were negative. Urine routine examination showed trace amount of albumin, red blood cells (RBCs) 2–4/HPF, UTP was 0.56 g/day, and serum creatinine, electrolytes and urine C/S were also normal. Viral markers were negative but serum iron and vitamin B12 level were deficient. Hb electrophoresis was normal. Thyroid function test was normal but ultrasonography (USG) of whole abdomen showed mild splenomegaly. Wound swab culture revealed growth of methicillin susceptible *Staphylococcus aureus*. Antinuclear antibody (ANA) and anti-double-stranded deoxyribonucleic acid (anti-dsDNA) both were positive. Rheumatoid factor (RA) and anti-cyclic citrullinated peptide antibody (ACPA) were also positive. But pANCA, cANCA and antiphospholipid antibody were negative. Finally, extractable nuclear antigen (ENA) profile was done and anti-ribonucleoprotein (RNP) antibody and SmD1 were found positive.

QUESTIONS

1. What is the likely diagnosis?
2. How should the patient be managed?

DISCUSSION

For this case, besides RA, we got several important clues like headache, blurring of vision, leg ulcer, melena, alopecia, psychosis and Raynaud's phenomenon. On examination, there were anemia, joint tenderness, leg ulcer, flame-shaped hemorrhage in fundoscopy and mild splenomegaly. Together with all these, our differentials were RA with systemic lupus erythematosus (SLE), or other overlap syndromes. After doing investigations, we found some positive results: microangiopathic hemolytic anemia with thrombocytopenia in PBF, slightly raised bilirubin and hugely raised LDH, slightly prominent spleen, positive ANA, anti-dsDNA, anti-CCP antibody and anti-RNP antibody give final diagnosis of mixed connective tissue disease (MCTD).

Final Diagnosis: Mixed Connective Tissue Disease

We treated her with tab hydroxychloroquine, methotrexate (MTX), steroid and other supportive measures; leg ulcer was treated with antibiotics and regular dressing, and she was discharged with improving symptoms.

Mixed connective tissue disease (MTCD)/Sharp's syndrome is an uncommon systemic inflammatory rheumatic disease. MCTD is a specific subset of the broader category of rheumatic "overlap syndromes", a term used to describe when a patient has features of more than one classic inflammatory rheumatic disease. These classic rheumatic diseases include SLE, polymyositis, scleroderma, and rheumatoid arthritis. MCTD patients have rheumatic overlap syndrome plus anti-RNP antibodies.[1] Individuals with an overlap syndrome may not meet complete diagnostic criteria for one (or more than one) classic rheumatic disease but must have a positive laboratory result for anti-RNP antibodies to be labeled as MCTD.[1]

The onset of MCTD can occur anytime from early childhood to elderly adulthood, but the average age of onset is 37 years. Approximately, 75% of individuals are female.[1]

Raynaud's phenomenon may precede the development of additional symptoms of MCTD. It occurs in approximately 90% of individuals with MCTD. Among patients with MCTD, patterns of organ targeting have been reported that suggest disease subtypes. Some patients have predominantly vascular manifestations, and have higher risk for pulmonary hypertension. Other patients have more myositis manifestations and have higher risk for interstitial lung disease. Some patients with more classic RA manifestations may have a lower risk of major internal organ damage.[1,2]

The treatment is based upon the specific symptoms that present in each case. Nonsteroidal anti-inflammatory drugs, hydroxychloroquine or very low doses of corticosteroids are given for mild illness. Corticosteroids and immunosuppressive drugs are indicated for moderate to severe illness.[3]

Despite treatment, MCTD worsens in about 13% of the people, causing potentially fatal complications. Causes of death include pulmonary hypertension and heart disease. The prognosis is worse for people who have mainly features of systemic sclerosis or polymyositis.[3]

REFERENCES

1. Mixed Connective Tissue Disease, Genetic and Rare Diseases Information Centre. Available from: https://rarediseases.info.nih.gov/diseases/7051/mixed-connective-tissue-disease#ref_8046
2. Szodoray Pl, Hajas A, Kardos L, Dezso B, Soos G, Zold E, Vegh J, Csipo I, Nakken B, Zeher M, Szegedi G, Bodolay E. Distinct phenotypes in mixed connective tissue disease: subgroups and survival. Lupus. 2012;21(13):1412-22. doi: 10.1177/0961203312456751.
3. Nevares AM. Mixed Connective Tissue Disease (MCTD). 2018. Available from: https://www.msdmanuals.com/home/bone,-joint,-and-muscle-disorders/auto immune-disorders-of-connective-tissue/mixed-connective-tissue-disease-mctd

CASE 53

CONFUSED BOY WITH JOINT PAIN AND FEVER

CASE SUMMARY

A 16-year-old immunized young student of low socioeconomic background, fifth issue of non-consanguineous marriage, resident of Birulia, Savar (central part of Dhaka) presented with low-grade fever, and severe pain in multiple joints for 8 days, followed by unconsciousness for several hours. His mother stated that, 8 days back, the boy developed low-grade fever (maximum-recorded temperature was 101°F), not associated with chills and rigor, and subsided with medication (paracetamol). It was associated with anorexia and generalized weakness, which was gradually increasing in severity. He also experienced asymmetrical severe joint pain especially in wrist, elbow and knee joints- not associated with swelling, redness or morning stiffness. Arthralgia was accompanied by generalized body ache. Then, several hours before admission in hospital, he became confused and subsequently lost consciousness. There was no history of convulsion, Raynaud's phenomenon, skin rash, or bleeding from any site. On query, the mother recalled that the boy had fever and joint pain one year back which subsided after symptomatic treatment.

On general examination, the patient was mildly anemic, and Glasgow Coma Scale (GCS) score was 6/15 (E1, M3, V2). Vital signs were normal except temperature was 100°F. On systemic examination, neck rigidity was absent, cranial nerves were intact and fundoscopic examination was normal. Plantar responses were bilaterally flexor with no weakness on any side of the body. Rheumatologic examination showed no features of synovitis. All other examination findings were normal.

Investigations showed complete blood count (CBC): Hemoglobin (Hb)—12.30 g/dL, white blood cell (WBC)—9,500/mm^3 (neutrophil—73%, lymphocyte—20%, eosinophil—2%, monocyte—2%), erythrocyte sedimentation rate (ESR)—10 mm/hr; platelet—110,000/mm^3; serum electrolytes—Na: 143 mmol/L, K—3.36 mmol/L, Cl—104 mmol/L, CO_2—25 mmol/L; serum creatinine—1.18 mg/dL; urine R/M/E—normal. Blood culture yielded no growth. Cerebrospinal fluid (CSF) study: appearance—clear; clotting in CSF: absent, cytology: WBC—02/mm^3 (lymphocytes—100%), red blood cell (RBC)—Nil, microbiological—acid-fast bacilli (AFB) stain: AFB not found, Gram-stain: bacteria not found; biochemical: protein—44.67 mg/dL (range—15-25), sugar—80.46 mg/dL (range—40-70).

QUESTIONS

1. What is the clinical diagnosis?
2. What investigation will you do for confirmation?

DISCUSSION

We retook elaborate history from the patient's attendant (mother) regarding the initial onset of fever and arthralgia, but she repeated that they did not visit any doctor at the very beginning of the symptoms. However, she mentioned a very important clue that many of the patient's neighbors had been suffering from chikungunya fever at that time. So, considering the history and examination, our provisional diagnosis was chikungunya encephalitis.

For confirmation, we went for the following investigations:
- Blood:
  - Chikungunya IgM (ICT): positive
  - Anti-dengue IgM: negative.
- Cerebrospinal fluid:
  - Reverse transcription (RT) polymerase chain reaction (PCR) for chikungunya: positive.
- Magnetic resonance imaging (MRI) brain: bilateral frontoparietal white matter lesions with restricted diffusion with no enhancement, which was described as an early sign of viral encephalitis.

Final Diagnosis: Chikungunya Encephalitis

Chikungunya fever is caused by an alphavirus in Togaviridae family and is transmitted by the bite of *Aedes* mosquitoes. It was first isolated in 1952-1953 when an epidemic occurred in East Africa. The name "chikungunya" came from Makonde language that means "which bends up," referring to the stooped posture resulting from severe joint pain. Apart from arthralgia, other symptoms are high fever, headaches, nausea and vomiting.

Symptomatic chikungunya virus (CHIKV) infections result in systemic febrile illness with rash and arthralgia, which is usually self-limiting. Although cases of severe disease, including meningoencephalitis and death, have also been reported. Central nervous system (CNS) complications of chikungunya fever are neurocognitive or behavioral disorders, acute disseminated encephalomyelitis (ADEM), acute encephalitis or encephalopathy, and Guillain-Barré syndrome.[1]

Considering the clinical presentation, CSF and MRI findings—we came to the diagnosis of chikungunya encephalitis in the patient though this is an atypical presentation. The patient was infected during an epidemic episode of chikungunya fever in Dhaka city and many of his neighbors also had developed the disease. CSF examination revealed increased protein with lymphocyte predominance, which is usually seen in viral encephalitis. The patient also tested positive for anti-chikungunya IgM in his serum and CHIKV real-time reverse transcriptase (rRT-PCR) was positive in CSF—making this a confirmed case. Though this young boy presented in a grave condition, after proper hospital management-he survived.

REFERENCE

1. Sam IC, Kümmerer BM, Chan YF, Roques P, Drosten C, AbuBakar S. Updates on chikungunya epidemiology, clinical disease, and diagnostics. Vector-Borne Zoonotic Dis. 2015;15(4):223-30.

CASE 54

DISORIENTED YOUNG MAN WITH FEVER AND ACUTE ABDOMEN

CASE SUMMARY

A 22-year-old young man presented with the complaints of high-grade, intermittent fever for the last 22 days. His maximum recorded temperature was 102°F, associated with chills and rigor, subsided with sweating with or without taking medication. Fever was associated with severe, constant and generalized headache with photophobia, phonophobia and vomiting. Moreover, he experienced relative constipation, abdominal pain and intractable vomiting. At first, he was admitted in Sadar Hospital (secondary healthcare center), where he was conservatively treated as a case of subacute intestinal obstruction in the surgery department. But following one episode of convulsion, he was referred to Dhaka Medical College and Hospital (DMCH) and got admitted in the medicine department. During hospital stay, he again developed two episodes of partial onset secondary generalized seizure. In addition, he developed severely painful right testicular swelling with burning micturition, nocturia, urgency and frequency. On query, his mother gave history of low-grade fever with evening rise of temperature associated with anorexia and generalized weakness and occasional headache for the last several months prior to this illness. There was no history of contact with known patient of pulmonary tuberculosis (TB).

On examination, the patient was disoriented, GCS score was of 10/15. He was febrile (T—101°F), without having any lymphadenopathy. Neurological examination could not be done properly but neck rigidity was present and plantar was bilaterally extensor. Fundoscopic examination was normal. Abdomen was soft, slightly distended and mildly tender. Bowel sound was present. There was mild swelling on the right side of scrotum. Rest of the systemic examination was unremarkable.

Investigations showed: hemoglobin (Hb)%—13.5 g/dL, white blood cell (WBC)—13,800/cumm (N—84%, L—10%, M—5%), platelets (PLT)—349,000/cumm, erythrocyte sedimentation rate (ESR) in 1st hour—8 mm, peripheral blood film (PBF)—nonspecific morphology, serum creatinine—0.9 mg/L, urine routine examination (RE)—normal, urine culture and sensitivity (C/S)—no growth, C-reactive protein (CRP)—less than 3.48 mg/L, procalcitonin—less than 0.1 ng/mL, MT—2 mm, prostatic smear: Gram stain—nil, acid-fast bacilli (AFB) stain—nil, C/S—*Escherichia coli* (sensitive to several antibiotics), serum electrolyte: sodium (118 mmol/L), potassium (2.7 mmol/L) and Cl (85 mmol/L), cerebrospinal fluid (CSF) study: total cell count—4 cells/cumm (N—0%, L—100%), glucose—99.31 mg/dL, protein—41.22 mg/dL, ADA—4.13 U/L, Gram stain—no organism seen, Z-N stain—AFB not found, CSF for GeneXpert—*Mycobacterium tuberculosis* (*MTB*) not detected, CSF for polymerase chain reaction (PCR) for MTB—positive. Chest X-ray (CXR) posteroanterior (PA) view—normal, ultrasonography (USG) of whole abdomen—moderate intra-abdominal collection, excessive bowel gas, USG of both testes—right-sided chronic epididymo-orchitis.

The patient was put on category 1 anti-TB chemotherapy with steroid. He showed excellent response and he started his daily activities.

About 15 days after initiating 2 fixed-dose combination (2FDC), he developed anorexia, malaise and lethargy. About 7 days after this, he developed relative constipation followed by nonprojectile, initially nonbilious then bilious vomiting and severe cramping diffuse abdominal pain. With these complaints, he readmitted in our care. Bowel moved with glycerin suppositories and fleet enema. Abdominal pain and vomiting subsided. On examination, he was dehydrated and afebrile. On abdominal examination, severe tenderness over right and left iliac and hypogastric region was present, with normal bowel sound.

Further investigation showed: Hb level—14.9 g/dL, WBC—4,500/cumm (N—75%, L—21%), PLT—290,000/cumm, ESR in first hour—5 mm, plain X-ray of abdomen—gas distended bowel loops suggestive of subacute intestinal obstruction, serum sodium and potassium level was persistently low which was corrected after replacement, alanine aminotransferase (ALT) level was high (ranging from 52 to 256 IU/L) on multiple reports. aspartate aminotransferase (AST) level was also high (ranging from 43 IU/L to 203 IU/L), serum bilirubin—0.6 mg/dL, hepatitis B surface antigen (HBsAg)—negative, hepatitis B e-antigen (HBeAg)—negative, anti-hepatitis E virus (HEV)—negative, serum creatinine—0.79 mg/dL, serum albumin—23 g/L, serum calcium—7.5 mg/dL, serum Mg—1 mg/dL, upper gastrointestinal tract (GIT) endoscopy—normal, USG of whole abdomen—excessive gas shadow in abdomen with otherwise normal findings. Colonoscopy was planned, but could not be done due to his poor general condition.

He was diagnosed as a case of disseminated TB with subacute intestinal obstruction with drug-induced hepatitis. Anti-TB medication was withheld. His nausea and vomiting subsided. But he became febrile. He was put on injection streptomycin (15 mg/kg) and tablet ethambutol (20 mg/kg), and tablet ciprofloxacin with steroid coverage. In the meantime, he developed resting tremor of both hands, eventually tremor involved his whole body, and developed choreiform movements as well. He became disoriented. On examination, temperature was 98°F, Glasgow Coma Score (GCS)—11/15, gross muscle wasting of all four limbs, power 3/5 in all four limbs, deep tendon reflexes were brisk with plantar flexor bilaterally, fundoscopic examination was normal. Slit-lamp examination: no Kayser-Fleischer (KF) ring.

After lowering down the liver enzymes to some extent, tablet rifampicin was started at challenging dose but had to stop due to elevation of liver enzymes. Tablet isoniazid was also withheld owing to elevation of the enzymes.

QUESTIONS

1. Do you want to change the previous diagnosis?
2. How do you manage this case?

DISCUSSION

We carried out further investigations: Magnetic resonance imaging (MRI) of brain—mild communicating hydrocephalus, serum NH_3—40 µmol/L, serum ceruloplasmin—25 mg/dL.

His tremor was improved after initiating tablet trihexyphenidyl and tablet tetrahydrobenazine. He was discharged with the above-mentioned anti-TB chemotherapy and advised for regular follow-up. He improved significantly after continuing ongoing medication for 2 months. His liver enzymes also became normal.

Our patient presented with fever, abdominal pain, vomiting and relative constipation, and was initially treated conservatively in the line of intestinal obstruction in the surgery department. But he developed convulsion and was transferred to medicine department. He also developed epididymo-orchitis. The diagnosis of disseminated TB was made on clinical background. Though CSF study was inconclusive but PCR for MTB came positive. Initiation of anti-TB chemotherapy along with steroid resulted in dramatical response. After a few days, the patient developed vomiting with raised transaminase level. Initially, we thought this event to be drug-induced hepatitis, however, no significant improvement was achieved even after stopping the medication. Also, we faced difficulty in readvocating the full dosage of medications. As it was a case of disseminated TB, we rescheduled the regimen, only continuing non-hepatotoxic drugs. Moreover, during hospital stay, he developed generalized tremor and choreiform movement on the top of anti-TB chemotherapy. In this difficult situation, we excluded the other possibilities like Wilson's disease. We continued the anti-TB regimen and subsequently he gradually improved with normal liver function test suggesting he also had hepatic involvement due to tuberculosis. On further follow-up, he recovered completely.

Final Diagnosis: Disseminated Tuberculosis [Central Nervous System TB, Intestinal TB, Hepatitis, and Right-sided Epididymo-orchitis]

The incidence of TB has been increasing globally; almost 2 billion people (one-third of the world's population) around the globe are infected with MTB.[1] Every year, around 80,000 Bangladeshis die of TB and about 190,000 new cases occur.[1] It can have a varied presentation, frequently mimicking other common and rare disease. Classical symptoms of prolonged cough and fever are insensitive predictors of TB. It commonly affects the lungs, but in up to one third of the cases involve other organs.

The clinical presentation of TB is variable with symptoms reflecting the underlying organ involved. It frequently presents as a nonspecific constitutional syndrome, with systemic manifestations, which can sometimes result in a diagnostic dilemma.

Abdominal TB is predominantly a disease of the young adult. The clinical presentation may be acute or chronic or acute-on-chronic. Even patient may be without symptoms. If a patient presents with intestinal obstruction, we should keep the possibility of TB in mind.

Tuberculosis of the central nervous system (CNS) is a highly devastating form of TB, which, even in the setting of appropriate antitubercular therapy, leads to unacceptable levels of morbidity and mortality.[2] Initial improvement of clinical symptoms may be obvious but may, in fact, briefly worsen despite appropriate anti-TB therapy.

Tuberculosis has nonspecific and diverse symptomatology. Careful approach and supportive results are required in order to reach the final diagnosis. If diagnosed early, it can be treated successfully with the conventional anti-TB drug.

REFERENCES

1. World Health Organization, Global tuberculosis report 2018. WHO, Geneva (2018).
2. Fanning A. Tuberculosis: 6 Extrapulmonary disease. Can Med Assoc J. 1999;160:1597–603.

CASE 55

YOUNG MALE WITH PASSAGE OF OFFENSIVE DARK-COLORED STOOL

CASE SUMMARY

A 30-year-old male migrant worker (resident of Dubai for the last 8 years) presented with passage of dark-colored stool for the last 3 months, and loss of appetite and generalized weakness for the same duration. He was reasonably well about 3 months back. Then he noticed passage of dark-colored stool with plenty of mucus. The stool was small in amount, offensive, soft in consistency and frequency was 8–10 times/day. The patient also complained of one episode of bloody diarrhea, offensive in smell, which lasted for 4 days. He also experienced loss of appetite and generalized weakness, which was associated with a weight loss of 13 kg in the last 3 months. He consulted with local physicians and was found severely anemic. He received one unit of blood transfusion and was prescribed folic acid, vitamin preparations and proton pump inhibitor (PPI). The patient mentioned that he underwent bone marrow aspiration twice. The patient did not give any history of fever, cough, abnormal pigmentation, gum bleeding, bone pain, abnormal swelling of the body or abdominal pain. He had an appendicectomy 3 years back. He was nonsmoker and nonalcoholic. He denied any extramarital sexual exposure or any history of intravenous (IV) drug abuse. None of his family members suffered from such type of illness.

On examination, patient was severely anemic. Other parameters of general examinations were normal, including BMI which was 20.5 kg/m^2. On abdominal examination, abdomen was nontender. Liver was palpable 7 cm from the right costal margin along the midclavicular line. Liver was firm in consistency, surface was smooth, and margin was sharp and nontender. There was no hepatic bruit. Spleen was palpable 8 cm from the left costal margin along its long axis, nontender, medial notch was present, firm in consistency. No other organomegaly, lymph node enlargement or mass was found. Stigmata of chronic liver disease were not found. Other systemic examinations revealed normal findings.

Investigations showed hemoglobin (Hb) level was persistently below 6 g/dL. Red blood cell (RBC): 2.9 million/mm^3, white blood cell (WBC): 3,600/mm^3, and platelet: 98,000/mm^3 with erythrocyte sedimentation rate (ESR): 89 mm in 1st hour. Peripheral blood film showed normochromic normocytic anemia, with mature WBC and eosinophilia, with thrombocytopenia. Bone marrow examinations revealed hypercellularity. Erythropoiesis was hyperactive, with both micronormoblastic and megaloblastic changes. Granulopoiesis was active and maturing into segmented forms. Megakaryopoiesis was normal. Plasma cells were increased, lymphocytes and histiocytes were seen. Trephine biopsy showed erythroid hyperplasia. Coombs' test was negative. Liver function test showed alanine transaminase (ALT)—39.5 U/L, aspartate transaminase (AST)—208 U/L, gamma-glutamyl transferase (GGT)—220 U/L, serum total protein: 55 g/L, serum albumin: 34 g/L, serum globulin—21 g/L, albumin to globulin (A:G) ratio—1.6:1, prothrombin time—16 seconds, international normalized ratio (INR)—1.23. Surface antigen of hepatitis B (HBsAg)—negative and anti-hepatitis C virus antibody (anti-HCVAb)-negative. Fasting plasma glucose—8.6 mmol/L. Plasma glucose 2 hours after glucose load—13.9 mmol/L. Fasting lipid profile: total cholesterol—250 mg/dL, triglycerides—180 mg/dL, HDL cholesterol—35 mg/dL, LDL cholesterol—165 mg/dL. Ultrasonography (USG) of whole abdomen showed hepatosplenomegaly suggestive of hepatic parenchymal disease and mild ascites. Endoscopy of upper gastrointestinal tract (GIT): grade-II/III esophageal varices. Mucosa of stomach looked pale. Colonoscopy: whole of colonic mucosa looked pale. Numerous punctate erythema on walls of transverse colon, descending colon, sigmoid and rectum. Histopathology—Chronic nonspecific colitis. MT—negative. Urine R/M/E, serum creatinine, serum electrolytes, and iron profile were normal. Serum ceruloplasmin level, and 24-hour urinary copper excretion were normal. Antinuclear antibody (ANA), anti-smooth muscle antibodies (ASMA), and antimitochondrial antibody-M2 (AMA-M2) were negative.

QUESTIONS

1. What next investigations do you want to do to approach further?
2. What is the diagnosis?

DISCUSSION

This young man came to us with hepatosplenomegaly and complications of portal hypertension. Investigations yielded no etiology, but moderately elevated hepatic enzymes, and paucity of other features of chronic liver disease brought consideration of nonalcoholic fatty liver disease (NAFLD) in mind.

Next investigation, fibroscan of liver, was done which revealed:
- Fibrosis score: 23.1 kPa
- Fibrosis stage: F4.

Liver biopsy could have been done for confirmation, but this invasive procedure was avoided on the patient's request. He was advised lifestyle interventions, and upper GI endoscopy was revised with variceal ligation.

Final Diagnosis: Nonalcoholic Steatohepatitis

Nonalcoholic steatohepatitis (NASH) is a component of NAFLD which is considered as a hepatic manifestation of metabolic syndrome due to its strong association with obesity, dyslipidemia, type 2 diabetes and hypertension. NAFLD comprises of simple steatosis, that usually follows a benign nonprogressive course; and NASH, in which there is steatosis with hepatocellular injury and hepatic inflammation that may progress to cirrhosis and hepatocellular carcinoma.[1-3]

While steatosis is usually asymptomatic, progressive NASH may manifest late in the natural history of the disease with complications of cirrhosis and portal hypertension, like variceal bleeding, or with hepatocellular carcinoma.[3]

NAFLD and NASH are diagnoses of exclusion. Liver biopsy remains the gold standard for diagnosis. Simple noninvasive scores for NAFLD/fibrosis, such as NAFLD fibrosis score (NFS), fibrosis index based on the 4 factors (FIB-4) score have been in use, but can be employed to calculate positive and negative predictive values for fibrosis/cirrhosis only. Supportive laboratory results include the reversal of normal AST : ALT ratio of < 1 in progressive NASH (AST : ALT > 1), non-specific elevations of GGT, low-titer antinuclear antibody (ANA) in 20-30% of patients and elevated ferritin levels. Ultrasound, CT, MRI or MR spectroscopy may give clue, but no routine imaging modality can yet differentiate between steatosis and NASH, or quantify fibrosis from cirrhosis.[2,3]

Patients diagnosed with NASH warrant screening for and treatment of cardiovascular risk factors. Treatment comprises of lifestyle modification by dietary changes and physical exercise. Sustained weight loss of 7-10% confers notable improvement in histological and biochemical NASH severity. Along with symptomatic management, coexistent insulin resistance, dyslipidemia and hypertension need treatment. Statins and fibrates (specifically bezafibrate) may be used to treat dyslipidemia. Specific insulin-sensitizing agents, like glitazones are promising.[3]

REFERENCES

1. Dyson JK, Anstee QM, McPherson S. Non-alcoholic fatty liver disease: a practical approach to diagnosis and staging Frontline Gastroenterology 3. 2014;5:211-8.
2. Hashimoto E1, Taniai M, Tokushige K. Characteristics and diagnosis of NAFLD/NASH. J Gastroenterol Hepatol. 2013;28 (Suppl 4):64-70. doi: 10.1111/jgh.12271.
3. Ralston SH, Penman ID, Strachan MWJ, Hobson RP. Davidson's Principles and Practice of Medicine. 23rd ed. Edinburgh: Churchill Livingstone/Elsevier; 2018. pp. 882-5.

CASE 56

TEENAGE GIRL WITH PROGRESSIVE LOW BACK PAIN

CASE SUMMARY

An 18-year-old girl presented with low back pain which was progressive for 3 months. Pain did not improve with analgesic. She gave a history of fall from chair 6 months back before this illness. For the last 2 months pain was so severe that patient was unable to move or walk. She also had fever which was intermittent in nature and was associated with generalized weakness. She gave history of 4 kg weight loss during this course of illness. Her mental development and motor function was normal for age.

On examination patient was moderately anemic, grossly emaciated, temperature was 98°F. Pulse 78 beats/min, blood pressure (BP): 120/80 mm Hg. Bony tenderness, and bleeding spots were absent. There was presence of lumbar spinal gibbus and tenderness over gibbus. No lymphadenopathy or organomegaly was found.

Investigations showed complete blood count (CBC): Hemoglobin 9 g/dL, WBC: 1.50×10^9/L, lymphocyte 85% without blasts, platelet count 22×10^9/L, PBF revealed pancytopenia. The X-ray of the spine showed diffuse vertebral body collapse and osteopenia (Fig. 1). Serum Ca: 9.3 mg/dL (reference range 8.4–10.2 mg/dL). Serum albumin: 37.5 g/L. Vitamin D: 26.1 ηg/dL. Parathyroid hormone (PTH): 3.57 pg/mL. Bone mineral density (BMD) showed: age matched Z-score—3.6. Ultrasonography (USG) of whole abdomen showed prominent intra-abdominal lymph nodes with splenomegaly.

QUESTIONS

1. What next investigations do you want to do?
2. What could be the final diagnosis?

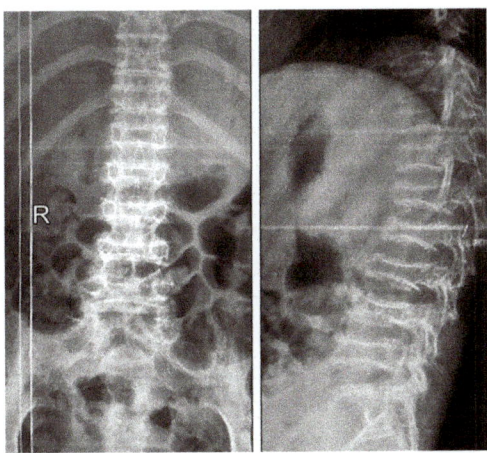

Fig. 1: Generalized osteopenia of spine and multiple vertebral compressions.

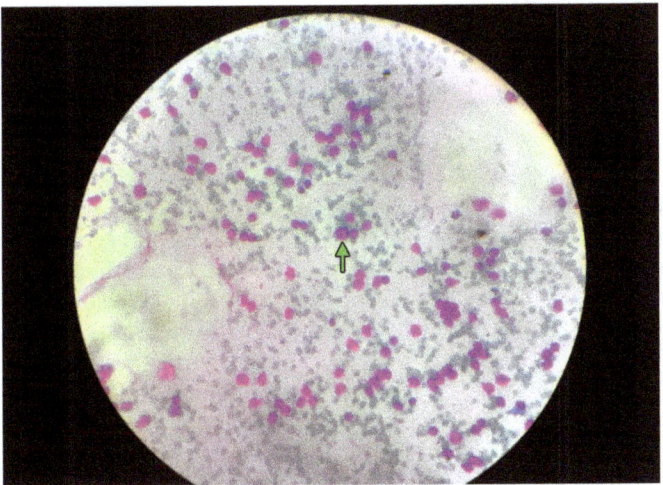

Fig. 2: Numerous lymphoblasts (arrow) in bone marrow smear.

DISCUSSION

To reach the diagnosis, next we did bone marrow examination: bone marrow aspirate showed acute lymphoblastic leukemia (ALL-L2) (Fig. 2).

Final Diagnosis: Acute Lymphoblastic Leukemia

Joint pain and bone pain can be presenting symptom in 25% patients in acute leukemia[1] but generalized osteopenia and vertebral complications are less common.[2] Children present with symptoms due to bone pains, cytopenia, lymphadenopathy and organomegaly. About 40-60% of patients may refuse to walk. The osteoarticular manifestations which are frequent in the ALL are osteopenia, lysis of bone, lesions of osteosclerosis and periosteal reactions.[3] There are very few cases of childhood ALL presenting with severe osteopenia. Childhood ALL commonly presents with fever, bony pain and symptoms related to cytopenias. Asymptomatic skeletal involvement may be present in ALL patients but presentation with pathological fracture is very rare. During course of leukemia radiological evidence of demineralization can be caused by the disease itself or it can be caused by inactivity, antileukemic drugs and steroids or due to abnormalities in mineral homeostasis.[4] Despite having normal peripheral blood counts spinal involvement can be presenting feature.[5,6] ALL which presents with constant severe bone pain, leukopenia and a long interval between the onset of symptoms and diagnosis, carries a poor prognosis. Vertebral compressions are a very rare presentation in a patient of ALL. Clinicians need to have a high index of suspicion to suspect ALL in these patients, especially if there is worsening back pain and associated vertebral compression with pancytopenia. Proper antileukemic drugs induce rapid symptomatic relief as well as radiographic evidence of bony remodeling.

REFERENCES

1. Vassilopoulou-Sellin R, Ramirez I. Severe osteopenia and vertebral compression fractures after complete remission in an adolescent with acute leukemia. Am J Hematol. 1992;39:142-3.
2. Cohn SL, Morgan ER, Mallette LE. The spectrum of metabolic bone disease in lymphoblastic leukemia. Cancer. 1987;59:346-50.
3. Reddy AP, Alok S, Suresh V. Osteoporosis and vertebral compression fractures as a presenting feature of childhood acute lymphoblastic leukemia. J Endocrinol Diabetes Obes. 2014;2(2):1021.
4. Pandya NA, Meller ST, MacVicar D, et al. "Vertebral Compression Fractures in Acute Lymphoblastic Leukaemia and Remodeling after Treatment,". Archives of Disease in Children. 2001;85(6):492-3.
5. Santangelo JR, Thomson JD. Childhood leukemia presenting with back pain and vertebral compression fractures. Am J Orthop. 1999;28(4):257-60.
6. Cherkaoui S, Hmimech A, Madani A, Benchekroun A. Vertebral Body Collapse at the Onset of Acute Lymphoblastic Leukemia. Pediatrics Research International Journal. 2014 Article ID 955855, DOI:10.5171/2014.955855.

CASE 57

YOUNG MAN WITH DIMNESS OF VISION, FACIAL NUMBNESS AND NASAL INTONATION

CASE SUMMARY

A 43-year-old male, smoker presented with gradual dimness of vision in both eyes for the last 14 months which was associated with left-sided headache. The headache was continuous, dull aching in nature. Initially he noticed blurring and double vision of both eyes. The dimness of vision gradually progressed to complete loss of vision in his left eye for last 4 months. He also noticed paresthesia in the left side of his face and nasal intonation of voice for 6 months. He had no complaints of fever, joint pain, oral or genital ulcer, cough, hemoptysis, chest pain, weight loss, unconsciousness or hemiparesis.

On examination, his left posterior auricular lymph node was enlarged, painless and fixed with skin. The cranial nerve examination revealed bilateral impairement of visual acuity [left eye—only perception of light (PL) present, right eye—hand movement]. Light reflex was absent in the left eye, and sluggish in the right eye. Accommodation reflex could not be evaluated due to impaired vision. Ocular movement was restricted in all directions. Fundoscopic findings were normal. There was reduced facial sensation and corneal reflex on left side. The palatal and tongue movements were also impaired on the same side with fasciculation of tongue muscles. Sensory and motor function examination revealed no abnormality. Signs of meningeal irritation were absent. Rest of the systems were normal.

All his baseline parameters were within normal limit including complete blood count (CBC), erythrocyte sedimentation rate (ESR), C-reactive protein (CRP) and diabetic profile. Thyroid stimulating hormone (TSH), and free T-4 (FT-4) levels were within reference range. Autoantibody and angiotensin-converting enzyme (ACE) levels were also normal. Magnetic resonance imaging (MRI) brain showed small infarct in left parietal lobe (Fig. 1). Cerebrospinal fluid (CSF) study was normal. Routine screening for malignancy including chest X-ray, ultrasound of abdomen showed no abnormality.

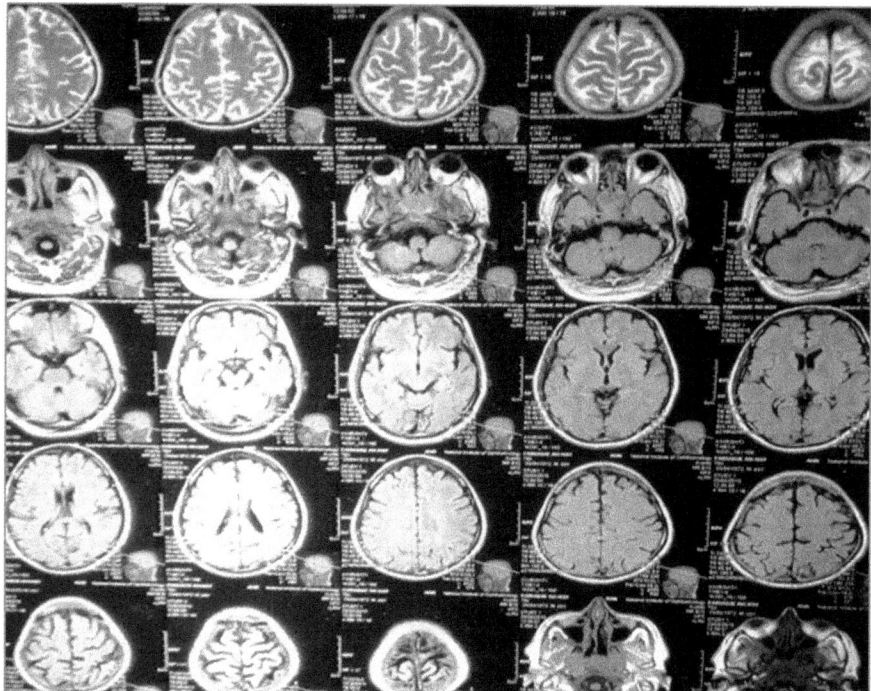

Fig. 1: MRI of brain showing small infarct in left parietal lobe.

QUESTIONS

1. What are the differential diagnoses?
2. What is the next step of investigation?

DISCUSSION

In this scenario, the patient presented with polyneuritis cranialis (bilateral second, third, fourth and sixth cranial nerves involvement and left-sided fifth, tenth, eleventh and twelfth cranial nerves involvement). So neurosarcoidosis, vasculitis, tuberculosis and paraneoplastic syndrome were taken into consideration. But normal findings in CBC, ESR, CRP, ACE level, and autoantibody profile made vasculitis and sarcoidosis unlikely. To find out the cause of his neurological abnormality, next we did CT scan and MRI of brain, which did not show any space-occupying, or inflammatory, or demyelinating lesion. We had another positive examination finding of posterior auricular lymphadenopathy-which was ventured into next. Fine needle aspiration cytology (FNAC) from the lymph node revealed poorly differentiated metastatic carcinoma.

The next step was a whole body screening to search the primary malignancy using computed tomography (CT) chest, abdomen and pelvis, prostate specific antigen (PSA) and alpha-fetoprotein (AFP) which yielded normal findings, except CT chest which revealed a small growth in his left lung with irregular margin. So in presence of a lung malignancy, polyneuritis cranialis due to metastatic brain or meningeal involvement, or due to paraneoplastic syndrome were the possibilities for this man's multiple cranial nerve palsy. No positive findings in physical examination, neuroimagings, and CSF study to support the former two conditions made paraneoplastic cranial neuropathy the most logical explanation.

Then we sent the patient to the oncology department for further evaluation. There, he was diagnosed with poorly differentiated adenocarcinoma of lung and prepared for subsequent oncological management.

Final Diagnosis: Paraneoplastic Syndrome (Cranial Neuropathy) due to Poorly Differentiated Adenocarcinoma of Left Lung with Metastatic Lymph Node

Paraneoplastic syndromes are symptom complexes that occur in patients with cancer and that cannot be readily explained by local or distant spread of the tumor or by the elaboration of hormones indigenous to the tissue of origin of the tumor.[1] Although the symptoms (endocrine, neuromuscular, musculoskeletal, cardiovascular, cutaneous, hematologic, gastrointestinal, renal or miscellaneous) of paraneoplastic syndromes might be associated with many types of malignancies, they are most commonly found with lung cancers. Adenocarcinomas are the most common lung cancers overall, but small cell lung cancer (SCLC) is considered to be the commonest culprit behind various paraneoplastic manifestations.[1,2]

Examples of paraneoplastic syndromes of the nervous system include:[3,4]
- Cerebellar degeneration
- Limbic encephalitis
- Encephalomyelitis
- Opsoclonus-myoclonus
- Stiff person syndrome
- Myelopathy
- Lambert-Eaton myasthenic syndrome
- Myasthenia gravis
- Neuromyotonia
- Peripheral and cranial neuropathy
- Dysautonomia.

In this case, the patient had cranial neuropathy—bilateral second, third, fourth, sixth cranial nerves; and left sided fifth, tenth, eleventh, and twelfth cranial nerves were impaired. Paraneoplastic cranial neuropathy is a rare entity and mostly found with SCLC, and those due to adenocarcinoma are extremely rare. Only a few cases associated with adenocarcinoma of different origins (breast, thyroid, ovary, lung, thyroid, pancreas, or prostate) have been found in literatures.[5,6] After ruling out all other possibilities, this patient's clinical features were only explainable with paraneoplastic syndrome due to underlying lung malignancy. Here lies the sad beauty of paraneoplastic syndromes that they might be the harbinger of the occult lesion, as in this case, since our patient did not have features suggestive of lung malignancy. Our sequential diagnostic approach lead to timely diagnosis. As most paraneoplastic disorders of the central nervous system are probably immune mediated, antineuronal antibodies in the CSF and serum should have been searched.[3-6]

Treatment of paraneoplastic syndrome is directed toward the treatment of primary disease; though prognosis is variable. However, occasionally intravenous immunoglobulin administration may improve the symptoms.[7]

REFERENCES

1. Kumar V, Abbas AK, Aster JC. Robbins Basic Pathology [StudentConsult.com]. 10th ed. Philadelphia, Pennsylvania: Elsevier; 2018. pp. 150-8.
2. McClelland MT. Paraneoplastic syndromes related to lung cancer. Clin J Oncol Nurs. 2010;14:357-64.
3. Graus F, Delattre JY, Antoine JC, Dalmau J, Giometto B, Grisold W, Honnorat J, Smitt PS, Vedeler Ch, Verschuuren JJ, et al. Recommended diagnostic criteria for paraneoplastic neurological syndromes. J Neurol Neurosurg Psychiatry. 2004;75:1135-40.
4. Dalmau J, Rosenfeld MR. Paraneoplastic syndromes of the CNS. Lancet Neurol. 2008;7(4):327-40. doi:10.1016/S1474-4422(08)70060-7
5. Camdessanché JP, Antoine JC, Honnorat J, Vial C, Petiot P, Convers P, et al. Paraneoplastic peripheral neuropathy associated with anti-Hu antibodies: A clinical and electrophysiological study of 20 patients. Brain. 2002;125(1):166-75. https://doi.org/10.1093/brain/awf006
6. Alabduljalil T, Behbehani R. Paraneoplastic syndromes in neuro-ophthalmology. Curr Opin Ophthalmol. 2007;18:463-9.
7. Ralston SH, Penman ID, Strachan MWJ, Hobson RP. Davidson's Principles and Practice of Medicine. 23rd ed. Edinburgh: Churchill Livingstone/Elsevier; 2018. pp. 1110-1.

CASE 58

YOUNG MAN WITH ABDOMINAL PAIN AND JAUNDICE

CASE SUMMARY

A 43-year-old man presented with abdominal pain for 3 months and jaundice for 1.5 months. The pain was in the upper abdomen, constant dull aching, mild to moderate in intensity, sometimes with radiation to back, with no aggravating or relieving factors. Jaundice was first identified by his wife as yellow eyes; later he noticed yellow skin, dark urine, and experienced nausea and itching. These complaints were accompanied by loss of appetite, weight loss and undue weakness. He did not have fever or cough and was not on any medication, except occasinal paracetamol intake. He had no history of trauma or of surgery. He was nondiabetic, normotensive, smoker, non-alcoholic; and none of his family members had similar or any other familial illness.

Examination revealed an icteric man with normal vital signs. Abdomen examination revealed diffuse tenderness without organomegaly or ascites.

Investigation revealed hemoglobin (Hb)—10 g/dL, erythrocyte sedimentation rate (ESR)—78 mm in the first hour, alanine aminotransferase (ALT)—108 U/L, serum bilirubin—7 mg/dL with direct bilirubin—5.3 mg/dL, serum alkaline phosphatase—650 IU/L, prothrombin time (PT)—15 seconds, viral markers were negative, fasting lipid profile—normal except low HDL, ultrasonography (USG) of W/A was unremarkable, serum amylase, serum lipase, carcinoembryonic antigen (CEA), and carbohydrate antigen 19-9 (CA 19-9) were noncontributory. Serum thyroid-stimulating hormone (TSH) was 9 mU/L. Endoscopy of the upper gastrointestinal tract (GIT) was unremarkable, but endoscopic retrograde cholangiopancreatography (ERCP) showed irregular narrowing of pancreatic duct. Computed tomography (CT) scan of the abdomen revealed diffused enlargement of pancreas without calcification, vascular encasement, peripancreatic fluid or lymphadenopathy.

QUESTIONS

1. What should be the next approach?
2. How to treat this condition?
3. How to monitor the condition?
4. What are the common association of this condition?

DISCUSSION

For this gentleman with jaundice and abdominal pain, we searched the common causes of jaundice and pancreatitis, and in doing so, discovered marvel findings in the imagings.

Based on the clinical features and imaging, we suspected autoimmune pancreatitis (AIP). Antinuclear antibodies (ANA) was positive, with negative anti-doudle-stranded DNA (anti-dsDNA). Serum immunoglobulin G4 (IgG4) level was 298 mg/dL. Diagnosis was confirmed by HISORt, Mayo Clinic Criteria for autoimmune pancreatitis which encompasses five cardinal features of AIP in **h**istology, **i**maging, **s**erology, **o**ther **o**rgan involvement, and **r**esponse to steroid **t**herapy-summarized in the mnemonic HISORt.

Final Diagnosis: IgG4-related Autoimmune Pancreatitis

This patient was given corticosteroid starting with 40 mg/day for 4 weeks, then gradually tapered within the next 8 weeks. He responded dramatically within 3 weeks.

The AIP is the pancreatic manifestation of a systemic IgG4-related fibroinflammatory disease which, along with pancreas, may also afflict the bile duct, salivary glands, retroperitoneum, and lymph nodes. *Organs affected by AIP have a lymphoplasmacytic infiltrate rich in IgG4-positive cells* (**h**istology and immunostaining). The inflammatory process *responds to steroid therapy*, but the intense fibrosis can lead to permanent structural and functional damage to pancreas.[1-5]

The AIP mimics carcinoma head of the pancreas in its presentation and imaging features. But lack of vascular encasement, pancreatic rim halo and narrow ducts are imaging features that favor *AIP* (**i**maging).[2]

Elevated titers of gammaglobulins, IgG, ANA, rheumatoid factor (RA), carbonic anhydrase, and lactoferrin may be found, however, elevated IgG4 is considered sensitive and specific marker of AIP (**s**erology).[2]

The AIP can be classified as type 1 and type 2 based on histological patterns and clinical features. *Type 1 might be associated with sclerosing cholangitis, retroperitoneal fibrosis, sclerosing sialadenitis, mediastinal lymphadenopathy, and type 2 can be associated with ulcerative colitis* (**o**ther **o**rgan involvement).

Treatment is with corticosteroids. Patients require monitoring of symptoms, serum IgG4 levels, liver function test (LFT), imaging of the pancreas and bile ducts.[1]

To identify the full spectrum of changes occurring in AIP, one needs to recognize its five cardinal features in histology, imaging, serology, other organ involvement, and its response to steroid therapy (HISOrt).[1]

REFERENCES

1. Chari ST. Diagnosis of autoimmune pancreatitis using its five cardinal features: introducing the Mayo Clinic's HISORt criteria. J Gastroenterol. 2007;42(18): 39-41. doi 10.1007/s00535-007-2046-8.
2. Hamano H, Kawa S, Horiuchi A, Unno H, Furuya N, Akamatsu T, et al. High serum IgG4 concentrations in patients with sclerosing pancreatitis N Engl J Med. 2001;344:732-8.
3. Kloppel G, Luttges J, Lohr M, Zamboni G, Longnecker D. Autoimmune pancreatitis: pathological, clinical, and immunological features. Pancreas. 2003;27(1):14-9.
4. Kamisawa T, Funata N, Hayashi Y, Eishi Y, Koike M, Tsuruta K, et al. A new clinicopathological entity of IgG4-related autoimmune disease. J Gastroenterol. 2003;38(10):982-4.
5. Irie H, Honda H, Baba S, Kuroiwa T, Yoshimitsu K, Tajima T, et al. Autoimmune pancreatitis: CT and MR characteristics. Am J Roentgenol. 1998;170(5):1323-7.

CASE 59

MIDDLE-AGED MALE WITH CHRONIC SINUSITIS AND WEIGHT LOSS

CASE SUMMERY

A 53-year-old man, plumber, reported that, about 8 months ago, his symptoms began with occasional red colored urine persisting during the entire urine stream without any passage of clot. It was associated with burning sensation and mild loin pain. He also had persistent dry cough associated with respiratory distress without any diurnal variation, relation with posture change, hemoptysis or chest pain. He also gave history of single episode of spontaneous epistaxis. These symptoms were associated with occasional fever and highest recorded temperature was 102°F. He had lost approximately 10 kg weight during this course of illness. He visited an ear, nose and throat (ENT) specialist for this and was labeled as a case of chronic sinusitis. He was treated with different antibiotics as an outpatient without any improvement.

Physical examination revealed ill-looking patient with mild anemia. His blood pressure was 150/90 mm Hg. There was no edema, cyanosis or clubbing. His breath sound was vesicular with prolonged expiration. Inspiratory fine crackles were heard in both mid and lower zones. Pleural rub was present in left mid-zone. On abdominal examination, mild tenderness was found in both loin area, but there was no palpable mass or organomegaly. All other systemic examinations revealed no abnormality.

Initial investigations revealed a marked inflammatory picture: erythrocyte sedimentation rate (ESR) was elevated at 83 mm/hr, C-reactive protein (CRP) was positive (60 mg/L). Urinalysis revealed trace protein, but numerous red blood cells per high power field. Serum creatinine was normal. X-ray paranasal sinus occipitomental (PNS OM) view revealed maxillary sinusitis. Posteroanterior (PA) view of chest X-ray showed features of bilateral pneumonitis. CT scan of chest revealed multiple nodules in both lungs in middle and lower zone. No abnormality was found in ultrasonography of whole abdomen. Antinuclear antibodies (ANA) were negative.

QUESTIONS

1. What investigations should be done?
2. What is the most likely diagnosis?
3. What are the management options?

DISCUSSION

The clue was involvement of both upper and lower respiratory tract along with renal involvement.

Due to the clinical presentation of multi-organ involvement, and presence of raised ESR and CRP, our initial diagnosis was primary vasculitis. Computed tomography (CT) chest revealed bizarre multiple nodules in both lungs, so our strong suspicion was granulomatosis with polyangiitis (GPA). We did some investigations which revealed:

- Cytoplasmic antineutrophil cytoplasmic antibodies (C-ANCA)[antibodies against proteinase-3 (PR3)] were positive
- Perinuclear antineutrophil cytoplasmic antibodies (P-ANCA) (specific for myeloperoxidase) were negative.

We planned for renal biopsy but unfortunately patient did not give consent.

Final Diagnosis: Granulomatosis with Polyangiitis

Granulomatosis with polyangitis is a small to medium sized vessel vasculitis.[1] It involves upper and lower respiratory tract and kidneys predominantly with granulomatous inflammation (necrotizing). Multiorgan involvement is possible.[2,3] It is also known as an autoimmune disease because of an association with ANCA against PR3 (C-ANCA).[3]

Usual findings are:

- Nose: runny nose, stuffy nose, bleeding from nose, crusting, nose deformity (saddle nose)
- Sinuses: sinusitis[4,5]
- Nodules and infiltrations in lungs (radiologically) and pulmonary hemorrhage in the form of hemoptysis
- Renal involvement in the form of glomerulonephritis
- Ocular involvement is also possible.[6]

Treatment options are, in nonsevere cases: glucocorticoid with, methotrexate. For more severe disease: glucocorticoid with cyclophosphamide or rituximab. Cyclophosphamide for 3-6 months, then switch to azathioprine or methotrexate to maintain remission.[7]

REFERENCES

1. Cavoli GL, Ferrantelli A, Bono L, et al. Kidney involvement in a Wegener granulomatosis case. Indian J Med Sci. 2012;66(9-10):238-40.

2. Heitkötter B, Kuhnen C, Schmidt S, et al. Granulomatosis with polyangiitis (Wegener's granulomatosis): a rare variant of sudden natural death. Int J Legal Med. 2018;132:243.
3. Takeuchi H, Kuroda I, Takizawa I, et al. Granulomatosis with polyangiitis (Wegener's granulomatosis) accompanied by dysuria. Case Rep Urol. 2016;2016:7812875.
4. Millet A, Pederzoli-Ribeil M, Guillevin L, et al. Antineutrophil cytoplasmic antibody-associated vasculitides: is it time to split up the group? Ann Rheum Dis. 2013;72(8):1273-9.
5. Kuan EC, Suh JD. Systemic and odontogenic etiologies in chronic rhinosinusitis. Otolaryngol Clin North Am. 2017;50(1):95-111.
6. Kubaisi B, Abu Samra K, Foster CS. Granulomatosis with polyangiitis (Wegener's disease): an updated review of ocular disease manifestations. Intractable Rare Dis Res. 2016;5(2):61-9.
7. Langford CA. Update on the treatment of granulomatosis with polyangiitis (Wegener's). Curr Treat Options Cardiovasc Med. 2012;14(2):164-76.

CASE 60

MEAT-LOVING YOUNG WOMAN WITH ABNORMAL STOOL

CASE SUMMARY

A 27-year-old woman presented with recurrent episodes of frequent passage of soft stool along with passage of worm-like whitish material during defecation for 3 years. It was associated with mild abdominal discomfort. On one occasion while defecation, she noticed passage of very large similar worm-like material through anus not mixed with stool. Later on, she experienced it multiple times while doing household works. Sometimes, she discovered moving segments on her clothing. Sometimes, she had to pull out the segment manually from anus (Fig. 1). The largest one was measuring about 1.5 cm. Afterward, the passage of segment was associated with mild cramping abdominal pain around umbilicus and perianal itching compelling here to go toilet. She used to take antihelminthics (albendazol and mebendazole) by herself with little relief, and similar symptoms recurred every 2–3 months. It became troublesome enough to hamper her daily activities. She did not give any significant negative history on systemic query. She never had acute attack of gastroenteritis during her period of illness for the last 3 years. She used to take different types of beef items very frequently, mainly kebab, chap, etc. from nearby restaurants as well as from the streets. On several occasions, she ate meat of lamb, camel, koyel and even pigeon. She denied eating any pork items because of religious purpose. She had no significant history of travel to area of diarrheal epidemics within or outside the country. She went to Saudi Arabia twice in 2007 (remained there for 1 month) and 2015 (stayed for 1.5 months). No family member had similar symptoms. She belonged to a decent family of upper class. Socioeconomic and sociobehavioral backgrounds were standard.

On examination, all findings were unremarkable except mild abdominal tenderness around umbilicus.

Investigation showed Hb%—13.10 g/dL, white blood cells (WBCs)—8,160/mm^3 (N: 55%, L: 40%, E: 2%), platelet (PLT) count—285,000/mm^3,

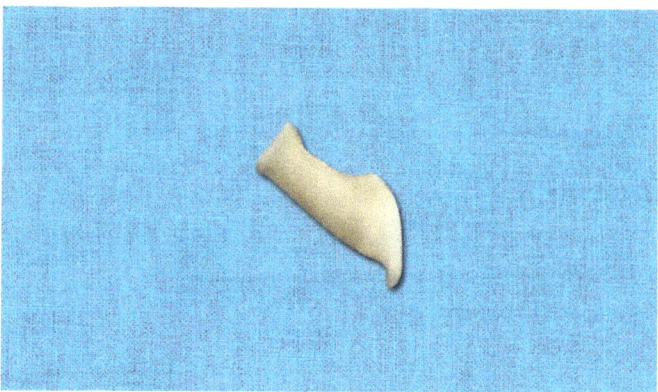

Fig. 1: Per anal discharge of whitish segments.

erythrocyte sedimentation rate (ESR) in the first hour—7 mm, circulating total eosinophil—160/mm^3, total immunoglobulin E (IgE)—82.08 IU/mL (reference: in adults <100), ultrasonography (USG) of whole abdomen—normal, X-ray of whole abdomen—normal.

QUESTIONS

1. What is the diagnosis?
2. How would you confirm this?
3. How will you treat the case?

DISCUSSION

The description and the stool findings of whitish segments are consistent with cestode infection (Fig. 1). Being a meat lover, she used to take uncooked meats (kebab especially) which may be responsible for her diagnosis of *intestinal taeniasis*. The differentials were:
- *Taenia saginata*
- *Taenia saginata asiatica*
- *Taenia solium.*

Subsequent investigations were done in this case:
Stool examination: It revealed presence of egg of *Taenia*. Fecal egg count showed presence of *Taenia* in moderate amount. Suspected parasite segment identification from stool revealed *T. saginata*.

Final Diagnosis: Intestinal Taeniasis due to *Taenia saginata*

Niclosamide tablet 2 g single dose was given. She was discharged with advice to maintain regular follow-up.

Taenia saginata (also called *Taenia rhynchus saginata*) is a beef tapeworm. It is found globally and most prevalently where cattle are raised and beef is consumed. It is relatively common in Africa, Europe, Southeast Asia, South Asia and Latin America.[1]

Taenia saginata infection is usually asymptomatic. The proglottids are motile and pass in the feces. Patients may have perianal discomfort during passage of proglottid. Abdominal pain or discomfort, nausea, appetite change and fatigue may occur. Heavy infection often results in weight loss, dizziness, abdominal pain, diarrhea, headaches, nausea, constipation, chronic indigestion and loss of appetite. Intestinal obstruction in humans can be alleviated by surgery. The tapeworm can also expel antigens that can cause an allergic reaction in the individual.[2] It is also a rare cause of pancreatitis, cholecystitis and cholangitis.[3] A fecal examination is helpful to find out parasite eggs. The eggs identify the family, not the species as different tainidae have similar eggs. Since it is difficult to diagnose using eggs alone, looking at the scolex or the gravid proglottids can help identify it as *T. saginata*.[4] Available serologic tests cannot provide any diagnostic clue. Eosinophilia and high levels of serum IgE may be found.

Taeniasis is easily treated with praziquantel (5-10 mg/kg, single-administration) or niclosamide (adults and children over 6 years: 2 g, single-administration after a light breakfast, followed by laxative after two hours.[2]

After either drugs, the proximal part of the worm disintegrates in the gut and the scolex cannot be found. Failure of proglottids to reappear within 3-4 months indicates cure.[5]

Adequate cooking (56°C for 5 minutes) of beef viscera destroys cerci. Refrigeration, freezing (-10°C for 9 days) or long periods of salting is lethal to cerci. Inspection of beef and proper disposal of human excreta are also important measures.[2]

REFERENCES

1. Eckert J. Helminths. In: Kayser FH, Bienz KA, Eckert J, Zinkernagel RM, editors. Medical Microbiology. Stuttgart: Thieme; 2005. pp. 560-2.
2. Taeniasis/Cysticercosis [online]. WHO Fact Sheet N°376. World Health Organization; 2013. [cited 2014 Feb 7].
3. Uygur-Bayramiçli O, Ak O, Dabak R, Demirhan G, Ozer S. *Taenia saginata* a rare cause of acute cholangitis: a case report. Acta Clin Belg. 2012;67(6):436-7.
4. Larry Roberts S, John Janovy Jr. Gerald D. Schmidt & Larry S. Roberts' Foundations of Parasitology. 8th ed. Boston (MA): McGraw-Hill; 2009.
5. Harrison LJ. Differential diagnosis of *Taenia saginata* and *Taenia solium* with DNA probes. Parasitology. 1990;100:459-61.

CASE 61

MIDDLE-AGED LADY WITH HEADACHE AND FACIAL NERVE PALSY

CASE SUMMARY

A 63-year-old woman, housewife, presented with a 4 months history of headache, which was throbbing in nature and severe enough to interfere with daily activities. It was initially located at the left side of the head involving left temporal region. She also complained progressive deafness on her left ear associated with intense ear pain, tinnitus and vertigo. It was not preceded by any aura and also not associated with any fever, eye pain, blurring of vision or vomiting. After several days, she noticed deviation of mouth on right side and her voice became hoarse. She also experienced difficulty in swallowing, which was painless, more marked for liquid, associated with nasal regurgitation and cough during deglutition.

On examination, she was ill-looking. Vital signs were within normal limit. Neurologic examination revealed left-sided facial (VII) nerve palsy which was lower motor neuron type. There was sensory neural deafness on her left ear evident by Rinne and Weber test. Both sensory and motor functions of trigeminal nerve were impaired on left side. IX, X, XII cranial nerve functions were impaired on left side. Fundoscopic examination revealed no abnormality. The remainder of the examination was normal.

All routine investigations including complete blood count report was normal except erythrocyte sedimentation rate (ESR), which was 38 mm in 1 hour. Chest X-ray, ultrasonography (USG) of whole abdomen reports were normal. Magnetic resonance imaging (MRI) of brain was also normal. Pure tone audiometry revealed left-sided sensory neural type of moderate hearing loss. Cerebrospinal fluid analysis (CSF) study report was normal. Vasculitis marker, both perinuclear anti-neutrophil cytoplasmic antibodies (P-ANCA) and cytoplasmic antineutrophil cytoplasmic antibodies (C-ANCA) were negative. Serum electrolytes, serum calcium, serum albumin, and angiotensin-converting enzyme (ACE) levels were normal.

QUESTIONS

1. What further history is pertinent in this case?
2. What further investigation should be done?
3. What is the most likely diagnosis?
4. What is the prognosis of this type of case?

DISCUSSION

As initial pattern of history revealed multiple cranial nerve palsies, but the locations of cranial nerves were highly diverse, so the differential diagnoses were primary central nervous system (CNS) vasculitis and neurosarcoidosis. All these differentials were excluded after investigation. Finally, after taking detailed history, we found that the patient developed this condition followed by an episode of vesicles around her left ear.

In our case, Varicella Zoster Virus IgG was positive. So, our diagnosis was Ramsay Hunt syndrome.

Final Diagnosis: Ramsay Hunt Syndrome

Ramsay hunt syndrome is a rare disease, occurs as a result of reactivation of varicella zoster virus usually in the VII cranial nerve. VIII cranial nerve involvement is also commonly reported. This disease usually presents with peripheral facial nerve palsy along with erythematous vesicular rash around the ear or mouth. Intense severe ear pain with tinnitus, vertigo, hearing loss, nausea, vomiting, nystagmus and rarely headache are recognized frequent symptoms. Typically rash and facial nerve palsy occur simultaneously, but rarely, facial nerve palsy can occur after rash or even without any history of rash.[1,2]

In some cases, multiple cranial nerve palsies (V, VII, VIII, IX, and X, XI, XII) have been reported.[3]

In our case, the presentation was atypical because multiple cranial nerve palsy occurred after several days of vesicular rash.

Diagnosis is mainly clinical by taking detailed history and identification of characteristic symptoms. *Varicella zoster* virus in vesicle fluid, saliva, middle ear fluid can support the diagnosis but not always necessary to establish the diagnosis. MRI and CSF study can be done to exclude other diseases.

Antiviral acyclovir and corticosteroid prednisolone are currently used and many studies showed treatment started earlier (within 72 hours) has better prognosis, whereas delayed treatment may cause incomplete recovery. So, it is important to suspect the symptoms promptly and atypical symptoms should be reported, so that physicians can be informed about the unusual symptoms.[4]

REFERENCES

1. Lustig LR, Smith HW. Herpes zoster oticus. Merck Manual Professional Version. [online]. Available from http://www.merckmanuals.com/professional/ear,-nose,-and-throat-disorders/inner-ear-disorders/herpes-zoster-oticus. [Accessed July 2016].
2. Sweeney CJ, Gilden DH. Ramsay Hunt syndrome. J Neurol Neurosurg Psychiatry. 2001;71:149-54.
3. Arya D, Bajaj T, Gonzalez J, et al. Ramsay Hunt syndrome with multiple cranial neuropathy in an human immunodeficiency virus (HIV) patient. Am J Case Rep. 2018;19:68-71.
4. Murakami S, Hato N, Horiuchi J, et al. Treatment of Ramsay Hunt syndrome with acyclovir-prednisone: significance of early diagnosis and treatment. Ann Neurol. 1997;41(3):353-7.

CASE 62

YOUNG HOUSEWIFE WITH PROLONGED FEVER AND JAUNDICE

CASE SUMMARY

A 25-year-old housewife hailing from Rajshahi (northern part of Bangladesh) presented with fever for the last 7 months. Fever was low to moderate grade, persisted most of the time and did not completely subside during first 3 months of illness. In later months, it subsided completely with sweating after taking antipyretic drugs. Maximum recorded temperature was 103°F. Fever was accompanied by loss of appetite and early satiety. For the last 3 months she experienced unintentional weight loss of 6 kg and developed yellowish coloration of eyes and urine, which was not associated with itching or color change of stool but accompanied with generalized weakness.

Examination revealed her to be a malnourished with moderate anemia and jaundice, liver was 4 cm from right costal margin in midclavicular line (MCL), smooth, nontender; spleen was 3 cm from left costal margin along its long axis.

Lab investigations confirmed anemia, leukopenia, thrombocytopenia, high erythrocyte sedimentation rate (ESR) (70 mm first hour). Mean corpuscular volume (MCV) was high (102 fl), serum bilirubin was high 9.3 mg/dL with indirect bilirubin 6.31 mg/dL. Reticulocyte count—4%, alanine aminotransferase (ALT)—171 U/L, Mantoux test (MT)—negative. Lactate dehydrogenase (LDH)—309 U/L, ultrasonography (USG) showed hepatosplenomegaly.

QUESTIONS

1. What are the differentials to be considered in this case?
2. What should be the next diagnostic workup?

DISCUSSION

At this point differentials of hemolytic anemia, disseminated tuberculosis, and visceral leishmaniasis (kala-azar) were considered. In this case, the patient was residing in kala-azar endemic area so we did rk39 test which came out reactive. Bone marrow examination also confirmed presence of intracellular *Leishmania donovani* (LD) bodies. To identify the nature of hemolysis, we performed direct Coombs test, which was also positive. Final diagnosis was labeled as visceral leishmaniasis with autoimmune hemolytic anemia. Patient was treated with liposomal amphotericin B which resolved all her problems.

Final Diagnosis: Visceral Leishmaniasis with Autoimmune Hemolytic Anemia

Visceral leishmaniasis (VL) (kala-azar) is an infectious disease which is caused by Leishmania Donovani (LD) complex. It is endemic in Bangladesh, India, South part of Europe, North Africa, Middle East, and South America.

Several hematological changes can be found in kala-azar. Most commonly anemia, associated with leukopenia, thrombocytopenia, almost complete absence of eosinophils, pancytopenia and intravascular coagulation.[1] Various causes are responsible for anemia, like sequestration and destruction of red cell in enlarged spleen, immune mediated mechanism and alteration in RBC membrane permeability. Hemolysis is a major cause of anemia, with plasma volume expansion associated with massively enlarged spleen.[2]

Autoimmune hemolytic anemia (AIHA) has been reported in few case reports of kala-azar previously.[1,3]

REFERENCES

1. Varma N, Naseem S. Hematological changes in visceral leishmaniasis/kala-azar. Indian J Hematol Blood Transfus. 2010;3:78–82.
2. Safi AES, Adm ASK, Hamza KM. Hematological Profile of Patients with Visceral Leishmaniasis at Al-Gaderf State - Sudan. J Clin Med. 2016;2(3):31–9. http://www.aiscience.org/journal/cmj ISSN: 2381-7631 (Print); ISSN: 2381-764X (Online)
3. Kabir A, Das A, Islam MS, Masud MS, Cader FA, Jahan S. Autoimmune haemolysis in visceral leishmaniasis: A Case Report & Review of Literature. Med J. 2014;14(2):198–200. https://doi.org/10.3329/jom.v14i2.19686

CASE 63

FEBRILE YOUNG GIRL WITH HEMIPARESIS FOLLOWED BY NECK SWELLING

CASE SUMMARY

A 19-year-old girl presented with a 3 days' high-grade continued fever with chills and rigor with preceding history of low-grade irregular fever and arthralgia involving large joints for the last 3 months. She was having skin rash, subconjunctival hemorrhage and episodes of spontaneous nasal as well as per vaginal bleeding for the last 3 days. Two days later, she developed sudden severe headache, alteration of consciousness followed by right-sided weakness. She had no history of trauma, convulsion, abdominal pain, alteration of bowel habit, alopecia, oral ulcer, photosensitivity, yellowish discoloration of sclera or urine, previous bleeding manifestations, contact with tuberculosis patients, travel to hill tracts or any history of unprotected sexual exposure.

Physical examination revealed toxic appearance with disorientation, Glasgow Coma Scale (GCS) score of 13/15 (E4M5V4), moderate anemia, bilateral posterior cervical and left supraclavicular tender lymphadenopathy, impalpable, nontender, pleomorphic purpura over right upper chest and right leg and ecchymoses over right elbow. Her pulse was 90/min, regular; blood pressure (BP) was 100/60 mm Hg; temperature was 102°F, and there were bilateral papilledema and retinal hemorrhage in left eye, right-sided upper motor neuron (UMN) type of hemiparesis, without signs of meningeal irritation. She had tender hepatomegaly about 4 cm from right costal margin, but no splenomegaly, no painful joint swelling, and no murmur was heard.

Investigation showed that hemoglobin (Hb) level was variable, but low. Erythrocyte sedimentation rate (ESR) was high (110 mm in 1st hour) and peripheral blood film (PBF) showed bicytopenia with few atypical-looking mononuclear cells. Reticulocyte count was 5%. The bleeding time and clotting time were normal. Bone marrow study showed hyperactive marrow and increased cellularity in all three cell lines. Liver function test revealed alanine aminotransferase (ALT) was 40 U/L, lactate dehydrogenase (LDH) was 296 U/L, C-reactive protein (CRP) was 4.02 mg/L (risk high > 3 mg/dL), and serum creatinine and electrolytes were normal. Mantoux test was negative and immunochromatographic test (ICT) for malaria and kala-azar was also negative. Triple antigen was nonsignificant. Antinuclear antibody (ANA), anti-double stranded deoxyribonucleic acid (anti-dsDNA) and anti-phospholipid antibodies all were negative. Urine routine examination showed trace albumin and red blood cells (RBCs) 15–20/HPF, and urine culture showed *Escherichia coli* (10^7 CFU/mL), though blood culture was negative. Chest X-ray finding was normal.

QUESTIONS

1. What differential diagnoses should be considered for this case?
2. What further investigations are needed to reach the final diagnosis?
3. What should be the management plan?

DISCUSSION

At this stage, our provisional diagnosis was sepsis [source: urinary tract infection (UTI)] with stroke with right-sided hemiparesis. But a young female with high-grade fever, bleeding episodes and having neurological manifestations led us to think of other possibilities like thrombotic thrombocytopenic purpura (TTP), acute leukemia with stroke with right-sided hemiparesis, systemic lupus erythematosus with vasculitis and tuberculosis with tuberculoma in brain, lymphoma, etc.

As she was having right-sided hemiparesis, we did computed tomography (CT) scan of the head, which showed large intracerebral hematoma occupying left parietal region. Ultrasonography (USG) of the whole abdomen showed mild hepatomegaly. Coagulation profile showed: prothrombin time (PT)—12 seconds, activated partial thromboplastin time (APTT)—30 seconds, fibrinogen degradation product (FDP)—10 µg/dL (normal <5 µg/dL), D-dimer—1.34 mg/IFEU (normal <0.55 mg/IFEU).

On admission, the girl was very much toxic, disoriented and anemic as well. Initially, she was resuscitated by intravenous (IV) fluid, IV hydrocortisone, IV ceftriaxone and antipyretics. After getting the reports of urine culture IV pivmecillinam was added. In the meantime, she was given four units of fresh frozen plasma (FFP) and two units of fresh whole blood.

Seven days after admission, we examined the girl again and found gradual improvement of her general condition. Fever was on remission. Skin rashes got faded, no further bleeding was seen but her lymph nodes were increasing in size.

Then follow-up investigation showed Hb level variable from low to normal, ESR was 50 mm in 1st hour, platelet count was better. PBF showed normocytic anemia and mild thrombocytopenia, urine routine examination was normal. PT, APTT and D-dimer were also normal. USG of whole abdomen showed mild hepatomegaly with normal-sized spleen (8.6 cm).

This young girl had all the features of sepsis and responded very well to antibiotics and supportive treatment; except her cervical lymph nodes were gradually increasing in size. As follow-up peripheral blood film was inconclusive, we planned for lymph node biopsy (right supraclavicular node). After biopsy, microscopic section showed caseation necrosis and granulomatous inflammation suggestive of tuberculosis.

Final Diagnosis: **Tuberculous Lymphadenitis with Acute Intracerebral Hemorrhage with Right-sided Hemiparesis due to Disseminated Intravascular Coagulation (DIC) due to Urosepsis**

Tuberculous lymphadenitis (or tuberculous adenitis) is one of the most common forms of tuberculosis infections that appears outside the lungs. Tuberculous lymphadenitis is a chronic, specific granulomatous inflammation of the lymph node with caseation necrosis, caused by infection with *Mycobacterium tuberculosis* or related bacteria.

Stages of tubercular lymphadenitis:
- Lymphadenitis
- Periadenitis
- Cold abscess
- 'Collar stud' abscess
- Sinus.

Tuberculous lymphadenitis is popularly known as collar stud abscess, due to its proximity to the collar bone and its superficial resemblance to a collar stud, although this is just one of the five stages of the disease. One or more affected lymph nodes can also be in a different body parts, although it is most typical to have at least one near the collar bone.[1]

The diagnosis of tuberculous lymphadenitis requires a biopsy. Other possible diagnostic steps include: positive tuberclin test, chest radiograph, CT scan, cytology/biopsy (FNAC), AFB staining, and mycobacterial culture.

Sometimes the diagnosis may not be straightforward like in our case where there was no typical systemic symptoms of tuberculosis; rather patient presented with sepsis and after improvement showed gradual enlargement of lymph nodes. Thus, tuberculosis is an imperative clinical subsistence which should be kept in mind, especially in developing countries.[2]

Incision drainage with proper evacuation of the fluid followed by antitubercular medication is the mainstay of treatment. Treatment with antitubercular medication normally lasts for six months to one year. Symptoms may temporarily get worse during the treatment.[3]

REFERENCES

1. William CC. International Encyclopedia of Public Health. Academic Press; 2016.p. 274.
2. Hegde S, Rithesh KB, Baroudi K, Umar D. Tuberculous lymphadenitis: early diagnosis and intervention. Jour Int Oral Health. 2014;6(6):96-8.
3. Bhat SR. SRB's Manual of Surgery. 5th ed. JP Medical Pub.; 2016. pp. 55-6.

CASE 64

YOUNG MAN WITH CHRONIC DIARRHEA

CASE SUMMARY

A 25-year-old man, autodriver by profession, presented with recurrent episodes of passage of loose stools for the past 5 years. The frequency of loose motion varied from 4 to 8 times per day, and the stool was bulky, greasy, pale in color, offensive and not mixed with blood. He also complained of generalized weakness and loss of significant weight during this time. According to his mother, he had similar episode of diarrhea at his 6 months of age which required hospitalization but the condition was not cured. About a year ago, he again got admitted into a tertiary care hospital with loose motion and low-grade fever and after performing many investigations, he was diagnosed as a case of chronic hepatitis B virus infection with suspected intestinal tuberculosis. During his stay in the hospital, he received multiple units of whole blood transfusions and was given Category-1 anti-TB treatment. After completion of the treatment, though frequency gradually decreased, his diarrhea persisted. Throughout his illness, he denied any history of jaundice, cough, chest pain, joint pain, red eye, oral ulcer, hematemesis or abdominal pain. The patient was a nonsmoker, nonalcoholic and never used any intravenous (IV) recreational drug. No similar illness among family members, no contact with TB patient and no history of unsafe sexual exposure.

On examination, the patient was ill-looking, emaciated, moderately anemic, and had sparse facial and body hair. The tongue was smooth and furrowed; and angular stomatitis, leukonychia and dehydration were present. Pulse—104/min; blood pressure (BP)—110/60 mm Hg; temperature—normal. Examination of the abdomen revealed no abnormality except excessive bowel sound. The remainder of the examination was normal.

Investigations showed hemoglobin (Hb): 6.2 g/dL, white blood cells (WBCs)—5,000/cumm (DC: N—81%, L—15%), platelet—100,000/cumm, erythrocyte sedimentation rate (ESR)—80 mm in the first hour. The mean corpuscular volume (MCV)—101 fL and peripheral blood film (PBF)—pancytopenia with fair number of hypersegmented neutrophils. Chest X-ray (CXR), urine R/E, serum creatinine and serum electrolytes were normal. The liver function test was normal except serum albumin—27 g/L and prothrombin time (PT)—26.6 seconds. Hepatitis B surface antigen (HBsAg) and hepatitis B e-antigen (HBeAg) were positive, anti-hepatitis B core antibody (HBcAb) and anti-hepatitis B e-antibody (HBeAb) were negative, hepatitis B virus (HBV) deoxyribonucleic acid (DNA)—1.2×10^4 IU/mL. Ultrasonography (USG) of W/A and computed tomography (CT) scan of abdomen showed gas distended bowel loops, otherwise normal study. Thyroid profile was normal, MT and HIV-1 and 2 were negative.

QUESTIONS

1. What are the three most likely diagnoses?
2. What investigations should be performed next?

DISCUSSION

The history of this young male patient was clearly suggestive of malabsorption syndrome. The underlying cause might have been intestinal TB, though he received Cat-I anti-TB treatment without any significant improvement. Celiac disease was an important consideration here, as the patient had the history of diarrhea just after weaning at his 6 months of age. Inflammatory bowel disease was another possibility though there was no history of joint pain, oral ulcer or any eye problem. No risky sexual behavior and negative human immunodeficiency virus (HIV) 1 and 2 also excluded the possibility of HIV infection.

The following investigations were done next:
- Fecal fat estimation: 10-20 droplets/hpf
- Serum folate assay: 1.1 ng/mL (reference value: 2.7-16.1 ng/mL)
- Serum vitamin B12 assay: 137.0 pg/mL (reference value: 239-931 pg/mL)
- Barium meal follow through: Normal study
- Colonoscopy: Normal
- Endoscopy of upper gastrointestinal tract (GIT): Possible villous atrophy of duodenal mucosa
- Histopathology of distal duodenal biopsy: Short and broad villi, moderate crypt hyperplasia. Increased intra-epithelial lymphocytes (30-100). Moderate number of lymphocytes in lamina propria.
- Tissue transglutaminase (tTG) immunoglobulin A (IgA): 145 U/mL (reference value: up to 50 U/mL).

Final Diagnosis: Malabsorption Syndrome due to Celiac Disease with Chronic Hepatitis B Virus Infection

Celiac disease, also known as celiac sprue or gluten-sensitive enteropathy, is a chronic disorder of the digestive tract that results in an inability to tolerate gliadin, the alcohol-soluble fraction of gluten. Gluten is a protein commonly found in wheat, rye and barley.[1]

When patients with celiac disease ingest gliadin, an immunologically mediated inflammatory response occurs which damages the mucosa of their intestines, resulting in maldigestion and malabsorption of food nutrients.[1]

The American College of Gastroenterology (ACG) recommends that antibody testing, especially IgA anti-tissue transglutaminase antibody (IgA tTG), is the best first test for suspected celiac disease, although biopsies are needed for confirmation.[2]

Other laboratory tests include the following:
- Electrolytes and chemistries—electrolyte imbalances; evidence of malnutrition
- Hematologic tests—anemia, low serum iron level, prolonged PT
- Stool examination—fat malabsorption
- Oral tolerance tests—lactose intolerance
- Serology—IgA antibodies.

Patients diagnosed with celiac disease should be examined for deficiencies, including low bone density.

The primary treatment of celiac disease is dietary. Removal of gluten from the diet is essential. A small percentage of patients with celiac disease fail to respond to a gluten-free diet. In those refractory cases, corticosteroids may be helpful.[3]

REFERENCES

1. Jameson JL, Kasper DL, Longo DL, Fauci AS, Hauser SL, Loscalzo J. Harrison's Principles of Internal Medicine. 20th ed. New York: McGraw Hill Education; 2018. pp. 2251-2.
2. Rubio-Tapia A, Hill ID, Kelly CP, Calderwood AH, Murray JA. ACG clinical guidelines: diagnosis and management of celiac disease. Am J Gastroenterol. 2013;108(5):656-76; quiz 677.
3. Woodward J. The management of refractory coeliac disease. Ther Adv Chronic Dis. 2013;4(2):77-90.

CASE 65

YOUNG MAN WITH SEVERE ANEMIA AND GENERALIZED EDEMA

CASE SUMMARY

A 38-year-old man presented with generalized weakness and significant weight loss followed by generalized swelling of the body for the past 3 months. His weakness gradually progressed to such extent that he developed difficulty to perform daily activities and it was associated with palpitation, dizziness and light-headedness. The patient became anorexic and lost one-third of his body weight within the last 3 months. He had generalized swelling for the past 22 days, starting with periorbital edema, followed by ascites and dependent edema. On query, he gave history of jaundice 2 months back, for which he took homeopathic medications and jaundice disappeared gradually. With these complaints, he got admitted at a local hospital, where he was found severely anemic and received 4 units of blood transfusion in 4 consecutive days, after which he was referred to Dhaka Medical College and Hospital (DMCH) as a case of anemia under evaluation. He denied any history of fever, cough, chest pain, itching, pale-colored stool, bleeding from any site, abnormal sleep pattern, skin rash, arthralgia, oliguria or hematuria, paresthesia, dysphagia, pigmentation, altered consciousness, convulsion or Raynaud's phenomenon. On the third day of hospital stay, the patient developed dry cough associated with sharp pain in the right lower chest. There was no paroxysmal nocturnal dyspnea or orthopnea. He had pulmonary tuberculosis 20 years back without any documentation.

On general examination, the patient was severely anemic and dyspneic with body mass index (BMI) 18.1 kg/m^2 with dependent edema. Pulse—120 beats/min, blood pressure (BP)—130/80 mm Hg, temperature—normal and respiratory rate—24 breaths/min. A bedside urine examination was normal. Abdomen and chest examinations revealed ascites and pleural effusion in right lower chest. Other systemic examination findings were normal.

Investigation showed that hemoglobin (Hb) level was 4.42 g/dL. Mean corpuscular volume (MCV) was 150.64 fl and erythrocyte sedimentation rate (ESR) was 80 mm in first hour and reticulocyte count was 31.46%. Renal function tests, serum electrolytes, and X-ray chest were normal. Electrocardiography (ECG) revealed borderline low-voltage tracing with sinus tachycardia. Echocardiography showed good left ventricular (LV) systolic dysfunction, ejection fraction (EF) 73%, and mild pericardial effusion (6 mm, posteriorly). Mantoux test (MT) was negative. Liver function test showed that serum bilirubin was 1 mg/dL, prothrombin time (PT) was 14 seconds and serum albumin was 1.5 g/dL. Random blood sugar (RBS) was 5.6 mmol/L and thyroid-stimulating hormone (TSH) was 1.64 IU/mL. Ultrasonography (USG) of the whole abdomen showed moderate ascites and right-sided mild pleural effusion. Stool occult blood test (OBT) was negative and upper gastrointestinal (GI) endoscopy revealed normal study. All the viral markers including human immunodeficiency virus (HIV) 1 and 2 were negative. Ascitic fluid study showed low albumin level and serum ascites albumin gradient (SAAG) was 0.84 g/dL. Serum vitamin B12 level was normal (376 pg/mL). Peripheral blood film (PBF) was suggestive of immune hemolytic anemia. Direct Coombs' test was positive and lactate dehydrogenase (LDH) level was 1,724 U/L. Then, antinuclear antibody (ANA) was done and it was found positive and anti-ds DNA was also positive.

QUESTIONS

1. What is the most likely diagnosis?
2. How should the patient be managed?

DISCUSSION

In our case, considering the history and physical findings, our provisional diagnosis was anemic heart failure as the patient was severely anemic and was in distress, had leg edema and features of pleural effusion. But normal jugular venous pulsation and absence of enlarged tender liver made the explanation of heart failure difficult. Our other differentials were decompensated chronic liver disease, intra-abdominal malignancy with metastasis, disseminated tuberculosis, nephrotic syndrome, connective tissue disease, etc. Absence of fever, lymphadenopathy, organomegaly, and no stigmata of chronic liver disease and normal urinary findings made those diagnoses unlikely. Then, we searched for the cause of anemia. Low Hb level, high reticulocyte count, high LDH level and positive Coombs' test led us to think of autoimmune hemolysis as the underlying cause of anemia. So, considering the simultaneous existence of autoimmune hemolytic anemia, polyserositis, positive ANA and positive anti-dsDNA, we connected the dots and reached the diagnosis of systemic lupus erythematosus (SLE).

Final Diagnosis: Systemic Lupus Erythematosus

Though our patient did not have the classical presentation of SLE, our focused investigations resulted in prompt diagnosis. He was treated with methylprednisolone and azathioprine, along with symptomatic management. We discharged him after resolution of polyserositis, with improving other symptoms.

The SLE has traditionally been considered a disease of women, yet, men may also be affected. Normal sex ratio is female: male = 9:1. However, male SLE patients often have more severe disease than females. Gender disparities have been reported in clinical manifestations and in serological and hematological indices as well.[1,2] Some reports suggest- men with lupus have a higher frequency of involvement of the lining of the lung and the heart—so called serositis.[2,3]

Worldwide, male patients of SLE presenting with an atypical phenotype face a delay in diagnosis, and hence, treatment as early symptoms of lupus are very nonspecific. The consequence is a greater burden of inflammation and subsequent damage over time. Once the diagnosis is established there are no major differences in antibody profiles or response to treatment.[2]

REFERENCES

1. Font J, Cervera R, Melvin N, et al. Systemic lupus erythematosus in men: clinical and immunological characteristics. Ann Rheumatic Diseases. 1992;51:1050-2.
2. Guy's and St Thomas' Charity 2019, Lupus Trust, London, UK [Internet]. Lupus in men. Available from https://www.lupus.org.uk/lupus-in-men.
3. Murphy G, Isenberg D. Effect of gender on clinical presentation in systemic lupus erythematosus. Rheumatology (Oxford). 2013;52(12):2108-15. Available from: https://doi.org/10.1093/rheumatology/ket160.

CASE 66

YOUNG FEMALE WITH ACUTE ABDOMINAL PAIN AND FEVER

CASE SUMMARY

A 20-year-old unmarried young lady presented to us with acute abdominal pain followed by several episodes of vomiting. Approximately about 2 week before admission initially she experienced mild, constant, dull aching lower abdominal pain. After about a week, the pain became generalized and more severe in right upper quadrant of abdomen which was aggravated during breathing and compelled her to visit the hospital. She also complained of fever with chills and rigor for last 4 days and highest recorded temperature was 104°F.

On examination, patient was severely anemic. All the vital signs were within normal limit except her body temperature was 101°F. Right upper quadrant of abdomen was tender. No organomegaly was found clinically. Ascites was evident by shifting dullness. All other systemic examinations revealed no abnormality.

Investigations showed her hemoglobin (Hb) was 5.1 g/dL and WBC count was elevated (17,000/mm^3) where neutrophil count was 82% and erythrocyte sedimentation rate (ESR) was 55 mm in 1 hour, and peripheral blood film was normal. Urinalysis was normal. Hepatic enzyme levels were not elevated. Fibrin degradation product (FDP) and D-dimer levels were within reference range. Blood and urine cultures yielded no growth. Ultrasonography (USG) of whole abdomen revealed bilateral prominent ovaries, moderate pelvic collection and mild ascites in lower abdomen and mild parenchymal enhancement of liver.

QUESTIONS

1. What next history is pertinent in this case?
2. What is the most likely diagnosis?
3. Name two common organisms that can cause this type of condition.

DISCUSSION

On detailed history taking, with proper privacy and after building a faithful relationship, the patient confessed that she had been sexually active for last 1 year. One month back she had a history of menstrual regulation (MR) with significant blood loss. She also admitted having foul smelling vaginal discharge for last 2 weeks, with recent increase in amount of discharge.

Along with history of MR, the pattern of abdominal pain initially at pelvic area followed by generalized pain and pelvic collection can be explained by pelvic inflammatory disease (PID) followed by peritonitis. So, to identify the cause of PID, Gram stain and culture of endocervical swab was sent and came out negative for *Gonococcus*.

More marked pain in right upper quadrant and parenchymal enhancement of liver with ascites with features of PID without evidence of sepsis in a woman of child bearing age ultimately lead us to diagnosis of Fitz-Hugh-Curtis syndrome (FHCS).

Most cases of PID and FHCS are caused by *Chlamydia trachomatis* and *Neisseria gonorrhoeae*. So, serological tests were done. Enzyme immunosorbent assay for *Chlamydia* was positive; and venereal disease research laboratory (VDRL), and *Treponema pallidum* hemagglutination assay (TPHA) were non-reactive. Laparoscopy is the gold standard imaging technique for better delineation of perihepatitis, but was not employed as ultrasonography had already demonstrated pelvic collection with acute hepatic involvement.

Final Diagnosis: Pelvic Inflammatory Disease Leading to Fitz-Hugh-Curtis Syndrome

Fitz-Hugh-Curtis syndrome is characterized by acute perihepatitis as a complication of pelvic inflammatory disease.

Usual sign, symptoms include fever, pain in lower abdomen with or without offensive vaginal discharge (pelvic infection symptoms) and right hypochondrium pain (suggestive of perihepatitis).[1]

Hematogenous/lymphatic or direct peritoneal spread of infection from pelvis to liver causes perihepatic capsular inflammation.[2]

Recommended treatment includes parenteral antibiotic—cephalosporin along with doxycycline or azithromycin.[1]

REFERENCES

1. Rueda DA, Aballay L, Orbea L, et al. Fitz-Hugh-Curtis syndrome caused by gonococcal infection in a patient with systemic lupus erythematous: a case report and literature review. Am J Case Rep. 2017;18:1396–400.
2. Ekabe CJ, Kehbila J, Njim T, et al. Monekosso GL. *Chlamydia trachomatis*-induced Fitz-Hugh–Curtis syndrome: a case report. BMC Research Notes. 2017;10:10.

CASE 67

YOUNG BOY WITH SKELETAL DEFORMITIES

CASE SUMMARY

A 17-year-old-boy presented with difficulty in walking for the last 1 year because of his leg deformity which developed insidiously over last several years. He also noticed a painless, nonreducible swelling in his scrotum for last few months. His mother mentioned that her son had delay in achieving developmental milestones, and suffered from repeated attacks of respiratory tract infections since childhood. His hearing was also impaired. He did not have any history of jaundice. One of his brothers died at the age of 18 due to kidney disease and another brother died at the age of 10 due to unknown cause. There was no consanguinity of marriage between parents. The boy was born normal and healthy, without any antenatal, intranatal or postnatal complications.

On general examination, the boy had dolichocephalic face, thick lips, macroglossia and maleruption of teeth. He was short-statured, and mildly anemic. Blood pressure was 120/90 mm Hg without any postural drop and other vital parameters were normal. Systemic examination revealed that he had pectus carinatum, bilateral knocked knees (genu valgum), pes cavus, inversion of foot and nontender hepatosplenomegaly, nonreducible scrotal swelling with get above the swelling possible and positive transillumination test. There was no neurological deficit except cranial nerve examination revealed bilateral conductive deafness. On ophthalmological examination, Kayser–Fleischer (KF) ring, and corneal clouding were absent. Fundoscopy was normal.

Complete blood count showed anemia and thrombocytopenia. Peripheral blood film showed bicytopenia with eosinophilia. Serum electrolytes were normal, serum creatinine was 3.46 mg/dL, serum calcium was 8.6 mg/dL and parathyroid hormone (PTH) was 60 pg/mL, alkaline phosphatase level was 100 U/L, serum albumin and inorganic phosphate were within normal limit. Vitamin D level was 32.4 ng/mL. Serum bilirubin was 8.7 µmol/L, alanine aminotransferase (ALT) and prothrombin time (PT) were in normal limit. All the viral markers were negative. X-ray of knee joints, ankle joints and foot (both) showed deformity. Ultrasonography of whole abdomen showed bilateral renal parenchymal disease and hepatosplenomegaly with coarse hepatic parenchyma. Computed tomography (CT) scan of head was normal.

QUESTIONS

1. What are the differentials?
2. What investigation could be done to reach a final diagnosis?

DISCUSSION

Our differentials were:
- Mucopolysaccharidosis
- Rickets with hydrocele
- Wilson's disease.

Short stature, skeletal deformity, hepatosplenomegaly with coarse hepatic parenchyma were explainable by Wilson's disease as it can cause metabolic bone disease (including rickets), various musculoskeletal manifestations and endocrine abnormality. But our patient never had jaundice or neuropsychiatric manifestations, and KF ring was absent. We did serum ceruloplasmin, and urinary copper levels which were normal; and D-penicillamine challenge test was negative.

Though the patient had deformity, but serum calcium and phosphate, parathyroid hormone (PTH), alkaline phosphatase (ALP) and vitamin D level—all were normal, which disfavored the possibility of rickets.

All the clinical manifestations such as typical facial features, short-stature, pattern of skeletal deformity, repeated respiratory tract infection and impaired hearing, presence of hepatosplenomegaly and hydrocele were pointing toward the diagnosis of mucopolysaccharidosis (MPS). So, we sent blood sample for genetic analysis, and the report was consistent with the diagnosis of Hurler syndrome (mucopolysaccharidosis I-H). Urinalysis for glycosaminoglycans and serum assays for lysosomal enzymes could have been done. As renal involvement is not usually present in mucopolysaccharidosis, our patient's raised creatinine level required renal biopsy for further explanation, but due to his parents' denial we could not proceed for it. Bone mineral density (BMD) and liver biopsy could not be done due to same reason.

Final Diagnosis: Mucopolysaccharidosis (Hurler Syndrome)

Mucopolysaccharidosis manifests as the defective activity of the lysosomal enzymes. It blocks degradation of mucopolysaccharides leading to abnormal accumulation of heparan sulfate, dermatan sulfate and keratan sulfate.[1] There are multiple subtypes of the disease, out of which MPS I includes Hurler (MPS I-H), Hurler-Scheie (MPS I-H/S), and Scheie (MPS I-S) syndromes. Patients with severe features were historically classified as Hurler syndrome.[2] MPS are autosomal recessive disorders in inheritance with the exception of Hunter syndrome (MPS II), which is a sex-linked recessive disorder.

Patients with MPS develop normally in early life. Though the presenting age of MPS is variable mostly present in the first few months after birth.

Mucopolysaccharidosis presents with multi-organ involvement mostly with the following features:[3]

- *Central nervous system (CNS) disease*: Hydrocephalus and cervical spine myelopathy
- *Cardiovascular disease*: Angina, valvular dysfunction, hypertension, and congestive heart failure
- *Pulmonary disease*: Airway obstruction, potentially leading to sleep apnea, severe respiratory compromise or cor pulmonale
- *Ophthalmologic disease*: Corneal clouding, glaucoma, chronic papilledema, and retinal degeneration
- *Hearing impairment*: Deafness
- *Musculoskeletal disease*: Short stature, joint stiffness, and symptoms of peripheral nerve entrapment.

Urinalysis focusing on glycosaminoglycans (e.g. dermatan sulfate, heparin sulfate and keratan sulfate) and serum assays for lysosomal enzymes (alpha-L-iduronidase, iduronate sulfatase, heparan N-sulfatase, N-acetylglucosaminidase, alpha-glucosamine-N-acetyltransferase, N-acetyl alpha-glucosamine-6-sulfatase, N-acetylgalactosamine-6-sulfatase, N-acetylgalactosamine-6-sulfatase, B-galactosidase, N-acetylgalactosamine-4-sulfatase, and B-glucuronidase) are the first choice of investigations for the disease.[4,5]

Also imaging studies such as plain radiography should be done to detect dysostosis multiplex. CT scan of head in order to help in diagnosing hydrocephalus and echocardiography to monitor ventricular function and size in MPS patients with cardiovascular disease should be done to figure out the extent of the disease involvement.[4,5]

The prognosis varies depending on the type of MPS. Most of these patients have shortened life spans with death in infancy.

REFERENCES

1. Jones KL, Jones MC, del Campo Avenelles M. Storage disorders. Smith's Recognizable Patterns of Human Malformation. 7th ed. Philadelphia: Elsevier Saunders; 2013. pp. 594–611.

2. Jones S, Wynn R. Mucopolysaccharidoses: clinical features and diagnosis. 2019. In Elizabeth T (ED), UpToDate, retrieved May 2019 from https://www.uptodate.com/contents/mucopolysaccharidoses-clinical-features-and-diagnosis.
3. Thumler A, Miebach E, Lampe C, et al. Clinical characteristics of adults with slowly progressing mucopolysaccharidosis VI: a case series. J Inherit Metab Dis. 2012;35(6):1071-9.
4. Bassyouni HT, Afifi HH, el-Awadi MK, et al. Mucopolysaccharidosis type I: clinical and biochemical study. East Mediterr Health J. 2000;6(2-3):359-66.
5. Martin R, Beck M, Eng C, et al. Recognition and diagnosis of mucopolysaccharidosis II (Hunter syndrome). Pediatrics. 2008;121(2):e377-86.

CASE 68

GENTLEMAN WITH BILATERAL LEG WEAKNESS AND GENERALIZED HYPERPIGMENTATION

CASE SUMMARY

A 46-year-old man was admitted in hospital through the outpatient department (OPD) with bilateral leg swelling, weakness with tingling sensation and generalized hyperpigmentation for 1 year. At first he noticed swelling of both legs, followed by darkening of skin of both feet and then leg. Gradually the hyperpigmentation spread all over the body. Besides these, he had been experiencing weakness and painful tingling sensation with numbness starting at both lower limbs for last 4 months. Gradually both upper limbs were also involved and the weakness restricted his mobility and he experienced difficulty in performing daily activities. He did not have fever, weight loss, headache, blurring of vision, epistaxis, back pain, bladder or bowel abnormality.

Examination revealed clubbed fingers and bipedal pitting edema. Skin was hyperpigmented, thickened and tightened especially in the distal part of the extremities. Neurological examination revealed reduced power 2/5 in lower limb bilaterally and 3/5 in the upper limbs. Deep tendon reflexes were absent even after reinforcement in both upper and lower limbs with flexor plantar responses bilaterally. Pain and temperature sensations were impaired as well. Abdominal examination revealed non-tender splenomegaly (about 5 cm from left costal margin).

Investigation revealed hemoglobin (Hb) 16.5 g/dL, erythrocyte sedimentation rate (ESR)—15 mm in first hour, platelet—553,000/mm^3, white blood cells (WBCs)—7,000/mm^3, red blood cell (RBC)—5.55 × 10^{12}/L. Serum creatinine, serum electrolytes, serum copper, serum prolactin, FSH, LH levels were normal. Serum TSH level was 30 mU/L, anti-TPO antibody was positive.

Antinuclear antibody (ANA), antibody profile against extractable nuclear antigens (ENA), and creatine kinase (CK) levels were normal. Serum vitamin B12 level was increased. Ultrasonography (USG) of whole abdomen revealed splenomegaly. Cerebrospinal fluid (CSF) study showed mildly raised protein. Serum albumin/globulin (A/G) ratio was 1.17. Serum protein electrophoresis and immunoelectrophoresis showed a monoclonal spike of IgG lambda. Urinalysis revealed no proteinuria and Bence Jones protein was not found. In skeletal survey X-ray skull lateral view, and X-ray chest P/A view revealed normal findings, but X-ray pelvis A/P and lateral view revealed two small osteosclerotic lesions at left ilium of pelvis. Bone marrow study revealed increased myeloid-erythroid ratio with megakaryocytic hyperplasia. Nerve conduction study was consistent with demyelinating motor sensory polyneuropathy with secondary axonal involvement. Histology from skin biopsy of the affected site was consistent with scleroderma.

QUESTIONS

1. What could be the final diagnosis?
2. What is the cause of edema in this case?

DISCUSSION

This patient's paraparesis could be explained by subacute combined degeneration of spinal cord, adrenomyeloneuropathy and copper deficiency. But, normal vitamin B12 and normal serum copper levels ruled out the possibilities. Adrenomyeloneuropathy is associated with brisk reflex and spasticity, which disfavored our patient's findings. Our patient had important features of chronic weakness (motor > sensory), absent deep tendon reflexes with flexor plantar response, skin changes (hyperpigmentation, thickening and tightening), peripheral edema, splenomegaly and investigations revealed thrombocytosis, hypothyroidism, demyelinating polyneuropathy, organomegaly, and monoclonal gammopathy. These brought **POEMS syndrome** (polyneuropathy, organomegaly, endocrinopathy, monoclonal gammopathy, skin changes) at the top of differentials. Matching our patient's features to the diagnostic criteria (Table 1) confirmed the diagnosis of POEMS syndrome.

Final Diagnosis: Polyneuropathy, Organomegaly, Endocrinopathy, Monoclonal Gammopathy, Skin Changes Syndrome

The POEMS syndrome, also known as polyneuropathy–endocrinopathy–plasma cell dyscrasia (PEP) syndrome or Crow-Fukase syndrome or Takatsuki disease, or osteosclerotic myeloma, is a paraneoplastic syndrome due to an underlying plasma cell neoplasm. The underlying cause of the disorder is poorly understood. It is a chronic disorder, with a median survival time of 8–14 years.[1]

Table 1: Diagnostic criteria for POEMS syndrome.[2]

Mandatory Criteria
- Polyneuropathy (typically demyelinating)
- Monoclonal plasma cell-proliferative disorder (almost always λ)

Major Criteria
- Castleman disease
- Sclerotic bone lesions
- Vascular endothelial growth factor (VEGF) elevation

Minor Criteria
- Organomegaly (splenomegaly, hepatomegaly or lymphadenopathy)
- Extravascular volume overload (edema, pleural effusion or ascites)
- Endocrinopathy (adrenal, pituitary, gonadal, parathyroid, thyroid and pancreatic)
- Skin changes (hyperpigmentation, hypertrichosis, glomeruloid hemangiomata, plethora, acrocyanosis, flushing and white nails)
- Papilledema
- Thrombocytosis/polycythemia

Diagnosis requires both mandatory criteria plus ≥1 major and ≥1 minor criterion

In this case, serum vascular endothelial growth factor (VEGF) level could have been done, as bipedal edema could be explained by raised VEGF level in POEMS syndrome.

There is no standard treatment; management depends on the underlying plasma cell disorder, for which radiation therapy, chemotherapy, and/or hematopoietic cell transplantation may be required. Radiation therapy directed to the sclerotic bone lesions produces substantial improvement of clinical symptoms in more than 50% cases. Unlike in chronic inflammatory demyelinating polyneuropathy (CIDP), neither plasmapheresis nor intravenous immunoglobulin (IVIG) produces clinical benefit.[1]

REFERENCES

1. POEMS syndrome. Derm Net NZ. September 13, 2014; http://dermnetnz.org/systemic/poems.html.
2. Dispenzieri A. POEMS syndrome: 2017 Update on diagnosis, risk stratification, and management. Am J Hematol. 2017;92:814-29. https://doi.org/10.1002/ajh.24802

CASE 69

MIDDLE-AGED MAN WITH ACUTE CONFUSIONAL STATE, HEMATEMESIS AND MELENA

CASE SUMMARY

A 65-year-old male presented with several episodes of hematemesis, two episodes of restlessness, and impaired consciousness for 5 days. These symptoms were preceded by several episodes of melena for 3 months, which were painless, persistent and of small amount. About 1 week after the last onset of melena, he became restless and started talking irrelevantly. With these complaints, he got admitted into the nearby hospital and was diagnosed as a case of "chronic liver disease with hepatic encephalopathy (grade-II) with variceal bleeding." After conservative treatment and blood transfusion, he was discharged. But his condition did not improve rather he gradually developed weakness of the left side of the body and nonprojectile vomiting, which initially contained undigested food particle, followed by only fresh blood. On query, patient's attendants gave a history of jaundice about 6 months back and patient had recurrent upper abdominal pain for 5/6 years and mentioned getting treatment for gastric ulcer with antiulcerant 3 years back. He had been taking nonsteroidal anti-inflammatory drugs (NSAIDs) for osteoarthritis for last 6 years. There was no history of abdominal distension or leg swelling, chest pain, fever, cough, breathlessness, headache, convulsion, blurring of vision, and rash or weight loss.

On examination, patient was semiconscious (GCS 8/15, E2 + M4 + V2), moderately anemic and nonicteric. Clubbing and palmar erythema were present. Pulse was 80 beats/min, blood pressure (BP): 100/60 mm Hg, temperature: 99°F and respiratory rate: 16 breaths/min. Abdominal examination revealed nontender hepatomegaly, which was about 4 cm from the right costal margin, smooth surfaced with regular margin, firm in consistency. Upper border of liver dullness was in right fifth intercostal space and there was no hepatic bruit. No splenomegaly, ascites or para-aortic lymphadenopathy

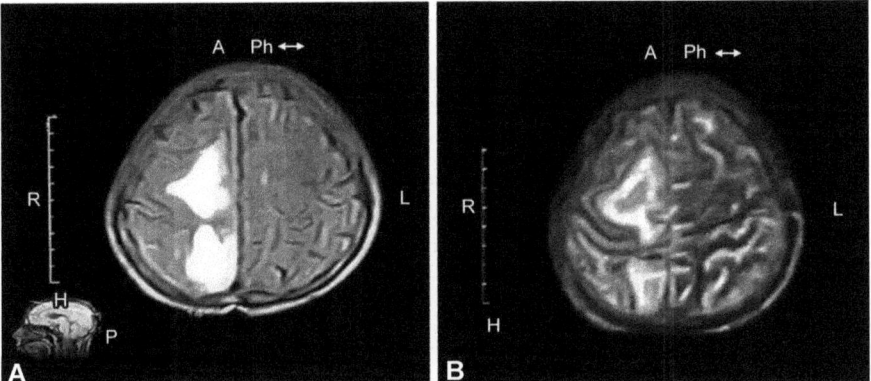

Figs. 1A and B: Magnetic resonance imaging (MRI) of brain. Multiple axial cuts showing hyperintensity at right-parietal region just adjacent to interhemispheric fissure.

was found. Nervous system examination showed left-sided hemiparesis. Other systemic examinations revealed no abnormality.

Investigations showed: Complete blood count (CBC): hemoglobin (Hb) was persistently low from 6.3 g/dL to 9.1 g/dL, platelet: 150 k/μL, white blood cell (WBC): normal, erythrocyte sedimentation rate (ESR): 68 mm in first hour. Peripheral blood film (PBF): red blood cell (RBC): Anisocytosis with anisochromia including macrocytes and microcytes with few number of target cells. Comment: Dimorphic anemia. *Liver function test*: Serum bilirubin: 7.4 μmol/L, alanine aminotransferase (ALT): 62 U/L, aspartate aminotransferase (AST): 55 U/L, alkaline phosphatase (ALP): 79 U/L, serum albumin: 24 g/L, prothrombin time (PT): 13.7 seconds, plasma ammonia: 93 μmol/L (N: 10-47). Viral markers: surface antigen of the hepatitis B (HBsAg): negative; anti-HBc (total) Ab: positive; hepatitis Be-antigen (HBeAg): negative; hepatitis B virus (HBV) DNA: undetected; anti-HCV Ab: negative; serum ceruloplasmin and urinary copper: normal. *Ultrasonography (USG)*: Slightly coarse liver parenchyma, prominent spleen and no ascites. Fibroscan of the liver: 16.8 kPa (fibrosis stage: F3-F4). Magnetic resonance imaging (MRI) of brain with contrast: Noncontrast enhancing T1W1 hypointensity and T2W1 and flair hyperintensity is noted at right-sided high parietal region just adjacent to interhemispheric fissure. Features suggestive of multifocal encephalitis (Figs. 1A and B).

QUESTIONS

1. What investigations should be done next?
2. What is the most likely diagnosis?

DISCUSSION

For this patient, the previous diagnosis of chronic liver disease with hepatic encephalopathy with variceal bleeding could explain the melena and irrelevant speech, but not the subsequent development of hemiparesis. Moreover, new-onset hematemesis and query regarding the recent status of gastric ulcer (which was diagnosed 3 years back) warranted further workup. We repeated endoscopy of upper gastrointestinal tract (GIT), which showed ulcerated growth at antrum and prepyloric area of stomach. Comment: Carcinoma stomach (Figs. 2A to D).

Gastric biopsy (by endoscopy): Microscopic examination showed fragments of gastric mucosa. They revealed adenocarcinoma, moderately differentiated in nature with chronic inflammatory cells infiltration. Diagnosis: Infiltrating adenocarcinoma, moderately differentiated.

Discovery of a malignancy compelled us to repeat neuroimaging to further delineate the nature of the cerebral lesions. *Computed tomography (CT) scan of brain showed*: diffuse ill-defined low-density area appearing as disproportionate edema is noted in right parietal region involving periventricular and supraventricular deep white matter. After intravenous (IV) contrast, no abnormal enhancement is seen. *Impression*: Suspected infiltrative lesion (? Carcinomatosis cerebri) in right parietal region involving periventricular and supraventricular deep white matter (Figs. 3A and B). Besides metastasis, this feature can also be explained by viral encephalitis, inflammatory or demyelinating lesion of brain. So, further confirmation warranted brain biopsy.

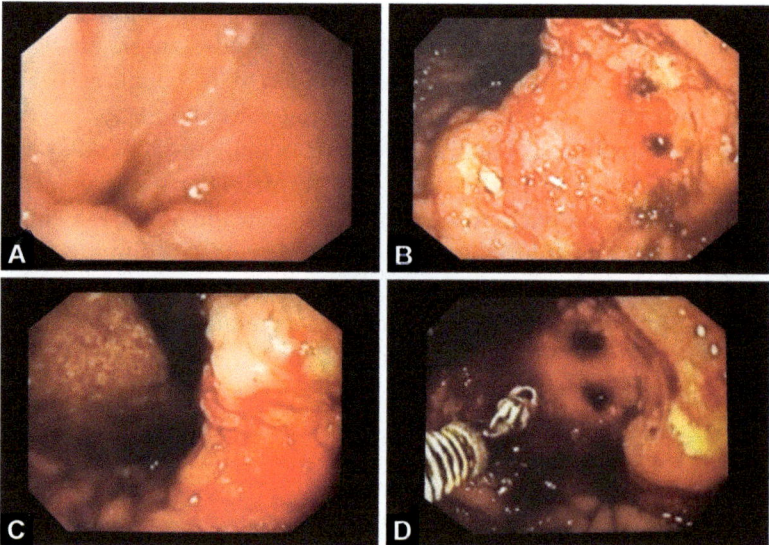

Figs. 2A to D: Endoscopy of upper gastrointestinal tract (GIT) showing ulcerated growth at antrum and prepyloric area of stomach.

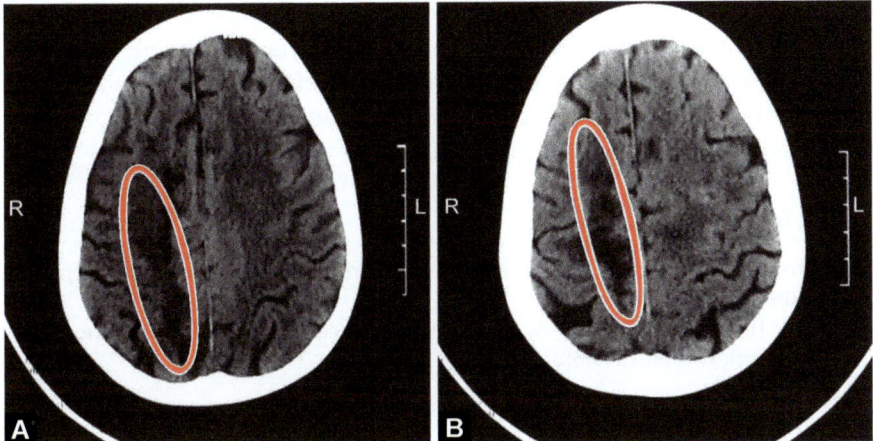

Figs. 3A and B: Computed tomography (CT) scan of the showing infiltrative lesion in right parietal region involving periventricular and supraventricular deep white matter.

Final Diagnosis: Infiltrating Adenocarcinoma of Stomach with Brain Metastasis with Chronic Liver Disease with Hepatic Encephalopathy

Gastric carcinoma is the fourth leading cause of cancer death worldwide, but there is marked geographical variation in incidence. It is most common in China, Japan, Korea, Eastern Europe and parts of South America. The overall prognosis is poor, with less than 30% surviving 5 years.[1] Virtually all tumors are adenocarcinomas arising from mucus-secreting cells in the base of the gastric crypts. Most develop upon a background of chronic atrophic gastritis with intestinal metaplasia and dysplasia. There are multiple risk factors for the development of gastric adenocarcinoma, among which most important is *Helicobacter pylori* infection.

The relation between peptic ulcer disease and gastric carcinoma is well established. Gastric ulcer is an important risk factor for development of gastric cancer. In our patient, we repeated the endoscopy of upper GIT considering his previous history of gastric ulcer disease, which helped us connect the missing dots and solve the case. Brain biopsy and histopathology could have further delineated the nature of cerebral involvement.

Over one-third of patients at the time of diagnosis of gastric adenocarcinoma are in advanced stages presenting with metastases to the peritoneum, lymph nodes, lung, liver or bones. Brain metastases from gastric adenocarcinoma are exceedingly rare. Prior studies revealed that only 0.47–0.70% patients with gastric cancer were identified to have brain metastases.[2]

Patients with brain metastases from GIT have poorer prognosis. Modern palliative chemotherapy and immunotherapy lengthen survival by a few months, and possibly the frequency of brain metastases from stomach cancer will rise; therefore, radiotherapy becomes an important treatment modality.

In this individual case, the patient's attendant refused to get chemotherapy. Later, he developed frequent episodes of hematemesis and melena; and after readmission, he died in the next morning.

REFERENCES

1. Crew KD, Neugut AI. Epidemiology of gastric cancer. World J Gastroenterol. 2006;12(3):354-62.
2. York JE, Stringer J, Ajani JA, et al. Gastric cancer and metastasis to the brain. Ann Surg Oncol. 1999;6(8):771-6.

CASE 70

MIDDLE-AGED LADY WITH RECURRENT FRACTURES

CASE SUMMARY

A 60-year-old lady presented with history of generalized bodyache for 4 years which was more marked in lower back with subsequent involvement of chest, both arms and thighs over the span of few months. The progression of the pain was so severe that she performed her daily activities with difficulties. One year back, she noticed deformity of both arms and 6 months back, she became unable to walk, and could not even stand from sitting or sit-up from supine position without any aids. There was no association of trauma, morning stiffness, joint pain or swelling. Also there was no history of significant weight loss, fever, rash, cough, bleeding from any site and urinary or fecal disturbance. She was diabetic (controlled) and hypertensive. She took various analgesics without significant improvement of pain. She was on menopause for last 14 years, was nonsmoker, nonalcoholic but occasionally chewed betel nuts. There was no significant family history.

On examination, patient was found to be mildly pale with average body built and nutrition. Bony tenderness was present with gross deformity of both upper arms bowing outwards. A palpable, tender, circumferential hard swelling was present over each deformity. There was no restriction of motion of joints but both the active and passive movements were painful. The rate and volume of distal pulses were normal. There was no redness or swelling of joints and no muscle wasting. The tone and power of the muscle and all reflexes of upper and lower limbs were normal. Sensory modalities were intact.

Investigations revealed complete blood count: moderate anemia (hemoglobin 9.7 g/dL) with normal ESR (5 mm in first hour) with normal total and differential WBC count. Peripheral blood film showed normocytic normochromic anemia with matured WBC with normal platelet count. Serum creatinine level was 0.7 mg/dL and urine analysis was also normal. Protein electrophoresis showed no abnormal accumulation of immunoglobulin molecule.

Bone marrow study showed normal active marrow. Further investigations revealed the following status:
- Serum calcium: 7.00 mg/dL (normal 8.1–10.4 mg/dL), with normal serum albumin level.
- Serum PO_4: 1.8 mg/dL (normal range 2.5–5 mg/dL)
- Serum PTH: 20.10 pg/mL (normal range 0–65 pg/mL)
- Serum alkaline phosphatase: 663 U/L (normal range 40–125 U/L)
- Serum magnesium: 2.00 mg/dL (normal level 1.82–2.43 mg/dL).

Radiography of chest, skull, both upper arms and sacroiliac joint revealed diffuse osteopenia in skull, clavicle, ribs, both humerus and femur. There was pathological old nonuniting fracture in upper one-third of both humerus and right femur. Bone mineral density (BMD) also showed osteopenia. T score was −1 to −2 U at various sites. Whole body bone scan showed increased tracer uptake in anterior end of left 3rd rib, shaft of both humerus and trochanteric region of both femur. Her serum electrolytes and ECG were normal. Echocardiography showed concentric left ventricular hypertrophy with good systolic functions (EF 61%). Thyroid function test was also normal.

QUESTIONS

1. What differential diagnoses can be considered for this case?
2. How should the case be managed?

DISCUSSION

Considering the history and clinical examination, our differential diagnoses were:
- Multiple myeloma
- Secondary tumours of bone

Then after doing initial investigations we considered additional differentials:
- Osteomalacia
- Osteoporosis
- Hyperparathyroidism.

Early in presentation, patient had bone pain with generalized bodyache. She was middle-aged and anemic, which made multiple myeloma a possibility. But normal ESR, normal findings in protein electrophoresis, normal bone marrow study, renal function test and decreased calcium and increased alkaline phosphatase level excluded the diagnosis of multiple myeloma. Secondary deposits to bone was another possibility but long history of illness with absence of suggestive clinical features for any possible primary tumor, lack of muscle wasting and whole body bone scan showing increased tracer uptake also made the diagnosis very unlikely.

Patient having low calcium and phosphate level and increased alkaline phosphatase made diagnosis of osteoporosis unlikely. Low serum calcium and phosphate concentration might be due to CKD, hypoparathyroidism, hypomagnesemia and also in vitamin D deficiency. Further investigation showing normal PTH level, normal renal function test (RFT) and normal Mg^{2+} level excluded all of the above, except vitamin D deficiency. The combination of hypocalcaemia, hypophosphatemia and raised alkaline phosphatase in this case pointed to a diagnosis of 'osteomalacia' either due to dietary deficiency of calcium, lack of vitamin D or intestinal disease with malabsorption such as tropical sprue. Osteomalacia is partiularly common among females having pigmentation of skin or wearing veils resulting in less endogenous synthesis of vitamin D due to lack of sun exposure. Our patient did not have any significant gastrointestinal disturbances but she used to wear veil (burka with hijab and niqab) while going out. We then decided to measure the 25(OH)-D status and it showed decreased level (25.0 nmol/L or 10 ng/mL). Therefore, finally we diagnosed our case as osteomalacia either due to vitamin D deficiency or vitamin D resistance.

We treated our case with injection vitamin D3 for 6 weeks. After getting the injection the patient showed signs of improvement gradually; patient could sit and could move her limbs and as her tenderness reduced, she allowed physical examination by doctors. There was an improvement of laboratory profile also. With these observations we diagnosed the case as osteomalacia due to vitamin D deficiency. The diagnosis could be further confirmed by bone biopsy, which would show the pathognomic features of increased thickness and extent of osteoid seams. However for being middle-aged, poor general condition and increased chance of fracture we did not go for bone biopsy.

Final Diagnosis: Osteomalacia Due to Vitamin D Deficiency

Undiagnosed vitamin D deficiency is not uncommon and 25-hydroxy vitamin D is the biomarker for vitamin D status not 1,25-dihydroxy vitamin D as it may be elevated or remains normal in vitamin D deficiency state due to secondary hyperparathyroidism.

Osteomalacia is the softening of the bones caused by inadequate bone mineralization.[1] The most common cause of osteomalacia is a deficiency of vitamin D which is normally derived from sunlight exposure, and to a lesser extent from the diet.[2] So, a detailed dietary history, lifestyle and any history of gastrointestinal pathology is mandatory. Investigation must include bone X-ray which may show demineralization and looser's zone, and serum 25-hydroxy vitamin D level.[2]

Treatment should begun with oral calcium and 1 alpha hydroxy vitamin D3. Besides adequate sun exposure, dietary supplementation of vitamin D and calcium are the measures that can be used to prevent osteomalacia.[2]

REFERENCES

1. Salmon B, Bardet C, Coyac BR, et al. Abnormal osteopontin and matrix extracellular phosphoglycoprotein localization, and odontoblast differentiation, in X-linked hypophosphatemic teeth. Connective Tissue Research. 2014;55(Suppl 1):79–82. doi:10.3109/03008207.2014.923864. PMID 25158186
2. Jameson JL, Kasper DL, et al. Harrison's Principles of Internal Medicine. 20th ed. New York: McGraw Hill Education; 2018.

CASE 71

MIDDLE-AGED MALE WITH RECURRENT ALTERED LEVEL OF CONSCIOUSNESS

CASE SUMMARY

A 65-year-old male presented with the complaints of generalized muscle weakness for the past 1 day and altered level of consciousness for the past several hours. His attendant stated that he complained of sudden onset of muscle weakness, which was associated with tingling sensation, followed by dizziness, after which, he vomited 3-4 times. Then he became unresponsive and confused, for which he was admitted in Dhaka Medical College and Hospital (DMCH). After rapid exclusion of hypoglycemia, further history was taken. Previously, he suffered from 3 episodes of similar symptoms in the last 2 months, and was treated for hyponatremia in a local hospital once and in the DMCH twice [serum electrolyte reports were available (Table 1)]. Patient did not have fever, weight loss, cough, respiratory distress, chest pain, convulsion, abdominal pain, or bowel-bladder involvement. He had been diabetic (controlled) for 9 years, and hypertensive for about 4 years (controlled with amlodipine).

On examination, he was ill-looking and disoriented, pulse—85 bpm, blood pressure—110/70 mm of Hg, temperature—normal, anemia and dehydration—absent, clubbing—absent, lymph node—not palpable. Nervous system revealed—GCS was 11/15. Higher psychic function could not be evaluated as patient could not follow command. Cranial nerves were intact. Motor examination showed muscle bulk—normal, tone—hypotonic, power—3/5 on admission, later 5/5. Reflexes were normal. Sensory modalities could not be evaluated properly. Cerebellar examination and other systemic examinations revealed normal findings.

Investigations showed, CBC—Hb—11 g/dL, ESR—97 mm/hr, WBC—11,740/, cumm; platelets—409,000/cumm; neutrophil—70%, lymphocyte—24%. PBF—anemia with chronic disorder with neutrophilic leukocytosis. RBS—4.6 mmol/L. CRP—24 mg/L (≤6 mg/L). Urine R/M/E—albumin— +, pus cells—2-3/HPF. Serum electrolytes showed mild hyponatremia and hypochloremia (Table 1).

Table 1: Serum electrolytes in mmol/L.

Time	During this episode	At third episode	At second episode	At first episode
Na⁺	130	130	126	119
K⁺	3.8	3.6	2.9	4.6
Cl⁻	94	94	86	88
TCO$_2$	26	24	25	26
Ca^{2+}	8.8	—	8.3	—

Blood urea—10.1 mg/dL. Urine electrolyte: U. sodium—49 mmol/L (40-100). U. potassium—27 mmol/L (12-62), U. chloride—62 mmol/L (55-125). Urinary osmolarity—310 mOsm/kg (60-1,400). Urine pH—5. Serum cortisol—34 nmol/L. Blood urea—2.6 mmol/L, serum creatinine—1.5 mg/dL. Serum TSH—2.29 µLU/mL. Serum ADH—2.2 pg/mL (1-4.8). Chest X-ray—no abnormality detected. USG of the whole abdomen—normal study. Endoscopy of the upper GIT—normal. CT scan of whole abdomen—normal study.

QUESTIONS

1. What further investigation can be done in this case?
2. What is the final diagnosis?

DISCUSSION

Our initial investigations demonstrated that the patient had euvolemic hyponatremia. He did not have history of polydipsia, or infusion of hypotonic saline, and hypothyroidism was excluded. But the underlying cause of this middle-aged man's recurrent hyponatremia was yet to be established—warranting additional work-up. Further investigations showed:

- *CT scan of chest:* Irregular infiltrate in right upper lobe—most likely pneumonia.
- *CT-guided FNAC:* The aspirate consisted of mostly blood, lymphocytes, histiocytes and polymorphs. A few tiny clusters of atypical bronchial epithelial cells were seen.
- *Open lung biopsy and histopathology:* Granulomatous change suggestive of tuberculosis.

Final Diagnosis: Syndrome of Inappropriate Antidiuretic Hormone Secretion due to Pulmonary Tuberculosis

The onset of symptoms of hyponatremia depends on the speed of development of hyponatremia, not on its severity. Pulmonary disorders that can cause syndrome of inappropriate antidiuretic hormone secretion (SIADH) include pneumonia, tuberculosis, malignancy and obstructive lung disease.[1] Our patient had no history of use of diuretics. So, on the background of clinical euvolemia, presence of low plasma osmolality, and absence of adrenal, thyroid, pituitary or renal insufficiency, SIADH due to pulmonary tuberculosis (PTB) was established.

Tuberculosis (TB) is commonly found in developing countries. Lung is predominantly affected while extrapulmonary tuberculosis (EPTB) is also encountered. The clinical features of EPTB can be nonspecific that mimics other diseases and is usually misdiagnosed. Even pulmonary TB can be nonspecific. In our case, the patient presented with recurrent loss of consciousness and his biochemical changes were suggestive of SIADH but there was no clinical or other evidence of pulmonary TB. Lung biopsy was done for high suspicion of TB and it revealed granulomatous changes. Hence, it is very important to have a high index of suspicion to rule out TB, as this disease is a curable disease. Late diagnosis or untreatable TB will lead to high morbidity and mortality.

REFERENCE

1. Ralston SH, Penman ID, Strachan MWJ, et al. Davidson's Principles and Practice of Medicine. 23rd ed. Edinburgh: Churchill Livingstone/Elsevier; 2018. pp. 357-8.

CASE 72

MIDDLE-AGED MAN WITH SWELLING OF LEGS AND ABDOMEN

CASE SUMMARY

A 50-year-old man, government officer in Qatar, hypertensive, nondiabetic presented with gradual swelling of legs and huge distension of abdomen for the past 7 months. There were several episodes of jaundice, each episode being associated with nausea, anorexia and weakness for the last 1 year. There was also history of significant oliguria. The patient noticed significant weight loss of approximately 12 kg in the last 1 year. Patient denied any history of itching, alteration of bowel habit or pale stool. There was no history of alcohol intake, intravenous (IV) drug abuse or blood transfusion. The patient was a known case of chronic kidney disease with chronic atrial fibrillation with dilated cardiomyopathy. There was a history of cardiac arrest with an episode of ventricular tachycardia followed by implantable cardioverter defibrillator (ICD) insertion 1 year back. With this illness, the patient had to stay in hospital for 6 months during which he developed progressive shortness of breath, abdominal and leg swelling also with paroxysmal nocturnal dyspnea and orthopnea.

On general examination, patient was ill-looking, undernourished, mildly anemic and icteric. Bipedal pitting edema was present. Flapping tremor was present, but there was no clubbing, palmar erythema, engorged neck veins or testicular atrophy. Cardiovascular system examination revealed hypotension without any postural drop and the apex beat was on the left fourth intercostal space, 14 cm from the midline and lateral to the left midclavicular line and heaving in nature. On abdomen examination, it was distended with full flanks and centrally placed, everted umbilicus. The liver was enlarged with regular margin, smooth surface and firm to soft consistency, and spleen was just palpable. Ascites was evident by shifting dullness. Bowel sound was normal without any hepatic rub or bruit. Other systemic examination revealed no abnormality.

Complete blood count (CBC): hemoglobin (Hb)—10.1 g/dL, white blood cell (WBC)—4.4 × 10^9/L (N—68%, L—23%, M—07%, E—02%), platelet count—150 × 109/L, erythrocyte sedimentation rate (ESR)—61 mm in the first hour, packed cell volume (PCV)—31%, serum bilirubin—2.9 mg/dL, aminotransferase (ALT)—19 U/L, serum albumin—22.8 g/dL, prothrombin time (PT)—18 seconds, international normalized ratio (INR)—1.6, activated partial thromboplastin time (APTT)—40.8 seconds, serum creatinine—1.9 mg/dL, serum electrolytes—normal, serum lipid profile—normal, except low high-density lipoprotein (HDL) cholesterol, thyroid function tests—normal, viral markers for hepatitis B virus (HBV) and hepatitis C virus (HCV) both were negative, B-type natriuretic peptide (BNP)—1832.40 pg/mL, troponin I—95 ng/L, creatine kinase-muscle/brain (CK-MB)—less than 5 ng/mL, urine microscopy was normal. Repeated chest X-rays showed cardiomegaly. There was normal ventricular paced electrocardiography (ECG). Computed tomography (CT) of thorax and abdomen with contrast (done 1 year back) showed cardiomegaly with right-sided heart failure and congestive changes of lungs with mild right-sided pleural effusion and basal atelectasis. Staghorn stone was in the right kidney and trace of fluid was in right iliac fossa and pelvis. Ultrasonogram of whole abdomen showed mild hepatosplenomegaly with engorged hepatic venous system with thick-walled gallbladder. There was moderate ascites and right-sided nephrolithiasis.

QUESTIONS

1. What could be the next investigations?
2. What is the probable diagnosis?
3. How the patient should be managed?

DISCUSSION

The patient presented with features of cirrhosis of the liver. There was also a history of chronic atrial fibrillation with dilated cardiomyopathy and cardiac arrest with an episode of ventricular tachycardia followed by ICD insertion earlier. To rule out the other causes of anasarca, next choice of investigations was echocardiography, fibroscan of liver and ultimately liver biopsy. Echocardiography in our patient showed permanent pacemaker implantation (PPI) leads in right atrium (RA) and right ventricle (RV), moderate global hypokinesia with reduced ejection fraction (EF) (35%), restrictive pattern of diastolic dysfunction, mild mitral regurgitation (MR), aortic sclerosis, moderate pulmonary regurgitation (PR) and mild pulmonary hypertension with minimal pericardial effusion. Fibroscan of the liver confirmed cirrhosis. Liver biopsy was not done.

Final Diagnosis: Cardiac Cirrhosis

Cardiac cirrhosis is the spectrum of hepatic derangements occurring in the setting of right-sided heart failure with the signs and symptoms of congestive heart failure dominating clinically.[1] Patients usually present with asymptomatic liver enzyme abnormalities, jaundice and right upper quadrant discomfort though fulminant hepatic failure have also been reported. Our patient presented with gradually increasing swelling of the legs and abdomen with episodes of jaundice and also with flapping tremor indicating the patient was in either cardiac or hepatic failure.

Treatment of cardiac cirrhosis is medical therapy and in resistant cases, surgical modalities. Diuresis is the cornerstone of initial medical therapy for symptomatic relief concentrating more on right heart failure treatment. Beta-blockers and angiotensin-converting enzyme (ACE) inhibitors should be added in left ventricular dysfunction when the patient is euvolemic. In New York Heart Association class III or IV, heart failure spironolactone should be considered. Surgical interventions such as coronary artery bypass surgery (CABG), tricuspid valve repair, pericardiectomy, transjugular intrahepatic portosystemic shunt (TIPSS) and ultimately cardiac transplantation are the definitive treatment of cardiac cirrhosis.[2]

REFERENCES

1. Moller S, Bernardi M. Interactions of the heart and the liver. Eur Heart J. 2013;34(36):2804-11.
2. Fouad YM, Yehia R. Hepato-cardiac disorders. World J Hepatol. 2014;6(1):41-54.

CASE 73

YOUNG MAN WITH RECURRENT FEVER AND RASHES

CASE SUMMARY

A 32-year-old man was transferred to Dhaka Medical College and Hospital (DMCH) for better evaluation of his illness. His illness started about 10 months ago with high-grade continued fever, without any chills and rigor, associated with pain and swelling of multiple small and large joints of both upper and lower limbs. At that time, he felt better with some medicine prescribed by a local doctor. Subsequently, he faced similar type of attacks several times and also developed flat red rash in different sites of his body, first appearing on his face then on his back, shoulder, anterior chest and also in his hands and lower limbs. Rash used to worsen after sun exposure. He also noticed swelling of his upper eyelids. With these complaints, he visited many hospitals and many investigations were done, though no definitive diagnosis was reached. He was prescribed corticosteroid which resulted in partial symptomatic improvement, and steroid was being tapered. The patient also developed intermittent cough with scanty mucoid sputum production with respiratory distress about 1 month before admission. He had lost about 15 kg weight during this course of illness.

On physical examination, his vitals were normal except respiratory rate was 22 breaths/min. Hyperpigmented maculopapular erythematous rashes were seen on forehead, nose, cheeks and on his back, anterior chest and lower limbs, and there was scaly eruption on his knuckles. Upper eyelids were slightly swollen. On musculoskeletal examination, proximal interphalangeal (PIP) joints were swollen and tender, and movement was restricted and knee joint was tender and swollen. On respiratory system examination, mild bibasal end inspiratory fine crackles were present. On neurological examination, muscle power, jerks and gait were normal. All sensory modalities were intact.

Laboratory investigations revealed hemoglobin (HB)—11 g/dL; erythrocyte sedimentation rate (ESR)—71 mm in the first hour. All other routine investigations, including liver and renal function tests were normal.

Ultrasonography (USG) of whole abdomen revealed no abnormality. X-ray chest P/A view showed bilateral chronic basal pulmonary infiltrate. High-resolution computed tomography (HRCT) of chest revealed reticulonodular shadow in lower zone of both lungs. Spirometric study of the subject showed moderate degree restriction. Sputum and blood cultures yielded no growth. The ferritin level was high (28,415 ng/mL). C-reactive protein (CRP) was slightly raised (12.4 mg/L) and creatine phosphokinase (CPK) was within normal range. Electromyography (EMG) and nerve conduction study (NCS) were negative. Previously done multiple antinuclear antibody (ANA) reports were negative, but when we repeated the test, ANA became positive.

Rheumatoid factor (RF) test, anti-cyclic citrullinated peptide (CCP) and anti-double stranded deoxyribonucleic acid (anti-dsDNA) were negative.

QUESTIONS

1. What is the most likely clinical diagnosis?
2. Give some differentials in this condition.
3. Name three investigations that can help to reach the diagnosis.

DISCUSSION

There were several clues in this case that point towards the diagnosis.

There was a long history of recurrent fever associated with arthritis of small and large joints, and photosensitive rash which responded to corticosteroid. All these indicate a connective tissue disorder.

He had some cutaneous features like *heliotrope rash* (upper eyelid swelling) (Fig. 1A), *Gottron's papule* (knuckle rash) (Fig. 1B) and *shawl sign* (rash on his back) (Fig. 2), which are pathognomonic for dermatomyositis. His respiratory involvement can be explained by diffuse parenchymal lung disease which can be associated with dermatomyositis. The patient did not give any history of muscle weakness or myalgia, CPK was normal and EMG was negative.

ANA came out positive on subsequent investigation and CRP was raised. So our differentials were systemic lupus erythematosus (SLE), dermatomyositis and overlap syndrome.

Our next levels of investigations were:
- Extractable nuclear antigens (ENA) profile
- Muscle biopsy
- Skin biopsy.

ENA profile revealed anti-Jo-1 antibody was positive.

Muscle biopsy findings were nonspecific. There was no inflammatory infiltrate or signs of myositis.

Skin biopsy was suggestive of dermatomyositis evidenced by mild atrophy of epidermis with lymphocytic infiltrate in epidermis.

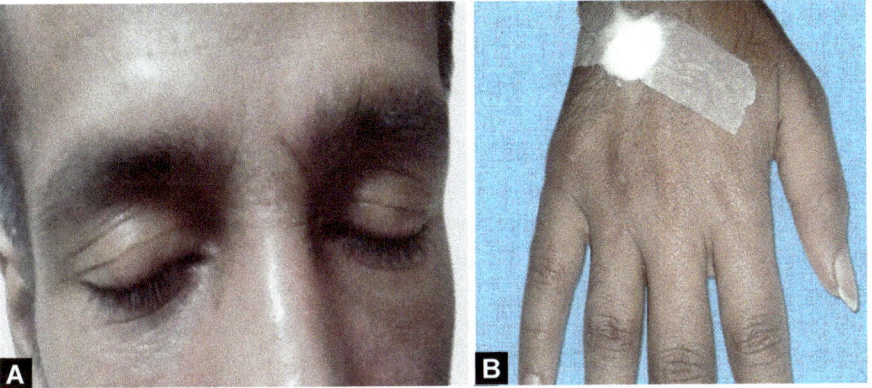

Figs. 1A and B: (A) Upper eyelid swelling; (B) Knuckle rash.

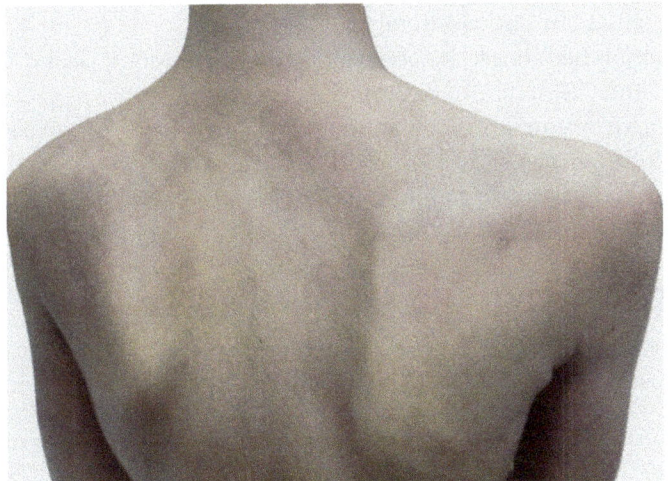

Fig. 2: Rash on the back.

So our final diagnosis was dermatomyositis without any muscle involvement, which is also known as *amyopathic dermatomyositis*.

Final Diagnosis: **Amyopathic Dermatomyositis with Diffuse Parenchymal Lung Disease**

Dermatomyositis is one of the inflammatory myopathies characterized by cutaneous manifestations and chronic muscle inflammation.[1]

Typically patient presents with symmetrical proximal muscle weakness manifested by difficulty in rising from a chair, climbing stairs and sometimes muscle pain. Though, in our case, the patient only presented with cutaneous manifestations without any muscle weakness or pain. Common systemic involvements are—fatigue, fever and weight loss.

Characteristic skin changes are Gottron's papule (scaly, erythematous or violaceous plaques over knuckles), heliotrope rash (eyelid swelling with violaceous coloration). Rash can occur in back, chest and shoulders in shawl distribution.

Respiratory and pharyngeal muscle involvement may occur and may cause aspiration and ventilatory failure.

In muscle biopsy, typical features are inflammatory cell infiltrate, fiber necrosis and regeneration but can also be normal as myositis may be patchy. To identify abnormal muscle, MRI may be needed before biopsy.[2]

On skin biopsy, characteristic features are perivascular lymphocytic infiltrate in dermis and mild atrophy of epidermis, which is difficult to distinguish from systemic lupus erythematosus (SLE).[3]

Electromyography is helpful for diagnosis. Creatinine kinase level is raised typically but may be normal, especially in amyopathic variety of dermatomyositis as in our case. Underlying malignancy can be associated, so screening should be done routinely.[2]

Autoantibodies should be checked. ANA is commonly found. Anti-Jo-1, anti-Mi-2, anti-TIF-1γ antibodies may be found.[4]

Treatment options are medication, physical therapy and exercise. Medications include corticosteroid, immunosuppressant such as methotrexate, azathioprine, cyclophosphamide, cyclosporine, tacrolimus. Intravenous immunoglobulin is helpful.[1]

REFERENCES

1. NINDS Dermatomyositis Information Page. National Institute of Neurological Disorders and Stroke (NINDS). August 2011; https://www.ninds.nih.gov/Disorders/All-Disorders/Inflammatory-Myopathies-Information-Page.
2. Ralston SH, Penman ID, Strachan MWJ, et al. Davidson's Principles and Practice of Medicine. 23rd ed. Edinburgh: Churchill Livingstone/Elsevier; 2018.
3. Miller ML. Diagnosis and differential diagnosis of dermatomyositis and polymyositis in adults. In: UpToDate, Post TW (Ed). UpToDate, Waltham, MA. (Accessed on March 1, 2016). www.uptodate.com
4. McHugh NJ, Tansley SL. Autoantibodies in myositis. Nat Rev Rheumatol. https://doi.org/10.1038/nrrheum.2018.56 (2018).

CASE 74

YOUNG GIRL WITH HEMIPARESIS AND EPILEPSY

CASE SUMMARY

A 15-year-old girl with a long 9 years' history of recurrent seizures presented with progressive weakness of the right side of the body for the last 3 months prior to admission. At her 6 years of age, her mother first noticed several episodes of blanking out 2-3 times daily when she abruptly stopped all activities for about 10 seconds followed by rapid return to full consciousness. The first generalized convulsion occurred 1.5 months later of this incidence which involved all four limbs, jerky in nature with upward rolling of eyeballs and frothy discharge from mouth. Each episode lasted for 1-2 minutes and she remained confused for about next 30 minutes but was never unconscious. For these complaints, she got admitted in Dhaka Medical College and Hospital (DMCH) about 2 years back and it was diagnosed as primary epilepsy and was discharged with antiepileptic drugs and was seizure-free for the next 6 months. At one point of time, she stopped taking all the medications and again started having convulsions which were of similar character as in the past. Seven months later, she became sick with development of high-grade continued fever with disorientation, irrelevant talk and double vision but her condition improved after a few days. Later, she was readmitted in the DMCH with progressive weakness of right side of her body. On query, she did not give any history of trauma, headache, nausea, vomiting, rash, bowel, bladder disturbances, abnormal movement, visual impairment, jaundice, weight loss or joint pain. She had normal developmental milestones and had been fully immunized as a child. Her age of menarche was 14 years and menstrual cycle was irregular. There was no family history of seizure disorder, or of any other familial illness.

On general examination, she was well behaved, cooperative, with average body build. Pulse rate was 72 beats/min and blood pressure was 130/80 mm Hg. There was a hypopigmented macule on lower part of the back 3 cm in size, ill-defined, nontender, non-itchy and not anesthetic (Fig. 1). Examination of nervous system revealed mini-mental state examination score 24 out of 30. Fundoscopy was normal as were the cranial nerves. Bulk

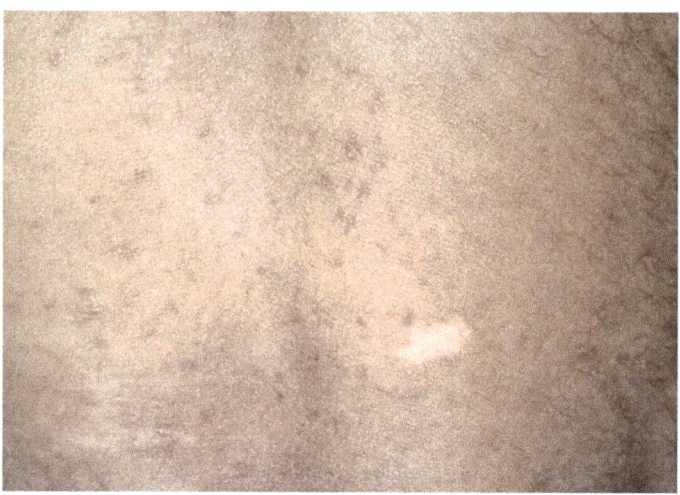

Fig. 1: Hypopigmented macule on lower part of the back.

of muscle was normal, tone increased in right side, power of muscle on right side of the body was 3/5, all reflexes in right side were exaggerated, clonus was absent, plantar response was extensor on right side, gait was of spastic variety. Sensory modalities were intact, cerebellar function test was normal; signs of meningeal irritation were absent. Examination of respiratory and cardiovascular systems was otherwise unremarkable.

Investigations showed, Hb—12.3 g/dL; peripheral blood film (PBF)—normocytic normochromic red blood cells with matured white blood cells and normal platelet counts; erythrocyte sedimentation rate (ESR) in first hour—5 mm; calcium—9.6 mg/dL, with normal albumin level; serum inorganic phosphate—4.9 mg/dL; serum creatinine—0.67 mg/dL, intact parathyroid hormone—19.6 pg/mL. Anti-phospholipid antibody and antinuclear antibody (ANA) were all negative. Computed tomography (CT) scan of head—multifocal calcified subependymal nodules in both lateral ventricles, diffuse asymmetrical deep white matter hypodensity in both (left> right) cerebral hemisphere with mild midline shift. Magnetic resonance imaging (MRI) of brain (Fig. 2)—intense gyral enhancement in both frontal and left parietal lobe with profuse perilesional edema causing ipsilateral ventricular compression and contralateral midline shift. Tiny subependymal signal void areas are noted along the outer wall of right lateral ventricle which corresponds with CT-detected calcified nodules.

QUESTIONS

1. What is the most likely diagnosis?
2. What further investigations should be performed to confirm the diagnosis?

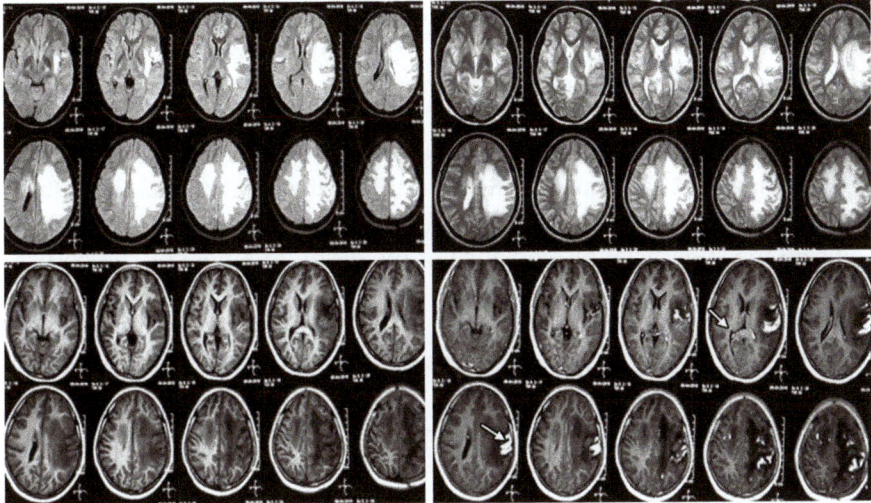

Fig. 2: MRI of brain: T1, T1 with contrast (below), T2 and FLAIR sequences (above) showing tiny subependymal signal void area along the outer wall of right lateral ventricle and intense gyral enhancement in both frontal and left parietal lobes.

DISCUSSION

If we consider the presentation of a young girl with a long history of repeated seizures, and right-sided hemiparesis, several differentials come in mind like intracranial space-occupying lesion, antiphospholipid syndrome (APS), systemic lupus erythematosus (SLE) and postencephalitic syndrome. But absence of other clinical clues, nonspecific finding in CBC and PBF, normal metabolic profile, negative ANA, anti-dsDNA and antiphospholipid antibody, ruled out all these possibilities.

There are several clues in this case: Epilepsy, presence of hypopigmented macule in back and subependymal nodule in the lateral ventricles in brain—suggesting tuberous sclerosis, a neurocutaneous disorder. Then we searched for other components of tuberous sclerosis.

Ultrasonography (USG) of the W/A—normal study of hepatobiliary system (HBS), kidneys, ureter and bladder—uterus-adnexa and retroperitoneal structures; electrocardiogram—normal. Echocardiography—a large heterogeneous mass in left ventricle apex suggestive of intracardiac tumor (rhabdomyoma). Wood's lamp exam of hypomelanotic macule reveals typical ash-leaf appearance.

Taking into consideration the radiological findings of CT scan and MRI of brain, cardiac rhabdomyoma on echocardiography and ash-leaf macule (or nevus depigmentosus) under Wood's light examination, the patient was diagnosed as a case of tuberous sclerosis.[1]

Final Diagnosis: Tuberous Sclerosis

Tuberous sclerosis (also known as tuberous sclerosis complex, TSC) is a multisystem genetic disorder affecting cellular differentiation, proliferation and migration early in development. It results in a variety of hamartomatous lesions to grow predominantly in the brain and also in other vital organs of the body such as the kidneys, heart, eyes, lungs and skin. In 1880, a French physician, Bourneville, first described the cerebral manifestations of this disorder applying the term "sclerose (hard) tubereuse (swelling)" to indicate the superficial resemblance of the lesion to a potato. The cortical manifestations may sometimes still be known by the eponym "Bourneville's Disease." TSC can present at any age and both sexes are equally affected.[2]

According to the Diagnostic Criteria Committee of the National Tuberous Sclerosis Association (USA):[3]

Major features of TSC include the following:
- Facial angiofibromas or forehead plaque
- Nontraumatic ungual or periungual fibroma
- Hypomelanotic macules (>3)—to be confirmed by Wood's light or UV light.
- Shagreen patch (connective tissue nevus)
- Multiple retinal nodular hamartoma
- Cortical tubers
- Subependymal nodule
- Subependymal giant cell astrocytoma
- Cardiac rhabdomyoma, single or multiple
- Lymphangioleiomyomatosis
- Renal angiomyolipoma.

Minor features of TSC include the following:
- Multiple randomly distributed pits in dental enamel
- Hamartomatous rectal polyps: Histologic confirmation is suggested.
- Bone cysts: Radiographic confirmation is sufficient.
- Non-calcified subependymal nodules
- Gingival fibromas
- Non-renal hamartoma: Histologic confirmation is suggested.
- Retinal achromic patch
- "Confetti" skin lesions
- Multiple renal cysts.

The following are the diagnostic criteria for TSC:[3]
- *Definite TSC:* 2 major features or 1 major feature plus 2 or more minor features
- *Possible TSC:* Either 1 major feature or 2 or more minor features.

Diagnosis should be possible in most cases using established clinical criteria. Molecular genetic testing is useful in uncertain or questionable cases, for pre-natal diagnosis and for screening family members of an affected individual. Under optimal circumstances, genetic testing identifies mutations in up to 75-80% of affected individuals. Therefore, a negative genetic diagnostic test result does not exclude the diagnosis. But the utility of molecular testing is limited by the cost.

There is no complete cure of tuberous sclerosis, although treatment is available for a number of symptoms. Antiepileptic drugs (AEDs) are the main-stay of therapy for patients with TSC. The choice of AED for treating seizures is based on the patient's seizure type, age of the patient, AED side effect profile and formulations available. In some rare cases, surgery may be required to remove the tumors if they begin to seriously affect the function of the heart or lung. Rapamycin or sirolimus may be effective to shrink the lung tumor.[4]

The prognosis of TSC is highly variable and depends on the severity of symptoms. Those individuals with mild symptoms usually do well and have a normal life expectancy. Individuals who are severely affected can suffer from severe mental retardation and persistent epilepsy. Of the severe cases, approximately, 30% die before the fifth year, 50-75% before attaining adult age.[5]

REFERENCES

1. Sarker P, Akhter S, Rahman MS, et al. A young girl with tuberous sclerosis presenting with recurrent episodes of convulsion & right sided hemiparesis. JOM [Internet]. 23Oct.2016 [cited 15Apr.2019];17(2):125–9. Available from: https://www.banglajol.info/index.php/JOM/article/view/30080
2. Ownes J, Bodenstener JB. Tuberous sclerosis complex: Genetics, clinical features and diagnosis. UpToDate: Updated 2015-06-16.
3. Franz DN, Thomas CW. Tuberous Sclerosis. Medscape: updated 2015-10-14.
4. Ishii M, Asano K, Kamishi N, et al. Tuberous Sclerosis diagnosed by incidental CT findings multifocal micronodular pneumocyte hyperplasia—a case report. J Med Case Rep; 2012. pp. 352–6.
5. Zarei M, Collins VP, Chandran S, et al. Tuberous sclerosis present in late adult life. J Neurol Neurosurg Psychiatry. 2002;73:436–40.

CASE 75

YOUNG MALE WITH FLUCTUATING FEVER AND MYALGIA

CASE SUMMARY

A 25-year-old male came to Bangladesh from Riyadh, Kingdom of Saudi Arabia, presented with fever for the past 3 months which was initially high grade, later became low grade in nature and was associated with chills and rigor and had two peaks in 24 hours. The first peak used to come around 2 pm and tended to persist for 2-3 hours. Another peak of fever usually came around 8:00 pm which persisted for 8-10 hours. Fever used to subside with profuse sweating. He consulted with a doctor in Saudi Arabia and received antipyretic and some antibiotics. He was afebrile for 5-6 days, but fever reappeared in the previous pattern. He also had nonspecific myalgia, anorexia, nausea, constipation, and weight loss of about 6 kg in last 3 months. On query, he mentioned about recurrent oral ulceration involving buccal mucosa and tip of the tongue for the last 5-6 years which resolved spontaneously after few days. But during this febrile period it became more frequent, severe and painful in nature, interfering with deglutition. The patient went to Saudi Arabia 5 years back. At first, he worked in an animal farm for 4 years where he used to work in processing of meat products of goat, cattle and chicken. Later, he worked in a restaurant as a cook for 7 months. Lately, he had been living in Saudi Arabia and running his own business of courier service there. He had no history of blood transfusion or intravenous (IV) drug abuse.

On examination, he was ill-looking, vitals were within normal limit except temperature was 101°F, two healed oral ulcers were present on buccal mucosa. Abdominal examination revealed 8 cm firm, nontender hepatomegaly 4 cm firm, nontender splenomegaly. The rest of the examination was normal.

Investigation showed, complete blood count (CBC) with erythrocyte sedimentation rate (ESR) was normal. Peripheral blood film (PBF); urine routine examination (R/E); serum creatinine; serum electrolyte; liver function test (LFT); chest X-ray (CXR) were normal. Blood and urine culture and sensitivity (C/S) showed no growth. Ultrasonography (USG) of the whole abdomen (W/A) showed hepatomegaly with homogeneous parenchyma and splenomegaly. Viral markers including HBsAg, anti-hepatitis C virus (HCV) antibody (Ab), anti-HIV 1 and 2 were negative. Serum antinuclear antibodies (ANA)—negative.

QUESTIONS

1. What is the most likely diagnosis?
2. What further investigations would you like to do to reach a final diagnosis?
3. How the patient should be treated?

DISCUSSION

This young man who came from Saudi Arabia, had prolonged fever, weight loss, used to work in meat processing and had hepatosplenomegaly; all raised strong suspicion of having brucellosis. So, further investigations done in this patient:
- Agglutination test for *Brucella abortus* and *Brucella melitensis*: 1:1280 and 1:1280.

Final Diagnosis: Brucellosis

The patient was treated by injectable gentamicin for 7 days and oral doxycycline for 6 weeks.[1] After starting antibiotics, regular follow-up of the patient was done to see the treatment response. After getting treatment for nearly 3 weeks, patient became afebrile, and his general condition improved. No organomegaly was found during physical examination.
- *Repeat USG* showed liver size had become normal, spleen was mildly enlarged.
- *Repeat agglutination test for Brucella abortus and Brucella melitensis:* 1:320.

Brucellosis is a zoonotic disease. It is caused by *Brucella* which is a gram-negative coccobacilli. There are four species responsible for human disease: B. melitensis (goat, sheep and camel), B. suis (pig), B. abortus (cattle) and B. canis (dog). It is called undulant fever as the fever rises and falls like a wave—typically in an undulant manner.

Transmission can occur by following ways: Through cuts and abrasions of the skin, ingestion of unpasteurized dairy products or raw meat, inhalation of infected aerosols and via the conjunctiva.

Symptoms of brucellosis are often nonspecific. Most commonly patient presents with fever. Other symptoms include malaise, sweats, anorexia, fatigue, arthralgia and weight loss.

For diagnosis, serum agglutination test is most commonly done. Titer above 1:160 is considered diagnostic if it is associated with compatible clinical picture. Cultures generally become positive after several weeks, as *Brucella* tends to grow slowly in conventional culture media.

Brucellosis can present with imprecise clinical symptoms, so diagnosis may become challenging. Early recognition and prompt treatment is necessary to prevent the complications.

REFERENCE

1. Ralston SH, Penman ID , Strachan MWJ, et al. Davidson's Principles and Practice of Medicine. 23rd ed. Edinburgh: Churchill Livingstone/Elsevier; 2018. p. 255.

CASE 76

YOUNG BOY WITH LAX SKIN

CASE SUMMARY

A 16-year-old young boy, second child of consanguineous marriage was admitted with complaints of swelling in the right armpit and over the right thigh for 9 months and wrinkling and laxity of skin for 1.5 months. The swellings were initially small and mobile but gradually increased in size. Two months later, he developed the same type of swelling in the left buttock. With these complaints, he was admitted in a tertiary care hospital and went through incision and drainage. Following the procedure, he developed multiple confluent papules mainly in both the armpits, flexural aspect of both elbow joints, groins, both thighs, upper part of both legs, both angles of lip and left side of the neck. They were painless but associated with itching. He also experienced wrinkling of the skin over the left thigh and laxity of the skin of both armpits, flexural surface of elbow joint and groins. There was hyperkeratosis involving upper part of both thighs but there was no scarring, cicatrization, discharge or bleeding. He gave no history of chest pain, abdominal pain, joint pain, visual disturbance or bleeding from any sites. No past history of tuberculosis or history of contact with tuberculosis (TB) patient. None of his family members is affected. Few years back he was surgically treated to remove mesenchymal tumor from right armpit and both elbow joints in abroad.

On examination, there was yellowish papulonodular skin lesion involving both angles of the lip. These yellow colored/erythematous papules coalesced to form larger plaque giving the skin a plucked-chicken appearance over the left lateral surface of the neck, axillae, antecubital fossae, groins, upper part of both thighs and legs. There were folds of loose skin over the axillae, antecubital fossae and groins sparing the neck area (Figs. 1A and B). There was wrinkling of the skin over the left thigh. Skin under the right thigh was found hard. There were scar marks over both the elbow joints suggesting previous surgery with evidence of impaired wound healing. There was a swelling in the upper

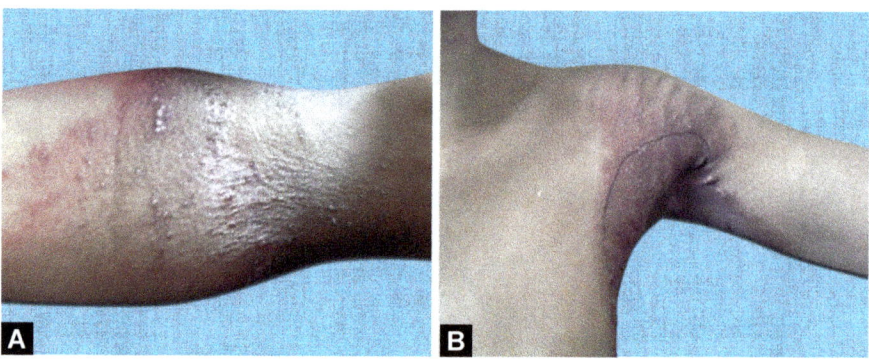

Figs. 1A and B: Plucked-chicken appearance over: (A) Antecubital fossa; (B) Folds of loose skin over the axilla.

part of left thigh near the anterior superior iliac spine which was nontender, ill-defined, approximately about 5 × 5 cm and soft in consistency; overlying skin was slightly erythematous. Another nontender, ill-defined swelling was noted in the left gluteal region measuring about 9 × 7 cm, which was firm in consistency. Fundoscopic examination revealed evidence of angioid streaks in both fundi. Other systemic examination findings were unremarkable.

Investigations showed: Hb%—70, erythrocyte sedimentation rate (ESR) in first hour—48 mm, white blood cells (WBCs)—13,000/mm^3 (N: 78%, L: 17%), platelet (PLT)—180,000/mm^3, hepatitis B surface antigen (HBsAg)—negative, antihepatitis C virus (anti-HCV) antibody—negative, MT—2 mm, chest X-ray (CXR) posteroanterior view—normal, ultrasonography (USG) of W/A—normal, pus from abscess for culture and sensitivity (C/S)—yielded no growth, electrocardiography (ECG), and echocardiogram were normal. Histopathology of skin from axilla—chronic abscess with dystrophic calcification, thigh tissue for histopathology—compatible with chronic abscess, bone scintigraphy—there were two big irregular area of increased radiotracer concentration noted in left upper thigh and right axillary region with adjacent upper part of right anterior chest wall suggestive of soft tissue uptake of bony tracer in primary lesions due to *dystrophic calcification.*

QUESTIONS

1. Is there any investigation which is needed further for this case?
2. What is the most likely diagnosis?
3. How would you follow up this case?

DISCUSSION

To confirm our clinical diagnosis, we decided to perform skin biopsy and color fundal photograph. Skin biopsy revealed perforating pseudoxanthoma

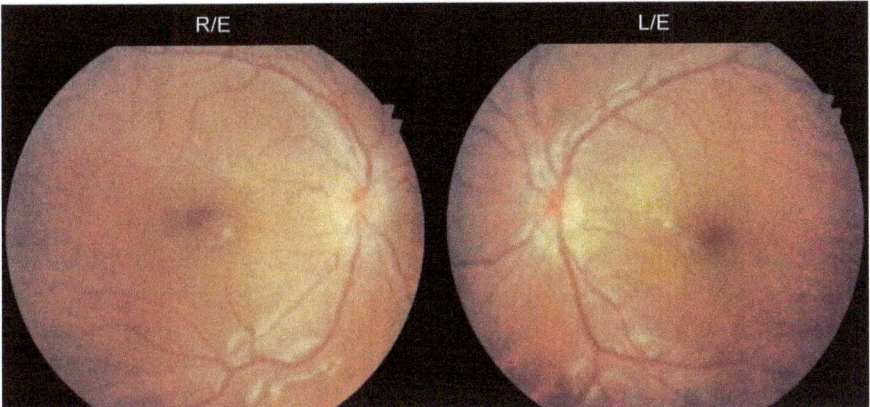

Fig. 2: Color fundal photograph showing angioid streaks.

elasticum (PXE), color fundal photograph and fundus fluorescein angiography revealed angioid streaks (Fig. 2).

Final Diagnosis: Pseudoxanthoma Elasticum with Mesenchymal Tumor

Pseudoxanthoma elasticum (also called Gronblad-Strandberg syndrome) is a hereditary multisystem disorder which is characterized by pathological calcification of the elastic connective tissue. It mostly affects the skin, eyes (Bruch's membrane of retina) and cardiovascular system.[1]

It follows autosomal dominant pattern in majority of the cases (about 90%). There is a mutation in gene *ABCC6* situated in the short arm of chromosome 16.

Pseudoxanthoma elasticum (PXE) is diagnosed by:
- Pathogenic mutations in the *ABCC6* or
- Ocular findings—angioid streaks >1 disk diameter (DD) or
- Peau d'orange in an individual <20 years of age together with characteristic pseudoxanthomatous papules and plaques on the neck or flexural creases in skin and diagnostic histopathological changes in lesional skin: calcified elastic fibers in the mid and lower dermis, confirmed by positive calcium stain.[2]

Our patient had eye findings along with skin findings making it a definite case of PXE.

Note that if definitive findings are present only in the skin or eyes, the presence of two pathogenic *ABCC6* mutations revealed by subsequent genetic testing would confirm the diagnosis of PXE even in the absence of a complete phenotype.

Without having met the above criteria, a patient could be considered to have "possible PXE."

It is suggested to do complete blood count (CBC) and occult fecal blood test every 6 months to 1 year to look for any gastrointestinal (GI) bleeding.

An ophthalmologic examination should be carried out at least once a year to detect early changes like retinopathy, angioid streaks or retinal hemorrhage.

Cardiovascular system should be examined with special attention to check out for any mitral valve insufficiency, coronary artery disease or peripheral vascular disease.

There is no definite treatment. Associated comorbid conditions, for example, diabetes mellitus, dyslipidemia and hypertension mainly due to premature atherosclerosis should be managed appropriately with care. Contact sports should be avoided and analgesics particularly nonsteroidal anti-inflammatory drugs (NSAIDs), aspirin and anticoagulants must be used with caution due to risk of hemorrhage. Smoking cessation should also be encouraged. Affected individuals must not take calcium more than their recommended daily allowance, particularly during childhood and adolescence.

REFERENCES

1. Bercovitch L, Terry P. Pseudoxanthomaelasticum 2004. J Am Acad Dermatol. 2004;51(1):13-4.
2. Marconi B, Bobyr I, Campanati A, et al. Intractable Rare Dis Res. 2015;4(3):113-22.

CASE 77

YOUNG BOY WITH RECURRENT BLEEDING DIATHESIS

CASE SUMMARY

An 18-year-old male student, first issue of a consanguineous marriage, presented with the complaints of hematemesis and melena for 2 days. He had history of excessive bleeding during attempted circumcision, on the background of spontaneous gum bleeding, epistaxis and easy bruising since childhood. With the course of time, bleeding increased in frequency and amount and the boy became pale and fatigued and received blood transfusion on several occasions. Then prior to admission, he suddenly developed hematemesis and melena 3 times in last 2 days, and subsequently, he became dizzy and weak. He denied history of hemarthrosis, muscle hematoma, hemoptysis, or hematuria. He did not have jaundice, fever, weight loss and loss of consciousness or any visual abnormality. He did not take any drugs such as aspirin, other nonsteroidal anti-inflammatory drugs (NSAIDs), clopidogrel, warfarin, or heparin prior to this incidence. There was no such illness in his family members.

On examination, he was ill-looking and severely anemic. His pulse was 104 beats/min, blood pressure: 90/60 mm Hg, temperature: 97°F, and respiratory rate: 20 breaths/min. There was no purpuric spot, lymphadenopathy or bony tenderness. Other systemic examinations findings were unremarkable.

The patient's complete blood count (CBC) on admission showed hemoglobin (Hb): 5.3 g/dL, mean corpuscular volume (MCV): 81.9 fL, mean corpuscular hemoglobin (MCH): 24 pg, hematocrit: 18.1%, white blood cell (WBC): 10,190/mm^3, platelet: 155,000/mm^3, erythrocyte sedimentation rate (ESR): 40 mm in first hour. The corresponding peripheral blood film (PBF) commented normocytic, normochromic anemia with plenty polychromatic cells. Iron profile revealed low-serum iron (60 µg/dL), ferritin: 80.1 µg/L, total iron binding capacity (TIBC): 246 µg/dL, transferrin saturation: 24.39%. His random blood sugar (RBS), urinalysis, creatinine, serum uric acid, serum electrolytes, abdominal ultrasonogram and upper gastrointestinal tract (GIT) endoscopy reports revealed no abnormality. Bleeding time (BT) was 15 minutes (prolonged), prothrombin time (PT): 12 seconds (normal), activated partial thromboplastin time (APTT): 28 seconds (normal).

QUESTIONS

1. What are the differential diagnoses?
2. Which investigations should be carried out to confirm the diagnosis?

DISCUSSION

Considering the history and physical examination and after doing initial investigations, our differentials in this case were:
- Von Willebrand disease
- Hemophilia
- Hereditary platelet functional disorder.

We went for coagulation factor assay: von Willebrand factor (vWF): 100%, factor VII: 80% and factor IX: 90%. Ristocetin cofactor was also normal. Though bleeding time was prolonged but normal vWF excluded the possibility of von Willebrand disease. Negative family history, normal APTT, and normal factor VIII level also excluded hemophilia as underlying cause.

Since no coagulation abnormality was found and bleeding time was prolonged, we searched for platelet function disorders and sent blood for clot retraction test; results revealed: there was *no retraction of clot observed in 1 hour, 2 hours, and 24 hours, note: suggestive of a platelet functional disorder—Glanzmann's thrombasthenia (GT) or due to antiplatelet drug.* Platelet aggregation test showed absence of both primary and secondary waves in response to all agonists: collagen, epinephrine and adenosine diphosphate (ADP); interpretation: *suggestive of Glanzmann's thrombasthenia.*

Final Diagnosis: Glanzmann's Thrombasthenia

Glanzmann's thrombasthenia (GT) is an exceptionally rare autosomal recessive coagulopathy affecting the megakaryocyte lineage resulting in failure of platelet aggregation. Here, there is qualitative or quantitative deficiency of integrin $\alpha IIb\beta 3$ [previously called glycoprotein IIb/IIIa (GpIIb/IIIa)] of platelets, which is an integrin aggregation receptor (also called the fibrinogen receptor). It is activated when the platelet comes in contact with collagen, ADP, epinephrine or thrombin. Integrin $\alpha IIb\beta 3$ is essential to blood coagulation, as when activated, it can bind fibrinogen (as well as vWF, fibronectin and vitronectin), which is key to fibrinogen-dependent platelet aggregation. As a result, in its absence the bleeding time is significantly prolonged.

Some patients of GT present with trivial bruising while others have drastic presentation. The site of bleeding is conspicuous: gingival hemorrhage, epistaxis, purpura and menorrhagia are almost constant features while bleeding from alimentary or urinary tracts is less frequent. Typically, as in our case, bleeding manifestations occur briskly after birth, but GT remains undiagnosed until later life.[1]

Glanzmann's thrombasthenia should be kept in mind for patients with mucocutaneous bleeding with a normal platelet count and morphology, but lack of platelet aggregation in response to all stimuli. Flow cytometry should be used to detect platelet $\alpha IIb\beta 3$ deficiency or nonfunction. Therapeutic management should include, if possible, local hemostasis and/or desmopressin (DDAVP) administration to avoid platelet alloimmunization. If these fail, or as per-operative safety preparation, transfusion of human leukocyte antigen (HLA)-compatible platelet concentrates may be given. Another increasingly used therapeutic alternative is recombinant factor VIIa. Though GT is a potentially life-threatening hemorrhagic disease, if we can provide vigilant supportive care, the prognosis is excellent.[2]

REFERENCES

1. Nurden AT, George JN. Hemostasis and Thrombosis, Basic Principles, and Clinical Practice. 6th ed. Philadelphia: Lippincott, Williams & Wilkins; 2005. pp. 987–1010.
2. Nurden AT. Glanzmann thrombasthenia. Orphanet J Rare Dis. 2006;1:10. [internet] Available from: https://doi.org/10.1186/1750-1172-1-10

CASE 78

YOUNG LADY HAVING RECURRENT LUMP IN THE ABDOMEN

CASE SUMMARY

A 26-year-old woman was admitted with complaints of recurrent episodes of feeling of lump in the upper abdomen for 6 years. Initially, she had a feeling of lump in the epigastrium which was gradually increasing in size. It was associated with right hypochondriac pain which was lancinating in nature, and persisted throughout the day without any radiation. She consulted with a registered surgeon and the lump was diagnosed as hepatic hydatid cyst; she underwent operation and was prescribed albendazole tablet twice daily for 3 months. Unfortunately, similar symptoms came back after 8 months. Again she was diagnosed as a case of hydatid cyst in the liver and went through operation named complete excision of hydatid cyst, endocystectomy with open cholecystectomy for the second time and discharged with albendazole tablet once daily for 3 months. A computed tomography (CT) scan of the whole abdomen was done which showed post operative state of hydatid cyst. Unfortunately, she became symptomatic again after 6 years. She experienced heaviness in the upper abdomen along with pain which was associated with anorexia and nausea. Other systemic queries and signs were unremarkable. She belonged to a lower middle-class family and there was history of handling dogs and cats around home.

On examination, there was an oblique scar in the upper part of the abdomen about 7 cm extending from epigastrium to right hypochondrium. There was non-tender hepatomegaly about 4 cm from right costal margin, firm in consistency, margin was regular, surface smooth and no hepatic bruit. Other findings were unremarkable.

Investigations showed Hb%—11.9 g/dL, white blood cells (WBCs)—8,000/mm^3 (N: 58%, L: 38%, E: 1%), platelet (PLT)—300,000/mm^3, erythrocyte sedimentation rate (ESR) in the first hour—40 mm, urine R/M/E—pus cell of 8-10/HPF with trace albumin, serum creatinine—0.9 mg/dL, serum bilirubin—0.72 mg/dL, alanine aminotransferase (ALT)—52 U/L, alkaline phosphatase—113 U/L, and this time ultrasonography (USG) of whole abdomen showed multiple hepatic cysts.

QUESTIONS

1. What are the further investigations?
2. How would you manage this case?

DISCUSSION

Based on the history, it was an obvious case of recurrent hydatid cyst. The main challenge remained on management part for this particular case. Subsequent investigations done to manage this case were as follows:

CT scan showed two hepatic cysts in both lobes of liver—suggestive of recurrence.

A conventional magnetic resonance imaging (MRI) showed one fluid signal intensity cystic lesion measuring about 4.4 × 3.6 cm in size in left lobe and 4.6 × 3.2 cm in size in right lobe of the liver—recurrence of hydatid cyst (Fig. 1A). Magnetic resonance cholangiopancreatography (MRCP) revealed no definite abnormality. Anti-*Echinococcus* antibody was positive.

Final Diagnosis: Recurrent Hepatic Hydatid Cysts

She was advised for surgery for the third time. However, she denied and looked for other options. We went for percutaneous aspiration-injection-reaspiration (PAIR) and, microscopic examination of aspirated fluid revealed brood capsule, scolex and hooklets (Fig. 1B). She was put on combination chemotherapy with praziquantel tablet 40 mg/kg body weight twice weekly

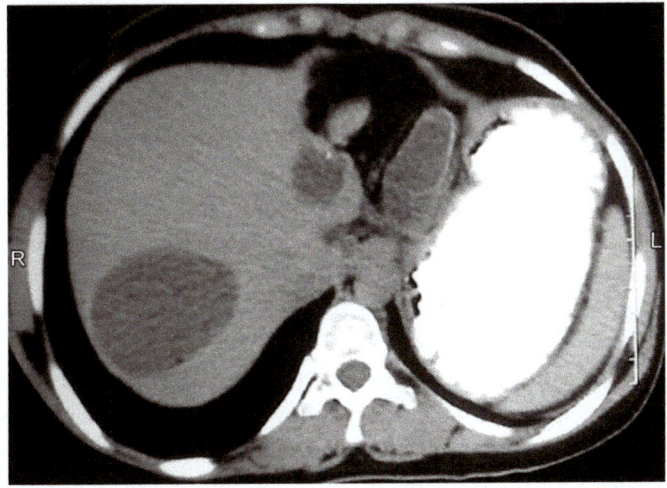

Fig. 1A

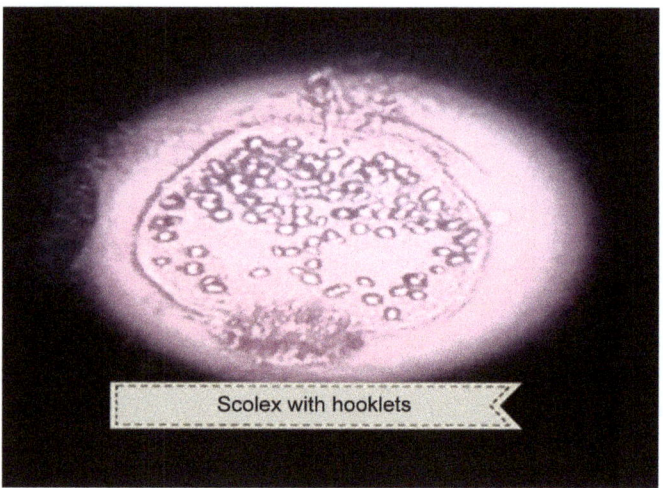

Fig. 1B

Figs. 1A and B: (A) Magnetic resonance imaging showing hepatic cyst; (B) Aspiration of cyst revealed brood capsule, scolex and hooklets of *Echinococcus granulosus*.

plus albendazole tablet 400 mg twice daily for 28 days for three cycles with 2 weeks gap in between. She was regularly followed up with USG of whole abdomen after completion of each cycle. It was noteworthy that she exhibited significant improvement without further recurrence.

Human hydatid disease or cystic echinococcosis (CE) is a parasitic infection caused by the larval form of cestode, *Echinococcus granulosus*. It primarily affects the population of developing countries.[1] In human, the most frequently affected organ is the liver. It is a challenging clinical problem throughout the world. Specially, recurrent hepatic hydatid cyst is one of the difficult entities to manage.

Thorough clinical history, meticulous clinical examination and serological testing (negative in 10–20% of cases) have pivotal role in reaching diagnosis.[1]

The routine blood tests are insignificant. Eosinophilia may be present. Hypogammaglobulinemia is present in 30% cases. Leukocytosis indicates cystic infection.[2]

Imaging studies like ultrasound, CT scan and MRI are the key tools for diagnosing hepatic hydatid cyst. The pathognomonic finding is that of daughter cyst within the larger cyst.[1,3,4]

Currently, ultrasound staging is recommended for *E. granulosus* infections for treatment purpose.

Surgical intervention is the primary treatment option for hydatid disease.

In our case, conservative surgery followed by chemotherapy was given twice. Unfortunately, she came up with the third recurrence. Overall, the recurrence rate appears to be high (4.6–22.0%) after surgical intervention.[1]

We preferred combination chemotherapy (albendazole plus praziquantel) in our case.

Disease recurrence can be reduced by combined therapy.[5] Intraperitoneal seeding of infection may develop by spontaneous spillage or during intervention (surgery or percutaneous procedures).

REFERENCES

1. Pakala T, Molina M, Wu GY. Hepatic echinococcal cysts: a review. J Clin Tran Hepatol. 2016;4(1):39-46. doi:10.14218/JCTH.2015.00036
2. Kasper DL, Fauci AS, Hauser SL, et al. Harrison's Principles of Internal Medicine. 19th ed. New York: McGraw Hill Education; 2015. pp. 1759-65.
3. Raymond A, Smego Jr. Treatment options for hepatic cystic echinococcosis. Int J Infect Dis. 2005;9(2):69-76.
4. Kumar A, Lal BK, Chattapodhay TK. Hydatid disease of the liver—non-surgical options. J Assoc Physicians India. 1993;41:437-43.
5. Fenton-Lee D, Morris DL. The management of hydatid disease of the liver. Part 2. Trop Doct. 1997;27:82-8.

CASE 79

YOUNG FEMALE WITH COUGH AND RAYNAUD'S PHENOMENON

CASE SUMMARY

A 40-year-old housewife presented with bluish discoloration of both hands and feet on cold exposure and water contact for last 2.5 years and cough with exertional dyspnea for 1 year. In the beginning, she noticed color change of both hands and feet on exposure to water and cold, usually starting from fingers and toes. On exposure, the fingers and toes became pale at first followed by bluish coloration that spread all over the hands and feet involving the hands more than the feet. Later, the bluish coloration turned into reddish either spontaneously or by rewarming with rubbing or hot compression. She also complained of recurrent episodes of large joint pain involving the upper limb more. The pain was symmetrical without any joint swelling and no axial involvement and usually subsided spontaneously or with medication. She also noticed occasional itchy cutaneous rashes on sun exposure in exposed areas of body including face and progressively increasing cough aggravated by eating or drinking. It was also associated with occasional exertional breathlessness but no history of hemoptysis, chest pain, any swallowing difficulty or skin change was found. Her bowel and bladder habits were normal. She was normotensive, nondiabetic, nonasthmatic and nonsmoker.

General examination of the patient was unremarkable except she had clubbing. Musculoskeletal system examination including gait, spine, Schober's test, and of all four limbs were normal. On respiratory system examination, the patient was dyspneic; respiratory rate was 20 breaths/min with symmetrical chest movement and expansibility. The chest was resonant on percussion but on auscultation there were fine crackles on both lower zones. Other system examinations were unremarkable.

Investigations showed complete blood count (CBC): Hemoglobin (Hb) 12.10 g/dL, erythrocyte sedimentation rate (ESR) 64 mm in first hour, white blood count (WBC) 7,000/mm^3 (N—70%, L—23%, M—03%, E—04%, B—0%), platelet count—312,000/mm^3, random blood sugar (RBS)—9.8 mmol/L, serum creatinine—0.9 mg/dL, urine routine examination (R/E)—normal except epithelial cell: 20–30/high-power field (HPF) and urinary total protein (UTP)—0.36 g/24 hours. Chest X-ray of the patient was suggestive of bilateral inflammatory pulmonary lesions. Ultrasonogram of whole abdomen was normal. Creatine phosphokinase (CPK), antinuclear antibody (ANA), and anti-double stranded DNA (anti-dsDNA) were done, where CPK was 49 U/L and ANA was positive but anti-dsDNA was negative.

QUESTIONS

1. What should be the next investigations to reach a diagnosis?
2. What would be the final diagnosis?

DISCUSSION

Considering the patient's clinical presentation, extractable nuclear antigen (ENA) profile was done where only the anti-Smith antibody was positive.

High-resolution computed tomography (HRCT) of the chest showed extensive area of reticulation and septal thickenings in posterior basal segments of both lower lobes and ground-glass appearance in both mid-zones. The final impression of the HRCT was interstitial thickening of both lower lobes, possibly early diffuse parenchymal lung disease (DPLD) (Figs. 1A and B).

Final Diagnosis: Systemic Lupus Erythematosus with Diffuse Parenchymal Lung Disease (DPLD)

Systemic lupus erythematosus (SLE) is a chronic inflammatory disease that has protean manifestations and follows a relapsing and remitting course. Ninety percent of patients are female and the peak age of onset is between 20 years and 30 years.

The most common initial manifestation of SLE is arthralgia or arthritis. The classic presentation of a triad of fever, joint pain, and rash in young women should lead investigations into the diagnosis of SLE. However, patients may present with constitutional, musculoskeletal, dermatologic, renal, neuropsychiatric, pulmonary, gastrointestinal, cardiac and hematological manifestations.[1]

Pulmonary involvement is common in SLE and occurs in up to 50% of patients.[2] Pulmonary involvement can affect the pleura, airway, pulmonary vasculature and parenchyma. Pleurisy or pleural effusion is the most common pulmonary manifestation of SLE occurring in 30–60% cases, usually in long-standing cases.[2]

The presence of DPLD in SLE is rare, occurring only in 3–13% cases. It usually follows a benign course with a subacute to chronic presentation.

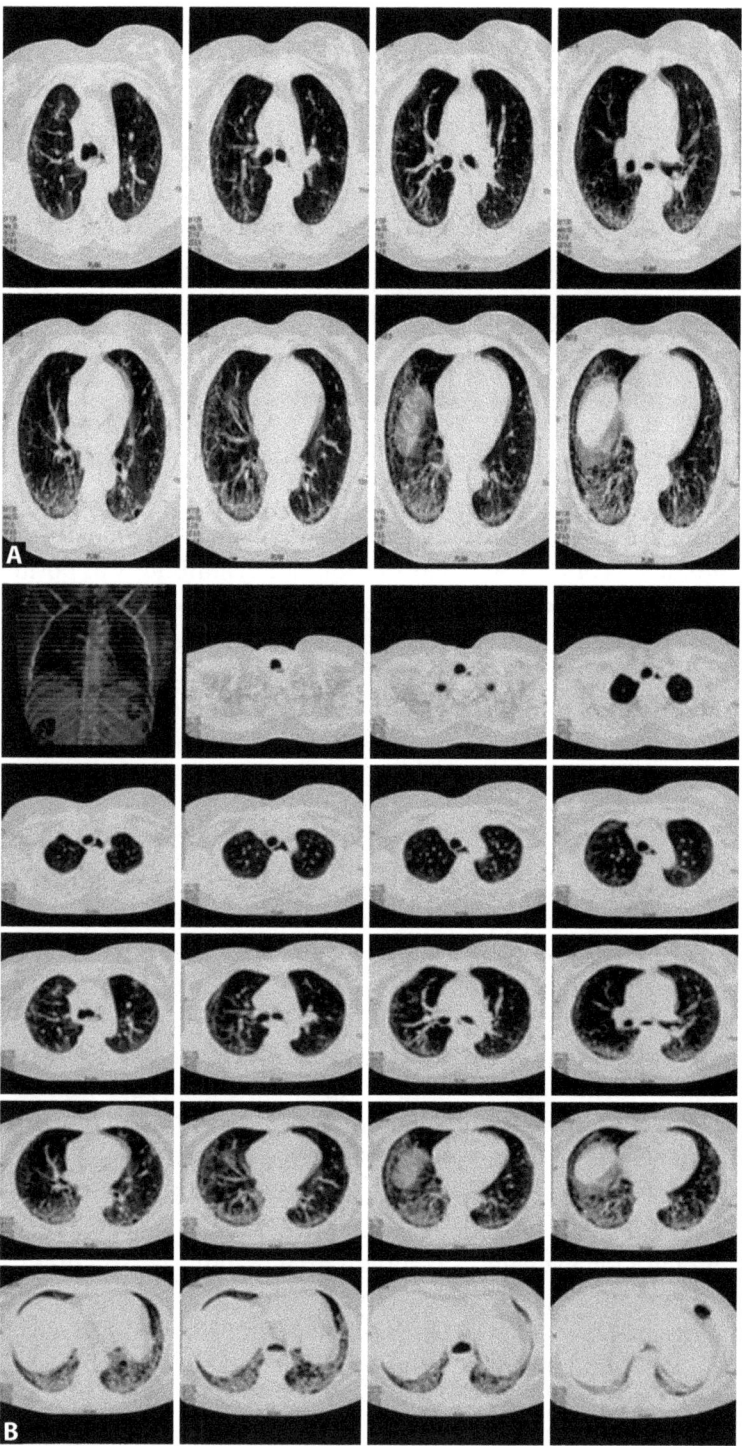

Figs. 1A and B: High-resolution computed tomography (HRCT) of chest showed interstitial thickening of both lower lobes, possibly early diffuse parenchymal lung disease (DPLD).

The onset is usually insidious, but it may be preceded by episode of acute pneumonitis. Patients present with chronic nonproductive cough, dyspnea, recurrent pleuritic chest pain and decreased exercise tolerance. Asymptomatic involvement is more common and abnormalities in pulmonary function tests are seen in the majority of patients with SLE in some studies.[2,3]

The presence of anti-Ro (anti-SSA) antibodies is considered to be a risk factor for SLE-associated chronic DPLD. In our patient, only ANA and anti-Smith antibody were positive.

HRCT may be extremely helpful in diagnosis of DPLD and two patterns are frequently seen: ground-glass appearance [consistent with biopsy showing cellular infiltrate, pattern of nonspecific interstitial pneumonia (NSIP)] or reticular appearance [consistent with biopsy showing fibrotic pattern, one seen in usual interstitial pneumonia (UIP)].[2-4]

An accurate diagnosis of the histopathological subtype of DPLD in SLE is important to guide prognosis and management. Although UIP and NSIP may be both responsive to corticosteroids, the prognosis in patients with NSIP is slightly better than UIP.

REFERENCES

1. Dubois EL, Tuffanelli Dl. Clinical manifestations of systemic lupus erythematosus. Computer analysis of 520 cases. JAMA. 1964;190:104–11.
2. Chakrabarti S, Pan K. First presentation of systemic lupus erythematosus as interstitial lung disease: A unique scenario. Saudi J Med Med Sci. 2015;3:84–7.
3. Clement A, Nathan N, Epaud R, et al. Interstitial lung diseases in children. Orphanet J Rare Dis. 2010;5:22. Published 2010 Aug 20. doi:10.1186/1750-1172-5-22
4. Cojocaru M, Cojocaru IM, Silosi I, et al. Manifestations of systemic lupus erythematosus. Maedica (Buchar). 2011;6(4):330-6.

CASE 80

MULTIPLE BEE STINGS WITH FATALITY IN A MIDDLE-AGED PATIENT

CASE SUMMARY

A 55-year-old male was admitted with a history of incurring multiple bee stings 7 days back followed by cessation of micturition, generalized swelling and breathlessness. After getting stung, he felt severe pain at the bite sites. He went to Upazila Health Complex (primary care hospital) and received injectable hydrocortisone, anti-histamine, pain killer and antibiotics. After 3 hours, he left the hospital willingly. On the first day, he developed swelling over the bite site. From the second day, he developed burning sensation on the skin, headache, weakness, dizziness, nausea and vomiting. On the fourth day, he had high colored scanty urine and generalized swelling.

On examination, he was restless, confused, dyspneic, had multiple sting marks all over the body, bite area were edematous, erythematous, severely tender and some sting marks healed up with scar formation (Fig. 1). He was

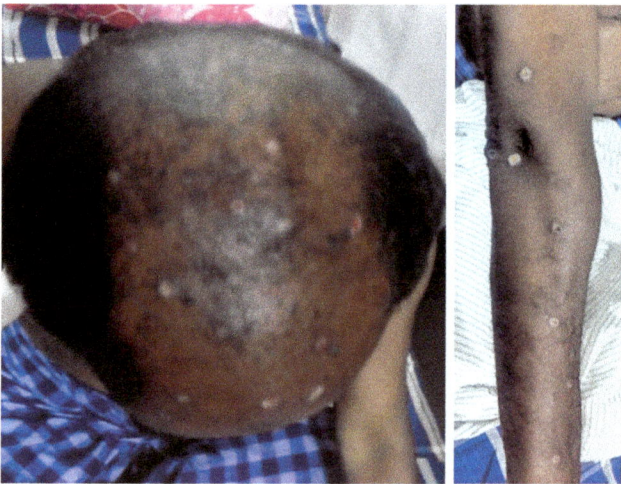

Fig. 1: Multiple sting marks, some healed-up with scar formation.

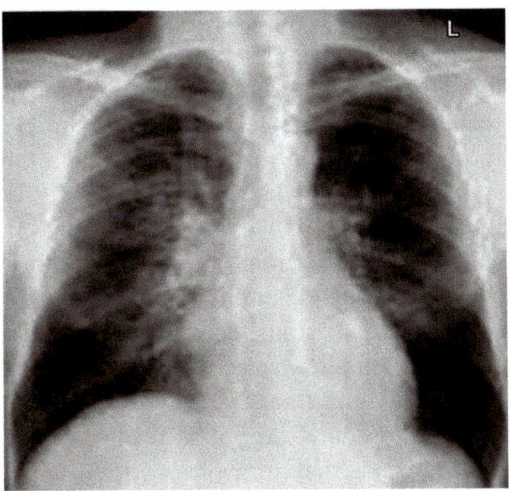

Fig. 2: X-ray chest P/A view showing pulmonary edema.

mildly anemic, bipedal pitting edema was present, febrile (temperature—100°F), pulse—110/min, feeble and blood pressure (BP)—nonrecordable.

Investigations revealed: white blood cells (WBCs)—17,490/mm^3; serum creatinine—15.6 mg/dL; creatine phosphokinase (CPK)—3353 U/L; serum electrolytes—sodium: 135 mmol/L, potassium: 5.3 mmol/L, chloride: 104 mmol/L; alanine aminotransferase (ALT)—255 U/L; aspartate aminotransferase (AST)—190 U/L; prothrombin time (PT)—19 seconds, chest X-ray (CXR) posteroanterior view—pulmonary edema (Fig. 2).

QUESTION

1. What would be the outcome of this case?

DISCUSSION

The patient was anuric throughout his hospital stay, and despite all our efforts, he succumbed to an unfortunate, but unavoidable death. He died on the third day of admission due to multiorgan dysfunction.

Final Diagnosis: Multiple Bee Stings with Acute Kidney Injury Due to Rhabdomyolysis with Acute Respiratory Distress Syndrome

In general, insects such as bees and wasps keep themselves away from human beings. They only sting for self-defense. Most of the time, one or a few stings are seen. Occasionally, a person may receive multiple stings due to disruption of a hive or swarm of bees.

Multiple bee stings can be a medical emergency. Particularly children, older adults and people having heart or respiratory problems are the high-risk group requiring immediate medical attention after getting multiple stings.

The venom produced by bee is responsible for clinical signs and symptoms. Gastrointestinal symptoms like nausea, vomiting and diarrhea, and neurological features like headache, vertigo, convulsion and dizziness are some noticeable manifestations.

Three main reactions are seen after bee venom accumulation. They are: (1) local reactions such as swelling and irritation, (2) anaphylactic reaction and (3) serum sickness like symptoms comprising hemolysis, disseminated intravascular coagulation, rhabdomyolysis and acute kidney injury (AKI).[1]

Several other clinically important features are observed after bee sting. They are: skin necrosis, bleeding, dropping of platelet count, pancreatitis, respiratory distress syndrome, rhabdomyolysis and AKI.

Our patient was attacked by multiple bees. He developed serious complications like AKI and acute respiratory distress syndrome (ARDS) leading to death.

Adults are the most vulnerable group to have severe reactions. They are more prone to die of anaphylactic reaction than children are.

Treatment depends on the severity of the condition. It should be noted that no specific anti-venom is discovered yet. Home treatment can be advocated for a single bee sting. But multiple bee stings can be life-threatening and prompt supportive treatment should be instituted early. For multi-organ failure, supportive treatment is necessary, though outcome may not be favorable.

REFERENCE

1. Deshpande PR, Farooq AK, Bairy M, et al. Acute renal failure and/or rhabdomyolysis due to multiple bee stings: a retrospective study. N Am J Med Sci. 2013;5(3):235-9.

CASE 81

YOUNG LADY WITH RECURRENT HEMATEMESIS

CASE SUMMARY

A 42-year-old nonalcoholic female attended the emergency department with several episodes of hematemesis. For the last 6 months, she had intermittent hematemesis for which endoscopy was done and multiple esophageal varices were found. Endoscopic variceal ligation (EVL) was performed. Despite EVL, she continued having hematemesis. She did not have history of previous jaundice, blood transfusion, unprotected sexual exposure, intravenous drug abuse, malignancy or any major surgery in the past. There was no abnormal bleeding from any other site. On repeated query, we did not find any positive history suggesting bleeding diathesis or thrombosis in her parents and siblings.

On examination, she was pale and there was mild splenomegaly. No stigmata of chronic liver disease were present.

Complete blood count showed pancytopenia. The liver function tests were normal. All viral markers were negative. Ultrasound of the abdomen showed normal hepatic parenchyma with splenomegaly with dilated portal vein. Fibroscan score was 5.8 kPa.

QUESTIONS

1. What is the diagnosis?
2. What investigation should be done next?
3. What are the possible etiologies of the disease?

DISCUSSION

This patient had developed non-cirrhotic portal hypertension as evidenced by her dilated portal vein. One of the common causes of non-cirrhotic portal hypertension is portal vein thrombosis (PVT).[1,2] Other causes might include extrahepatic portal vein obstruction (EHPVO) and congenital hepatic fibrosis (CHF). As the ultrasound ruled out the possibility of extra-hepatic portal vein obstruction at first instance, we performed the doppler ultrasound of her abdominal vessels which confirmed intrahepatic PVT.

This patient had no visible risk factor of venous thrombosis. She was mobile, no previous surgery was done and she was not using oral contraceptive pills. Malignancy screening was negative. Though there was no significant family history, considering her age and sex-we decided to screen for thrombophilia before starting warfarin. Her protein C and protein S were very low. Protein C was 19% and protein S was 59%. We treated her with low molecular weight heparin and warfarin. The tests should have been repeated after 2 weeks for further confirmation. But as warfarin therapy was started, we could not repeat the tests. Thus we diagnosed the case as **portal vein thrombosis** due to protein C and protein S deficiency. Gene sequencing to detect mutation could have further confirmed hereditary deficiency.

Final Diagnosis: Portal Vein Thrombosis due to Protein C and Protein S Deficiency

Protein C and protein S are vitamin K-dependent natural anticoagulants. Protein C and S deficiencies may be inherited or acquired. When inherited as autosomal dominant traits, they are mostly due to heterozygous missense mutations. Patients present with recurrent venous thromboembolism in unusual sites, such as cerebral sinus venous thrombosis, mesenteric vein thrombosis, portal vein thrombosis, and suprahepatic vein thrombosis (Budd-Chiari syndrome), and is associated with inherited thrombophilia in young individuals.[3,4]

Investigations needed to reach the diagnosis include measurement of the levels and activity of protein C and S. Testing should be done at least several weeks after an acute clotting episode and at least 3–6 weeks after stopping warfarin or heparin. Repeat testing should be done to confirm abnormal results, since false-positive results are common.[5]

Since only a few cases of PVT may be due to hereditary anticoagulant protein deficiency, this can only be confirmed by careful history taking and investigation of family members, preferably including both parents, or by screening siblings—which could be used for both diagnostic and counseling purposes. Gene sequencing to detect anticoagulant protein gene mutations may demonstrate whether such anticoagulant deficiencies in PVT are truly primary or not.[6]

Symptomatic protein C and S deficiencies are commonly treated with warfarin, but it must be given initially with an additional injectable anticoagulant (usually heparin, low-molecular-weight heparin, or a similar drug) until the warfarin is fully effective. Patient must never receive warfarin without first receiving another anticoagulant at the same time, as warfarin inhibits invivo protein C and S production which may result in precipitating a new clot or skin necrosis. It is safe to take only warfarin after 5 or more days of concurrent treatment with heparin, low-molecular-weight heparin, or a related drug, such as fondaparinux.[5]

REFERENCES

1. Trebicka J, Strassburg CP. Etiology and complications of portal vein thrombosis. Viszeralmedizin. 2014;30(6):375-80.
2. Plessier A, Rautou PE, Valla DC. Management of hepatic vascular diseases. J Hepatol. 2012; 56 (Suppl 1):S25-38.
3. Rodríguez-Leal GA, Morán S, Corona-Cedillo R, et al. Portal vein thrombosis with protein C-S deficiency in a non-cirrhotic patient. World J Hepatol. 2014;6(7):532-7.
4. Wypasek E, Undas A. Protein C and protein S deficiency - practical diagnostic issues. Adv Clin Exp Med. 2013;22(4):459-67.
5. Lipe B, Ornstein DL. Deficiencies of natural anticoagulants, protein C, protein S, and antithrombin. Circulation. 2011;124:e365-e368.
6. Johnson NV, Khor B, Van Cott EM. Advances in laboratory testing for thrombophilia. Am J Hematol. 2012;87 (Suppl 1):S108-S112.

CASE 82

YOUNG MALE WITH CONSTANT ABDOMINAL PAIN

CASE SUMMARY

A 21-year-old male presented with right upper abdominal pain and nausea for the last 6 months. Pain was constant, dull aching with no radiation and no aggravating factor but relieved with nonsteroidal anti-inflammatory drugs (NSAIDs). Pain was accompanied by nausea without vomiting and was associated with weight loss of about 3 kg in the last 6 months. He had no history of fever, jaundice or bowel—bladder disturbance. There was no previous history of tuberculosis or any contact with tuberculosis patient. He was nonsmoker and nonalcoholic.

General examination and systemic examination were unremarkable other than mild tenderness in right hypochondriac region.

Laboratory data revealed normal serum hemoglobin (Hb)—13.6 g/dL, erythrocyte sedimentation rate (ESR)—80 mm in the first hour, white blood cell count—11.000/cumm, differential count: polymorph—60%, lymphocyte—20%, eosinophil—14%, monocyte—6% and circulating eosinophil—1,540/cumm. Chest X-ray posteroanterior (PA) view was normal. Ultrasonography (USG) of whole abdomen revealed normal-sized liver with small hypoechoic focal lesion in the anterior inferior and lateral segment of left lobe, measuring 1.7 × 1.1 cm. Rest of the liver parenchyma appeared normal. Features suggestive of space-occupying lesion. Liver function tests were normal. Computed tomography (CT) of upper abdomen pre- and postcontrast revealed liver was mildly enlarged. Multiple small rim-enhanced well-defined rounded hypodense areas were seen in the hepatic parenchyma (Fig. 1). At 6 minutes delayed postcontrast scan, most of the hypodense areas became isodense to hepatic parenchyma.

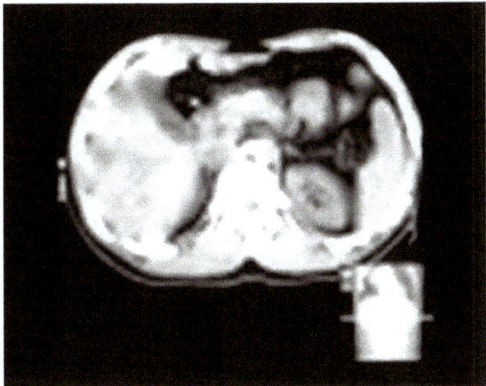

Fig. 1: Computed tomography (CT) scan of abdomen showing hypodense shadow in liver.

QUESTIONS

1. What are the possibilities?
2. What next investigations will you do to reach your diagnosis?
3. What is the plan of management?

DISCUSSION

From the above scenario, possibilities were:
- Inflammatory lesions/microabscess
- Atypical hemangioma
- Secondaries.

We did the following investigation to reach the diagnosis:
- Fine needle aspiration cytology (FNAC) done from liver mass (USG-guided) revealed: clusters of epithelioid cells, many lymphocytes, some histiocytes and clusters of normal hepatocytes. Background showed blood and small amount of caseous necrotic material. No malignant cell seen. Comment: granulomatous inflammation, suggestive of tuberculosis.

Final Diagnosis: Isolated Hepatic Tuberculosis

As isolated hepatic tuberculosis is a rare condition and liver involvement is clinically silent; initially, it is difficult to find the cause of presenting complaints. Broadly speaking, hepatic tuberculosis presents in three forms. The most common form is the diffuse hepatic involvement, seen along with pulmonary or miliary tuberculosis in 50–80% of patients dying of pulmonary tuberculosis. Despite the diffuse involvement of the liver pathologically, symptoms of liver disease are absent. The second form is diffuse hepatic infiltration with small granulomas (less than 2 mm) without recognizable pulmonary involvement (granulomatous liver disease). The third much rarer form presents as a focal/local tuberculoma or abscess. Isolated hepatic tuberculoma (synonyms: nodular hepatic tuberculosis and macronodular hepatic tuberculosis) is perhaps the rarest form of local hepatic tuberculosis.[1-4] Tubercle bacilli reach the liver by way of hematogenous dissemination; the portal of entry in the case of miliary tuberculosis is through the hepatic artery; whereas, in the case of focal liver tuberculosis, it is via the portal vein. Irrespective of the mode of entry, the liver responds by granuloma formation. Tuberculous granulomata are most frequently found in the periportal areas (zone 1 of Rappaport), but may occasionally occur in zone 3.[5]

Constitutional symptoms in the form of fever, anorexia and weight loss are present in 55-90% of the patients. Our patient had significant weight loss of 3 kg in 6 months. Abdominal pain is present in 65-87% of patients, but jaundice is uncommon.[6,7] Hepatomegaly and splenomegaly are the most common findings, being present in 70-96% and 25-55% of patients, respectively.[8,9] Our patient had mild hepatomegaly that was observed on CT scan of abdomen.

Usually liver function tests are within normal limit. Magnetic resonance imaging (MRI) and CT findings of liver tuberculosis reveal different stages of disease, varying from granulomatous tubercles with or without caseation necrosis to fibrosis and calcification in the healing stage.[10] USG findings of hepatic tuberculosis usually show hypoechoic lesion.[11] In our case, USG revealed hypoechoic lesion, but CT scan precontrast revealed hypoechoic but postcontrast revealed isodense lesion. So it is a quite difficult finding for a radiologist to reach a confirm diagnosis. Histopathological examination of the specimens from lesions is essential for exact diagnosis.

Infectious and noninfectious diseases which can cause caseating or noncaseating hepatic granulomatous reaction such as leprosy, sarcoidosis, Hodgkin's disease, brucellosis, infectious mononucleosis, inflammatory bowel disease, drug-induced liver damage and syphilis should be considered in the differential diagnosis of hepatic tuberculosis. Chronic active hepatitis may also mimic tuberculosis of the liver.[12]

Hepatic tuberculosis is treated like any other extrapulmonary tuberculosis. Chemotherapy with standard antituberculosis drugs remains the cornerstone of treatment. This is true for both diffuse and the local forms of the disease.

After getting category 1 antituberculosis regimen for 2 months, our patient came for follow-up with repeat ultrasonography report. Patient's general condition was improved and there was no right hypochondriac pain. On ultrasonography, there was also no space-occupying lesions in the liver. We then started continuation phase of anti-TB chemotherapy.

REFERENCES

1. Chen HC, Chao YC, Shyu RY, et al. Isolated tuberculous liver abscesses with multiple hyperechoic masses on ultrasound: a case report and review of the literature. Liver Int. 2003;23:346-50.
2. Johri BS, Kane MP, Mudbhatkal NS. Isolated tuberculosis of the liver. Indian J Med Sci. 1970;24:15-21.
3. Singbeil BA, Bickford AA, Stoltz JH. Isolation of *Mycobacterium avium* from ring-necked pheasants (Phasianus colchicus). Avian Dis. 1993;37:612-5.
4. Lim EJ, Johnson PD, Crowley P, Gow PJ. Granulomatous hepatitis: tuberculosis or not? Med J Aust. 2008;188:166-7.
5. Reynolds, TB, Campra, JL, Peters RL. 'Hepatic granulomata'. In: Zakim D, Boyer TD (eds.). Hepatology - A Textbook of Liver Disease, 2nd ed. WB Saunders: Philadelphia; 1990. p. 1098.
6. Oliva A, Duarte B, Jonasson O, Nadimpalli V. The nodular form of local hepatic tuberculosis. J Clin Gastroenterol. 1990;12:166.
7. Hersch C. Tuberculosis of the liver. South Afr Med J. 1964;38:857.
8. Alvarez SZ, Carpio R. Hepatobiliary tuberculosis. Dig Dis Sci. 1983;28:193.
9. Maharaj B, Leary WP, Pudifin DJ. A prospective study of hepatic tuberculosis in 41 black patients. Quart J Med. 1987;63:517.
10. Kawamori Y, Matsui O, Kitagawa K, Kadoya M, Takashima T, Yamahana T. Macronodular tuberculoma of the liver: CT and MR findings. Am J Roentgenol. 1992;158:311-3.
11. Jain R, Sawhney S, Gupta RG, Acharya S. Sonographic appearances and percutaneous management of primary tuberculous liver abscess. J Clin Ultrasound. 1998;27:159-63.
12. Rangabashyam N. Oxford Textbook of Surgery. Vol II. Abdominal Tuberculosis. Oxford: Oxford University Press; 1994. p. 2491.

CASE 83

YOUNG HOUSEWIFE WITH SEVERE ABDOMINAL PAIN AND DISTENSION

CASE SUMMARY

A 43-year-old housewife presented with swelling of abdomen for the past 5 days. Five days ago, she noticed gradual swelling of her abdomen which was progressive, associated with discomfort, heaviness, and shortness of breath while lying on her back. Seven hours before admission, she experienced severe abdominal pain which was central, reached peak within 2 hours of onset, then became constant, with no radiation. No apparent aggravating or relieving factor was there. But pain was accompanied by two episodes of vomiting of recently ingested food materials. She had no bowel movement for last 36 hours prior to admission. She did not report of having fever, weight loss, previous jaundice, bleeding from any site or similar illness. There was no history of taking nonsteroidal anti-inflammatory drugs (NSAIDs) or oral contraceptives.

Examination revealed dyspneic patient resting in propped-up position with three pillows. Her pulse rate was 90 beats/min; blood pressure (BP) was 90/60 mm Hg; temperature was 98°F; respiratory rate 22 breaths/min. Abdomen was massively distended with full flank and everted umbilicus. Abdomen was tender to touch, fluid thrill was present. Bowel sound was sluggish. Lungs were clear bilaterally.

Investigation showed hemoglobin (Hb) 11 g/dL, erythrocyte sedimentation rate (ESR) 35 mm in 1 hour, total count of white blood cells (WBC) was 11000/mm^3 with 84% polymorphs, platelet count 78,000/μL, C-reactive protein (CRP) titer of 36 mg/dL, random blood sugar, serum electrolyte, urine routine examination, chest radiograph, electrocardiogram, and echocardiography were normal. Abdominal X-ray showed distended bowel loops with mucosal thumb printing (Fig. 1A). Ascitic fluid study showed 25 WBCs/cumm with 100% lymphocyte, protein 3.5 g/dL, sugar 88.4 mg/dL. Adenosine deaminase (ADA) 14 IU/L. Acid-fast bacilli (AFB) or other bacteria were not found. Carcinoembryonic antigen (CEA), and

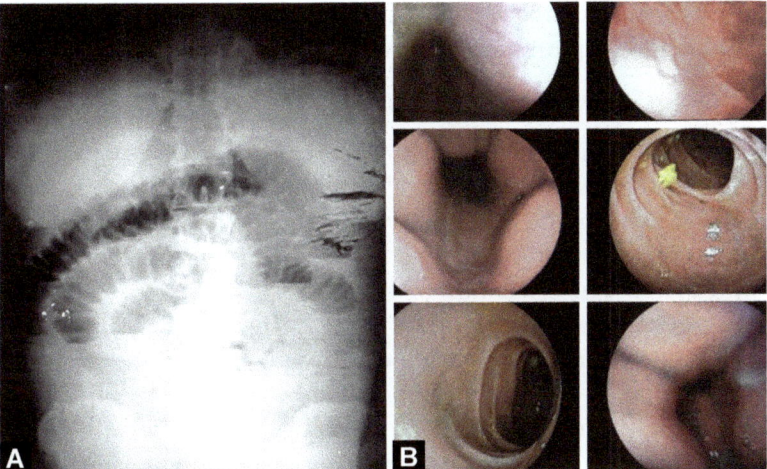

Figs. 1A and B: (A) X-ray of abdomen showing distended bowel loops with mucosal thumbprinting; (B) Endoscopy of upper gastrointestinal tract showed diffused hemorrhagic gastritis, erosive duodenitis with hemorrhagic change.

oncotic cytology were negative. Ultrasonography (USG) of whole abdomen showed huge ascites with mild hepatomegaly with uniform echotexture. Endoscopy of upper gastrointestinal tract showed diffused hemorrhagic gastritis, erosive duodenitis with hemorrhagic change (Fig. 1B).

QUESTIONS

1. What next investigations can be done to reach the diagnosis?
2. How would you further evaluate mucosal thumbprinting found in abdominal X-ray?

DISCUSSION

Rapid onset ascites followed by intestinal obstruction-like features coupled with exudative ascites with mucosal thumb printing and thrombocytopenia, is definitely a challenging situation to make a diagnosis. We performed antinuclear antibody (ANA) which was positive, and serum C4 level was low; later anti-double stranded deoxyribonucleic acid (anti-dsDNA) and anti-Sjögren's syndrome-related antigen antibody (anti-SSA Ab) came out reactive. Finally, the case was diagnosed as systemic lupus erythematosus (SLE). Our patient had the interesting finding of mucosal thumbprinting in abdominal X-ray, which indicated mucosal edema. So, keeping lupus enteritis in mind, we went for CT scan of abdomen (gold standard test); and it revealed diffuse wall thickening, dilatation of the lumen, enhancement of the mucosa and serosa (target sign)—suggestive of inflammatory enteritis.

Patient was given prednisolone 60 mg/day and hydroxychloroquine 250 µg per day and her symptoms were improved within 1 month.

Final Diagnosis: Systemic Lupus Erythematosus (Lupus Enteritis)

Peritoneal involvement is uncommon in SLE and SLE with ascites as the first manifestation is extremely rare.[1] It should be considered as diagnosis of exclusion, demanding an extensive investigation for the more common causes of exudative ascites. Though the diagnosis is difficult but treatment is easy with a fair prognosis in most of the cases.

Cause of acute abdomen in SLE involves lupus enteritis, urinary tract infection, acute gastroenteritis, pancreatitis, cholecystitis, inferior vena caval thrombosis.

Lupus enteritis underlies a broad spectrum of processes which includes mesenteric arteritis, intestinal vasculitis, lupus peritonitis, and abdominal serositis.[2] Patients who have complaints of abdominal pain should be evaluated carefully as overlooking the diagnosis and delaying treatment can result in bowel ischemia and perforation. The diagnosis of lupus enteritis is based on classical CT findings (bowel wall edema with target sign, mesenteric abnormalities and ascites) as histopathology seldom confirms the diagnosis.

REFERENCES

1. Liu R, Zhang L, Gao S, et al. Gastrointestinal symptom due to lupus peritonitis: a rare form of onset of SLE. Int J Clin Exp Med. 2014;7(12):5917-20.
2. Sran S, Sran M, Patel N, et al. Lupus enteritis as an initial presentation of systemic lupus erythematosus. Case Rep Gastrointest Med. 2014;2014:962735. doi:10.1155/2014/962735.

CASE 84

AN UNUSUAL PRESENTATION OF CHYLOUS ASCITES

CASE SUMMARY

A 30-year-old male presented to us with hugely distended abdomen. It was severe enough to cause respiratory distress. About 6 months back, he noticed gradual abdominal distension which was associated with dull aching abdominal pain. Before and after admission, repeated paracentesis was done for diagnostic and therapeutic purpose, but every time there was recurrence of marked ascites. He also mentioned having low-grade fever, associated with night sweats. He had lost around 20 kg weight in this ailment.

On examination, the patient was severely ill-looking; mildly anemic, bipedal edema was present. Abdomen was hugely distended and tender. Ascites was evidenced by fluid thrill. Deep palpation was impossible because of huge distension and tenderness. Scrotal edema was present but testes were normal in size and consistency. Stigmata of chronic liver disease were also absent. Digital rectal examination revealed nothing abnormal.

Investigations showed all the routine blood reports including complete blood count and peripheral blood film were normal except hemoglobin (Hb), which was 10 g/dL. Renal function test and thyroid function test revealed no abnormality. Liver function test revealed serum albumin level was low (2.5 g/dL). All viral markers were negative. Ultrasonography (USG) of whole abdomen revealed hepatosplenomegaly with marked ascites with normal doppler study of portal vein. Abdominal magnetic resonance imaging (MRI) showed para-aortic lymphadenopathy and hepatosplenomegaly with marked ascites. Abdominal paracentesis revealed milky, creamy cloudy fluid. Triglyceride was elevated in the fluid (3,840 mg/dL). Protein level was elevated and amylase level and adenosine deaminase (ADA) level was normal. No malignant cell was found. Computed tomographic (CT)-guided fine needle aspiration cytology (FNAC) from para-aortic lymph node was done, but the report was inconclusive. Diagnostic laparoscopy and histopathology were also done and unfortunately report was inconclusive with no granuloma, no malignant cell, only some lymphocytes. Exploratory laparotomy and biopsy were done and histopathology from mesenteric and para-aortic lymph node revealed atypical lymphoid hyperplasia.

QUESTIONS

1. Give some causes of chylous ascites.
2. What next investigation can be done to reach the final diagnosis?

DISCUSSION

Chylous ascites: It is due to lymph accumulation in the abdomen as a result of interruption in the lymphatic system. Diagnosis can be made when triglyceride concentration is greater than 200 mg/dL in the ascitic fluid.[1]

Common causes:
- Intra-abdominal malignancy: Most commonly lymphoma
- Infections: Abdominal tuberculosis, filariasis
- Cirrhosis
- Postoperative (Abdominal)
- Trauma (Abdominal)
- Congenital abnormality in lymphatic system
- Radiation therapy (Abdominal, pelvis).[1]

Our patient had hepatosplenomegaly with para-aortic and mesenteric lymphadenopathy along with chylous ascites.

To evaluate the current state, next step of investigation was immunohistochemistry (IHC). In our case, IHC report of biopsied mesenteric and para-aortic lymph node revealed:
- Positive for CD10 in follicles
- Positive for CD20 in both follicles and interfollicular area
- Positive CD3 for small number of cells in interfollicular areas
- CD5: Negative
- Ki-67: 5–10% in interfollicular area (Cell proliferation marker: It has prognostic value).

All these findings were consistent with low-grade follicular lymphoma.

Final Diagnosis: Low-grade Follicular Lymphoma

Follicular lymphoma is a subtype of non-Hodgkin lymphoma, which is clinically indolent. Most commonly present with painless peripheral lymphadenopathy. Widely disseminated disease can occur with involvement of spleen, liver and bone marrow. Systemic symptoms (fever, night sweats, weight loss) can present in 20% of patients.

Follicular lymphoma can be diagnosed histologically by tissue biopsy (lymph node). Genetic studies and immunohistochemistry can support the diagnosis. Bone marrow can also be done for staging. Histologically, this tumor has nodular growth pattern. The tumor cells express CD19, CD20, CD10, BCL6 and negative for CD5, CD23.[2]

Treatment options depend on staging and histological grading, ranging from wait and observe to radioimmunotherapy, combination chemotherapy, monoclonal antibody (rituximab) and hematopoietic stem cell transplantation.

Some common combination therapies are:

- R-Chop – Rituximab+ Chop (cyclophosphamide, doxorubicin, vincristine, prednisone)[3]
- R-CVP –Rituximab+ CVP(cyclophosphamide, vincristine, prednisone)[4]
- Bendamustine + rituximab.[5]

REFERENCES

1. Almakdisi T, Massoud S, Makdisi G. Lymphomas and chylous ascites: Review of the Literature. The Oncologist. 2005;10(8):632–5.
2. Freedman AS, Aster JC. Clinical manifestations, pathologic features, diagnosis, and prognosis of follicular lymphoma. In. Lister A, ed. UpToDate. Waltham, MA: UpToDate; 2014. pp. 1–16.
3. Hiddemann W, Kneba M, Dreyling M, et al. Frontline therapy with rituximab added to the combination of cyclophosphamide, doxorubicin, vincristine, and prednisone (CHOP) significantly improves the outcome for patients with advanced-stage follicular lymphoma compared with therapy with CHOP alone: results of a prospective randomized study of the German Low-grade Lymphoma Study Group. Blood. 2005;106(12):3725–32.
4. Marcus R, Imrie K, Belch A, et al. CVP chemotherapy plus rituximab compared with CVP as first-line treatment for advanced follicular lymphoma. Blood. 2005;105(4):1417–23.
5. Rummel MJ, Niederle N, Maschmeyer G, et al. Bendamustine plus rituximab versus CHOP plus rituximab as first-line treatment for patients with indolent and mantle-cell lymphomas: an open-label, multicentre, randomised, phase 3 non-inferiority trial. Lancet. 2013;381(9873):1203–10.

CASE 85

MIDDLE-AGED MAN WITH RECURRENT LIMB WEAKNESS

CASE SUMMARY

A 52-year-old male presented to us with difficulty in walking for the last 5 months. It initially started while working in the field. He felt weakness of both upper and lower limbs, but more marked in lower limbs. At that time he was able to do his daily activities and he noticed that weakness improved on exertion. These symptoms became progressively worse with development of swallowing difficulty after 3 months of onset of disease. Swallowing was more marked for liquid than solid and sometimes associated with nasal regurgitation. There was also difficulty in speech with nasal intonation. Two months later, patient developed drooping of upper eyelids and excessive blinking of eyes. His limb weakness worsened so much that he felt difficulty in rising from a chair and also incurred multiple falls. He lost about 5 kg weight in last 3 months. There was no history of fever, persistent cough, shortness of breath but he complained of occasional chest pain on right side. He was a cigarette smoker (20 packs/year).

On examination, he was ill-looking. All the vital signs were within normal limit and there was no postural drop of blood pressure. There was excessive blinking of eyes and bilateral partial ptosis with diurnal variation. Ice on eyes test was positive (3 mm increased). On neurological examination, there was dysarthria with nasal intonation. Motor system examination of the upper and lower limbs revealed, muscle power was 4/5 in all limbs. Muscle tone was normal. Both knee and ankle reflexes were diminished, plantar was bilateral flexor. Hoffman's sign was negative. Examination of cerebellar system was normal. Gait was waddling. All sensory modalities were intact. Joint examination was also normal and there was no muscular atrophy.

Laboratory findings showed normal blood counts. Chest X-ray and ultrasonography (USG) of whole abdomen were normal. Computed tomography (CT) scan of chest showed soft tissue mass in right hilar region with mediastinal lymphadenopathy and inflammatory changes in right lung with a tiny nodule in medial segment of middle lobe with right apical pleural thickening. Magnetic resonance imaging (MRI) of the brain showed microvascular chronic ischemic changes with mild cerebral cortical atrophy.

QUESTIONS

1. What is the most likely diagnosis?
2. Give some differential diagnoses.
3. What investigation do you want to do next?

DISCUSSION

The case history indicated proximal muscle weakness along with bilateral ptosis. Ice pack test was positive. So, our diffrentials were neuromuscular junction disorders such as myasthenia gravis (MG) and Lambert-Eaton myasthenic syndrome (LEMS).

In our case, symptoms started with limb weakness which improved after exercise, associated with subsequent development of dysphagia, and ptosis. Also, on query, the patient complained of dry mouth for the last 2 months. Examination revealed hyporeflexia, so our strong suspicion was Lambert-Eaton myasthenic syndrome.

Single fiber electromyography (EMG) and high-frequency repetitive nerve stimulation test finding was consistent with LEMS and CT-guided fine needle aspiration cytology (FNAC) from the mass lesion in right hilar region revealed small cell lung carcinoma.

Final Diagnosis: Lambert-Eaton Myasthenic Syndrome Associated with Small Cell Lung Carcinoma

Lambert-Eaton myasthenic syndrome is a neuromuscular junction disorder, associated with malignancy. Though both MG and LEMS have similar type of symptoms; LEMS is rarer and can be differentiated by the following points:
- Many studies have showed that in case of MG, initial muscle weakness involves extraocular muscles and bulbar muscles, whereas in LEMS, usually first involvement is limb weakness.
- Usually, MG develops craniocaudally, whereas LEMS develops in opposite direction.[1]
- In case of LEMS, weakness improved after exercise, whereas in MG, muscle weakness initiated or increased after exercise.[2]
- In LEMS, there may be some features of autonomic dysfunction, most commonly dry mouth and postural drop. This is not seen in MG.
- LEMS is associated with cancer, most commonly small cell lung carcinoma. Long-term smokers showed more risk.[3]

Eletrodiagnostic study can help to diagnose LEMS. At first, routine NCS study and needle EMG should be done. Diagnosis can be confirmed by either high frequency repetitive nerve stimulation (RNS) test or exercise test. Single fiber EMG should be done in case of any doubt, though it is less specific. Also presence of anti-voltage-gated calcium channel (VGCC) antibody is diagnostic.

Post-exercise increase in compound muscle action potential (CMAP) amplitude (at least 60%) compared with pre-exercise baseline value or a similar increment on high-frequency repetitive nerve stimulation without exercise is confirmatory for LEMS.[4]

Treatment is 3,4–diaminopyridine; if not tolerated, the alternative is guanidine and immunosuppression and most importantly treatment of underlying malignancy.[5]

REFERENCES

1. Wirtz PW, Sotodeh M, Nijnuis M, et al. Difference in distribution of muscle weakness between myasthenia gravis and the Lambert–Eaton myasthenic syndrome. J Neurol Neurosurg Psychiatry. 2002;73:766–8.
2. Simon JI, Herbison GJ, Levy G. Case report: a case review of Lambert-Eaton myasthenic syndrome and low back pain. Curr Rev Musculoskelet Med. 2011;4(1):1–5.
3. Tarr TB, Wipf P, Meriney SD. Synaptic pathophysiology and treatment of Lambert-Eaton myasthenic syndrome. Mol Neurobiol. 2015;52(1):456–63.
4. Weinberg DH. (2018) Lambert-Eaton myasthenic syndrome: Clinical features and diagnosis. In: Eichler AF (ED). UpToDate. Retrived April 2019, from https://www.uptodate.com/contents/lambert-eaton-myasthenic-syndrome-clinical-features-and-diagnosis.
5. Weinberg DH. (2019). Lambert-Eaton myasthenic syndrome: Treatment and prognosis. In: Eichler AF (ED). UpToDate. Retrieved April, 2019, from https://www.uptodate.com/contents/lambert-eaton-myasthenic-syndrome-treatment-and-prognosis.

CASE 86

YOUNG MAN WITH PURPURA AND HEMATURIA

CASE SUMMARY

A 20-year-old young man presented with the complaints of multiple painless pin-headed red spots on skin all over the body for the past 20 days and passage of red-colored urine for the past 7 days. Initially, red spots appeared in the arms and neck, and then subsequently involved all over the body including face and oral cavity; skin spots were initially red and then became black after few days. He also complained of passage of red-colored urine for the past 7 days with occasional passage of clot in the urine and episodes of spontaneous gum bleeding for 1 day. He mentioned having generalized weakness for the last 1.5 months. On query, he recalled that before appearance of red cutaneous spots, he had undocumented low-grade fever occurring only at night which subsided spontaneously without taking antipyretics. Later on, he developed high-grade fever which lasted for 2 days—maximum recorded temperature was 103°F with chills and was subsided with antipyretics. There was no history of jaundice, arthralgia, bloody diarrhea, palpitation, sore throat, neurological complaints, exposure to any chemicals or radiation. Before admission, he was treated with injectable antibiotics, oral steroid by a local doctor and received two units of blood transfusion. Then he was admitted into urology department and treated conservatively and later transferred to our department for further evaluation. On query, he gave history of recent unsafe sexual exposure. During the hospital course, after 12 days of admission, he suddenly developed headache and slurring of speech without any limb weakness. Immediate computed tomography (CT) scan showed intracerebral hemorrhage (Fig. 1). That time he received nine units of whole blood and one unit of platelet concentrate.

On examination, he was moderately anemic, there were palpable non-tender lymph nodes—one in right posterior cervical chain about 0.5 × 0.5 cm, another in right axillary lymph node (central group) measuring about 1.5 × 1.25 cm, another one in the left inguinal area measuring about 0.5 × 0.5 cm.

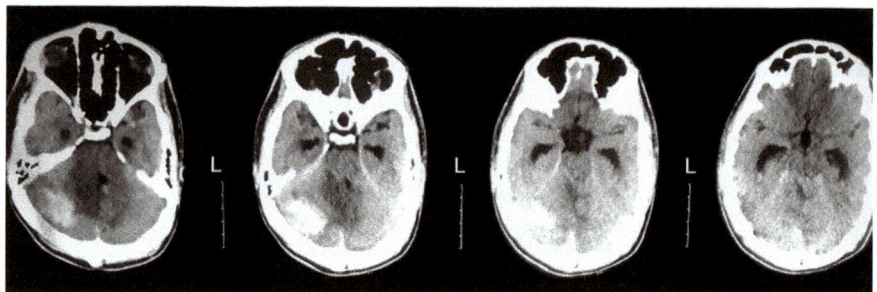

Fig. 1: Computed tomography (CT) scan of head showed acute intracerebral hemorrhage.

On skin survey, multiple purpuric spots were found all over the body which were nontender and did not blanch on pressure. Also bleeding spots were observed over the palate, tongue and rest of the oral cavity. Fundoscopic examination showed hemorrhage with exudate (3 o'clock position of left eye). Other systemic examination findings were unremarkable.

Investigation showed Hb level was persistently low (5.9, 5.2 and 8.2 g/dL), white blood cells (WBCs) counts were high with predominant neutrophilia (17,300/cumm; 16,980/cumm; 15,500/cumm), platelet (PLT) counts were low (3,000/cumm; 3,000/cumm; 11,000/cumm), erythrocyte sedimentation rate (ESR) in the first hour—30 mm, reticulocyte count was high—16%, peripheral blood film (PBF)—leukoerythroblastic blood picture with thrombocytopenia. Serum creatinine—0.90 mg/dL, alanine aminotransferase (ALT)—26 U/L, aspartate aminotransferase (AST)—54 U/L, serum creatinine—normal, urine R/M/E—plenty of red blood cells (RBC), pus cells—6 to 8/HPF, urine C/S—growth of *E. coli*, blood C/S—no growth. Chest X-ray (CXR) posteroanterior view—normal, X-ray of kidney, ureter, and bladder (KUB)—normal, ultrasonography (USG) of the whole abdomen showed mild hydronephrosis (left), multiple focal thickenings of bladder wall—possibly neoplasm or chronic cystitis, blood clot within the bladder lumen. Serum bilirubin—total: 1.34 mg/dL (direct: 1.14 mg/dL, indirect: 0.20 mg/dL); HBsAg, anti HCV Ab, anti-HIV 1 and 2 Ab—negative. Serum lactate dehydrogenase (LDH)—577 U/L; Coombs' test: direct—positive, indirect—negative; prothrombin time (PT)—13 seconds; international normalized ratio (INR)—1.04; activated partial thromboplastin time (APTT)—28 seconds; fibrinogen degradation product (FDP)—15 mcg/mL; D-dimer—1 mcg/mL; anti-leptospira antibody—negative.

QUESTIONS

1. What are the possible differential diagnoses for this case?
2. How should this patient be managed?

DISCUSSION

Based on history, clinical examination and investigations, our differential diagnoses were:
- Sepsis
- Acute leukemia
- Leptospirosis.

Normal PT, APTT, FDP and D-dimer made the diagnosis of sepsis less likely. Absence of blast cell in PBF disfavored the diagnosis of acute leukemia. Negative anti-leptospira antibody did not favor the diagnosis of leptospirosis as well. Then we searched for alternative diagnosis. We established the diagnosis of autoimmune hemolytic anemia based on positive Coombs' test and high reticulocyte counts. Persistent thrombocytopenia along with autoimmune hemolytic anemia clinched the diagnosis of Evans syndrome. Then, the question was whether it was primary or secondary Evans syndrome. We had made every possible effort to find out secondary causes. Negative lab results [antinuclear antibody (ANA)—negative, anticardiolipin antibody and lupus anticoagulant—negative, bone marrow—reactive marrow], persistent low hemoglobin level with positive Coombs' test and persistent low platelet count which responded to steroid therapy led us to make the diagnosis of primary Evans syndrome. It was a diagnosis of exclusion. Infection was considered as one of the risk factors for Evans syndrome.

Final Diagnosis: Primary Evans Syndrome

Evans syndrome is an autoimmune condition that presents with two or more cytopenias, which commonly include autoimmune hemolytic anemia (AIHA) and immune thrombocytopenia (ITP), with or without immune neutropenia (only in 15% of cases according to a report).[1]

The etiology of Evans syndrome remains unknown. Autoantibodies are directed against antigens specific to RBCs, platelets or neutrophils, but these autoantibodies do not cross-react.[2]

Evans syndrome exhibits myriad presentations. Patients may present with clinical features of thrombocytopenia, anemia, neutropenia and pancytopenia. Jaundice may indicate hemolysis.[2]

Potential complications of Evans syndrome include: hemorrhage with severe thrombocytopenia and serious infection in patients with neutropenia.[2] Our patient experienced intracerebral hemorrhage owing to thrombocytopenia.

The characteristic clinical course of Evans syndrome includes periods of remission and exacerbation.[2]

Treatment is not that much satisfactory with occasional fatal consequences.

Systemic lupus erythematosus (SLE) and lymphoproliferative disorder should be ruled out before making a diagnosis of Evans syndrome. Sometimes, AIHA and autoimmune thrombocytopenia (AITP) are found in patients with selective immunoglobulin A (IgA) deficiency or common variable immunodeficiency. These disorders must be excluded.[1]

In our day-to-day clinical practice, it is paramount to distinguish between primary and secondary Evans syndrome because it affects the outcome and management of the disease.

Corticosteroids and intravenous immunoglobulin (IVIG) remain the mainstay of treatment. Rituximab is considered as second-line option. Splenectomy, danazol and immunosuppressants may be used.[2]

REFERENCES

1. Michel M, Chanet V, Dechartres A, et al. The spectrum of Evans syndrome in adults: new insight into the disease based on the analysis of 68 cases. Blood. 2009;114(15):3167–72.
2. Shaikh H, Mewawalla P. Evans syndrome. [Updated 2019 Mar 16]. In: StatPearls [Internet]. Treasure Island (FL): StatPearls Publishing; 2019 Jan-. Available from: https://www.ncbi.nlm.nih.gov/books/NBK519015/

CASE 87

YOUNG MAN WITH UNEXPLAINED JAUNDICE AND FEVER

CASE SUMMARY

A 19-year-old male student presented with jaundice for the past 2.5 months, fever for same duration, and abdominal swelling for the past 2 months. Jaundice was not associated with passage of pale or dark-colored stool, itching or scratch marks. Fever was intermittent, high-grade, and subsided by taking medications with no diurnal variations and not associated with chills and rigor. Patient had abdominal distension associated with constant localized, dull aching pain in right hypochondrium, epigastrium and left hypochondrium. He also had anorexia and lost moderate amount of weight. Patient had a history of sudden neck swelling 3 years back, associated with mild cough and fever. The available medical documents showed, that time chest X-ray reported bilateral hilar lymphadenopathy, and biopsy and histopathology of cervical lymph node revealed granulomatous lymphadenitis. But no further evaluation was done at that time due to the patient's refusal.

On general examination, the young man was icteric, temperature—normal, pulse—72/min, BP—100/70 mm Hg. Generalized lymphadenopathy was present and there were multiple subcutaneous nodules at upper back, bilaterally medial to scapula. On abdominal examination, tender hepatomegaly and splenomegaly were found. Other systemic examination did not reveal any abnormality.

Investigation showed *complete blood count (CBC)*: hemoglobin (Hb)—6.92 g/dL, erythrocyte sedimentation rate (ESR)—140 mm in first hour, white blood cell (WBC)—15,000/mm^3 (N: 80%, L: 18%, E: 1%), peripheral blood film (PBF)—microcytic hypochromic anemia, leukocytosis, fair number of target cells. *Liver function test*: Serum bilirubin—12.11 mg/dL, alanine aminotransferase (ALT)—131 U/L, aspartate aminotransferase (AST)—322 U/L, serum alkaline phosphatase (ALP)—1,058 U/L, prothrombin time (PT)—25.6 seconds, international normalized ratio (INR)—2.10; surface antigen of hepatitis B (HBsAg), anti-HCV, HIV 1 and 2—negative.

Ultrasonography: Hepatosplenomegaly with para-aortic lymphadenopathy and dilated biliary tree. Endoscopy of upper gastrointestinal tract (GIT)—duodenal nodular lesion, bone marrow study—features were consistent with lymphoproliferative disorder.

QUESTIONS

1. What are the differential diagnoses you should consider?
2. What other investigations will you carry out for confirmation?

DISCUSSION

Considering the history, physical examination and investigations, we initially put the following differential diagnoses.
- Lymphoma
- Disseminated tuberculosis (TB).

For confirmation of the diagnosis and exclusion of the differentials, we went for *further investigations*:
- *Fine-needle aspiration cytology from cervical lymph node*: No granuloma or malignant cell was seen. Follicular lymphadenitis.
- *Lymph node biopsy*: Specimen—left epitrochlear lymph node. Sections showed multiple epithelioid granulomata, rounded fungal bodies within the granulomata and giant cell. No evidence of malignancy was seen. *Comment*: Fungal granuloma, suggestive of blastomycosis. Slides were reviewed in two separate laboratories and both laboratories showed same result of fungal lymphadenitis (blastomycosis) and immunohistochemistry was suggested for further confirmation.
- Special [Gomori Methenamine-Silver Nitrate (GMS)] stain of lymph node specimen confirmed the presence of yeasts and few hyphae of fungal elements. Specific species could not be determined in that material.

Final Diagnosis: Disseminated Fungal Infection (Blastomycosis)

Blastomycosis is an uncommon, chronic granulomatous and suppurative pulmonary and systemic mycosis. It is geographically restricted and the causative organism is fungus *Blastomyces dermatitidis*. This is a dimorphic fungus, which exists as a nonpathogenic mold in mycelial form in nature and converts to pathogenic yeast at body temperature. Inhalation or inoculations are the routes of acquisition of the infection.

Blastomycosis can produce a wide variety of illness, ranging from subclinical infection to progressive disseminated disease. Pulmonary infection can mimic bacterial pneumonia, while chronic infections mimic lung cancer or tuberculosis. Most common extrapulmonary site of disease is skin, followed by bone, central nervous system and prostate.[1]

Diagnosis is made by visualization of the yeast in tissue or confirmation by culture. Drug of choice is itraconazole; and in life-threatening cases, amphotericin B is indicated.

REFERENCE

1. Bradsher WR. Histoplasmosis and Blastomycosis. Clin Infect Dis. 1996;22(2): 8102–11.

CASE 88

YOUNG MAN WITH HEADACHE AND BLURRED VISION

CASE SUMMARY

A 27-year-old man was brought to hospital with headache and blurring of vision for the past 15 days and with one episode of convulsion. Headache was gradual in onset, located in right side, severe in intensity and described as the worst headache ever experienced. It was persistent and progressive but not associated with fever, vomiting, aura, photophobia or phonophobia. It was unchanged with posture. Persistent blurring of vision was there without any scotoma. Later on, he developed generalized tonic-clonic seizure which was associated with tongue biting and soiling of clothes, followed by postictal amnesia.

All the examination findings were normal, except for lacerations in left knuckles and bite mark on lateral border of tongue. Fundoscopy revealed early changes of papilledema. Blood pressure was 135/90 mm Hg, and other vitals were within normal limit.

Routine investigations such as complete blood count (CBC), random blood sugar (RBS), renal function test (RFT), liver function test (LFT), lipid profile, electrocardiography (ECG) and echocardiography were normal. Mild hyponatremia (131 mmol/L) was there. Magnetic resonance imaging (MRI) of brain revealed subacute infarcts at right temporal, occipital regions and at thalamus (Fig. 1).

QUESTIONS

1. Based on the clinical features and imaging, what investigations should be done next?
2. What might be the underlying causes of stroke at this age?

DISCUSSION

As the infarct region did not correspond to any arterial territory, we thought of venous stroke. Magnetic resonance venography (MRV) of brain revealed nonvisualized right transverse sinus and right sigmoid sinuses due to

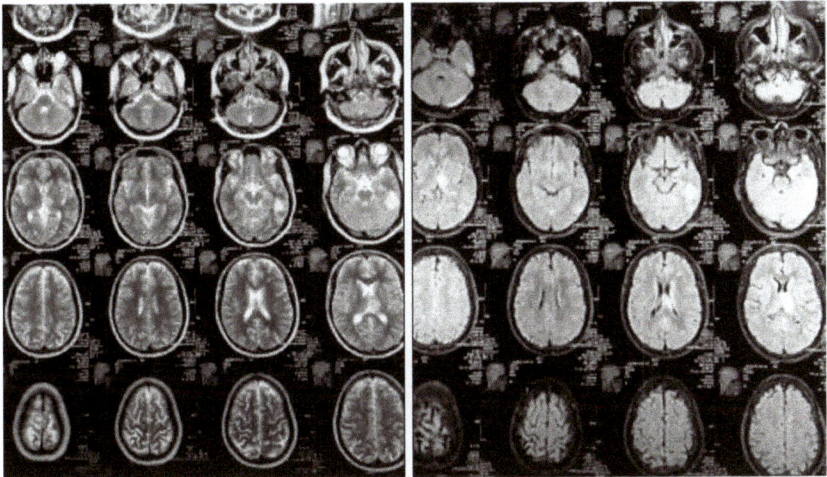

Fig. 1: Magnetic resonance imaging (MRI) of brain showing subacute infarcts at right temporal occipital regions and at thalamus.

thrombosis. Later, we explored the causes of thrombophilia which revealed reduced serum protein S level (24%). As false positive result is very common, this test needs repeatation after 2 weeks for confirmation of the diagnosis, provided the patient is not on warfarin therapy. Serum homocysteine, serum protein C, antithrombin-III, and antiphospholipid levels were noncontributory. The patient responded and recovered completely with anticoagulation.

During this period, we enquired about the predisposing factors which revealed that the patient had to work hard in an industry in hot humid environment for the last couple of weeks without adequate fluid replacement.

Final Diagnosis: Cerebral Venous Sinus Thrombosis due to Protein S Deficiency

Cerebral venous sinus thrombosis (CVT) can present with headaches due to isolated intracranial hypertension or focal deficits and seizures; or confusional states and lethargy owing to diffuse encephalopathy.[1]

Common predisposing factors are severe dehydration, in female—last trimester of pregnancy, puerperium, or because of genetic disorders of the clotting cascade, such as protein S or protein C deficiency, or the presence of factor V Leiden mutation.[2]

Even in the presence of hemorrhage, anticoagulation is the treatment of choice in CVT.

REFERENCES

1. Bousser MG. Cerebral venous thrombosis. In: Welch KMA Caplan LR, Reis DJ (Ed.). Primer on cerebrovascular diseases. Academic Press; 1997. pp. 385-9.
2. Deschiens MA, Conard J, Horellou MH, et al. Coagulation studies, factor V Leiden, and anticardiolipin antibodies in 40 cases of cerebral venous thrombosis. Stroke. 1996;27:1724-30.

CASE 89

YOUNG MAN WITH POLYARTHRITIS AND RENOMEGALY

CASE SUMMARY

A 27-year-old male, nondiabetic, normotensive *madrasa* teacher got admitted with the complaints of joint pain for the last 4 months and fever for 3 months. The patient stated that, 4 months back, one night he suddenly developed severe right elbow joint pain which awakened him from sleep. The pain was not associated with any swelling or redness and subsided gradually after taking medications. About 2 weeks later, he suddenly developed polyarthritis including metacarpophalangeal (MCP), proximal interphalangeal (PIP) and wrist joints of both upper limbs and metatarsophalangeal (MTP), ankle and knee joints of both lower limbs—associated with swelling, redness, and significant morning stiffness. Pain aggravated after a period of immobility and relieved after activities and taking analgesics. He also had arthralgia in shoulder and elbow joints. Patient also complained of recurrent bouts of fever for last 3 months. Each episode lasted for 5-6 days, and was continued in nature, not associated with chills, rigor or night sweats and subsided after taking paracetamol. Highest recorded temperature was 103°F. Fever was not accompanied by cough or alteration of bowel-bladder habits. Patient also reported hair loss, recurrent painless oral ulcers and significant weight loss of about 10 kg within last 4 months. He did not have any rash, photosensitivity, convulsion, abdominal pain or back pain. For joint pain, he was prescribed nonsteroidal anti-inflammatory drugs (NSAIDs), disease-modifying antirheumatic drugs (DMARDs) and steroid. He was the second issue of non-consanguineous marriage, and there was no history of similar illness, or any other significant illness in his family.

On examination, the patient had anemia, diffuse non-scarring alopecia and cervical lymphadenopathy involving both posterior chain and post-auricular region, largest one measuring about 1.5 × 1 cm, mildly tender, firm, and mobile, without any discharging sinus. Pulse—90 beats/minute, regular; BP—130/80 mm Hg, no postural drop; temperature—103°F; respiratory rate—20 breaths/minute. Musculoskeletal system examination revealed swelling,

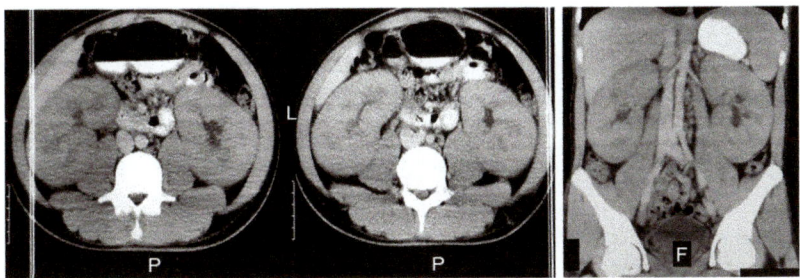

Fig. 1: CT scan of abdomen with oral and IV contrast, showing diffuse enlargement of both kidneys.

redness, tenderness and restriction of both active and passive movements in MCP, wrist, PIP, MTP, ankle and knee joints. Examination of abdomen revealed just palpable liver and bilaterally palpable and ballotable kidneys, which were firm, nontender without any bruit.

Investigations showed hemoglobin—8.4 g/dL, WBC count—17,000/mm^3, (neutrophils: 40%, lymphocytes: 51%), platelets—95,000/mm^3, ESR—70 mm in first hour, PBF—bicytopenia with lymphocytic leukocytosis. Urine R/M/E and serum electrolytes were normal. Serum creatinine—1.8 mg/dL. Ultrasonography of the whole abdomen—mild hepatomegaly (liver 15 cm, homogeneous echotexture, no focal abnormality), both kidneys were enlarged (right kidney: 17 cm, left kidney: 15 cm), corticomedullary differentiation was mildly impaired, cortical echogenicity was increased, no focal lesion was found. CT scan of abdomen with contrast demonstrated mild hepatomegaly with bilateral diffusely enlarged kidneys (Fig. 1). RA factor, anti-CCP antibody, ANA, anti-HIV antibodies were negative. Serum LDH—3,138 U/L, uric acid—12.80 mg/dL.

QUESTIONS

1. What are your differential diagnoses?
2. What findings do you expect in histopathology of lymph node and bone marrow studies?

DISCUSSION

For this young nondiabetic febrile patient with oral ulcers, photosensitivity, polyarthritis, significant weight loss and hepatomegaly—rheumatoid arthritis, systemic lupus erythematosus, and overlap syndrome were important considerations—though all these failed to explain presence of bilateral huge renomegaly. Moreover, RA factor, anti-CCP, ANA and anti-dsDNA, all were negative. So, keeping lymphadenopathy and renal involvement in mind, we had the following differential diagnoses: lymphoma, acute leukemia, polycystic kidney and liver, disseminated tuberculosis, bilateral renal cell

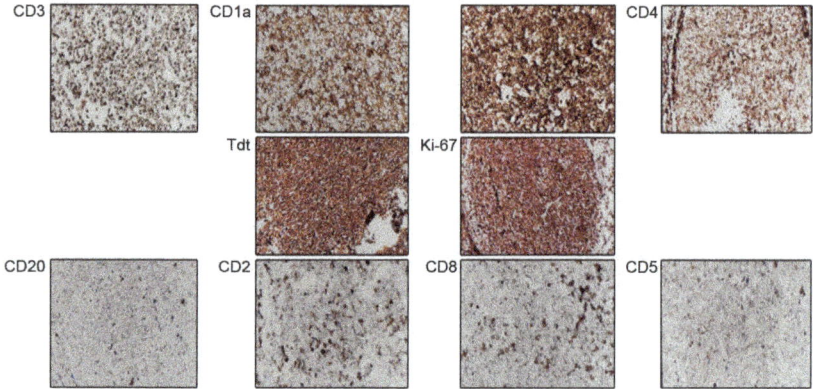

Fig. 2: Immunohistochemistry showing CD3, CD1a, CD7, CD4, Tdt (EP-266) diffusely positive and Ki-67 expression: 85–90%; with negative CD20, CD2, CD8 and CD5.

carcinoma (RCC) with metastasis, and HIV nephropathy. Since the images clearly demonstrated that there were no cysts or hydronephrotic changes, rather the kidneys had diffuse enlargement, hence polycystic kidney disease was unlikely. Bilateral large RCCs commonly produce asymmetric renal swelling, renal dysfunction and hematuria, which were absent in this case. Other initial investigations disfavored HIV and tuberculosis. Further invasive investigations were needed to reach the diagnosis. So, we did the following:

- *Excision biopsy and histopathology of lymph node:* Loss of nodal architecture with diffuse infiltration of large round cells, mitoses were noted. Findings were consistent with *diffuse large cell non-Hodgkin lymphoma, high grade.*
- *Bone marrow study:* Some cellular elements were visible; majority cells were blasts having scanty cytoplasm; nuclear:cytoplasmic (N:C) ratio—high; coarse chromatin and inconspicuous nucleoli resembling lymphoblast. These features were suggestive *of acute lymphoblastic leukemia.*
- *Immunohistochemistry (lymph node):* CD3, CD1a, CD7, CD4, Tdt (EP-266) diffusely positive and Ki-67 expression was 85–90%. CD20, CD2, CD8 and CD5 were negative. Diagnosis was consistent with *adult T-cell lymphoblastic leukemia/lymphoma* (Fig. 2).

Final Diagnosis: Adult T-cell Lymphoblastic Leukemia/Lymphoma

According to the World Health Organization classification, acute lymphoblastic leukemia (ALL)/lymphoblastic lymphoma (LBL) is a lymphoblastic neoplasm committed to either T-cell or B-cell lineage and involves bone marrow and blood.[1] Conventionally, *"lymphoma"* denotes neoplastic process confined to a mass lesion with absent or minimal involvement of peripheral blood and bone marrow; whereas *"leukemia"* is used when there is extensive peripheral blood and bone marrow involvement. LBL accounts for approximately 2% of all lymphomas.[2]

Lymphomas usually present as painless lymphadenopathy with or without systemic symptoms like fever, weight loss, night sweats, itching and hepatosplenomegaly. LBL can be an extranodal disease, with a predilection to involve mediastinum, skin, bone, liver, spleen, testis and central nervous system.[1] There is variation in clinical presentation of its subtypes. B-cell LBL commonly involves the skin, bone, soft tissue, lymph nodes, ovaries, retroperitoneum and tonsils. Contrarily, T-cell LBL usually presents as a mediastinal mass; or with cervical, supraclavicular and axillary lymphadenopathy.

Renomegaly with arthritis as initial manifestation of lymphoma is very uncommon. Also, lymphomatous infiltration in kidneys is a rare phenomenon, whereas kidney as a sole site of involvement is even rarer, with less than 100 reported cases of renal lymphoma diagnosed by percutaneous kidney biopsy.[3-6] Interestingly, as kidneys do not have identifiable lymphatic channels, there is considerable doubt among pathologists over renal involvement of lymphoma. Some think it is a disseminated malignancy, because in 10–20% of cases lymphoma affects both kidneys[7]—as was found in our patient. Mucosa-associated lymphoid tissue renal lymphoma is the probable underlying mechanism.[8] Diffuse large B-cell lymphoma is the most common subtype reported and precursor LBL/ALL accounts for fewer cases.[3,9,10] Renal involvement usually occurs late in the course of lymphoma and is typically clinically silent, but may rarely manifest with nonspecific hematuria, fever, flank pain and oliguria. It poses difficulty in diagnosis, and carries a very poor prognosis.[11]

Contrast-enhanced CT is the preferred method for diagnosing renal lymphoma, but due to its risk of nephrotoxicity, magnetic resonance imaging (MRI) is being recommended lately, especially in patients with renal failure.[10,12] The imaging findings can vary from unilateral to bilateral, single to multiple masses or diffuse parenchymal infiltration.[7] B-LBL/ALL is morphologically indistinguishable from precursor T-LBL/ALL on light microscopy, and differentiation requires the detection of lineage-specific markers by immunophenotyping.[13]

We diagnosed our patient based on histology and immunohistochemistry of lymph node, and bone marrow study with flow cytometry. Fine needle aspiration or core renal biopsy would have been the best method to establish diagnosis with high specificity and sensitivity,[8] but was not carried out, as the diagnosis was already established by lymph node and bone marrow studies, and also due to patient's general ill-health.

Treatment of acute T-cell lymphoblastic lymphoma/leukemia with renal involvement is controversial as pathogenetic mechanisms are unclear. Role of radiotherapy in treatment of bilateral diffuse lymphoma infiltration is not established. And whether it should be treated by chemotherapy alone, or in combination with radiation, is equally unclear due to lack of therapeutic trials. This uncertainty compels clinicians to adopt a practical approach and treat according to histological grade. Since most renal lymphoma cases are high-grade, they are treated by cyclophosphamide, doxorubicin, vincristine, prednisone (CHOP) or other chemotherapy regimen with or without radiotherapy.[6,7] However, results are usually unsatisfactory owing to rapid disease progression and treatment resistance.[8]

The patient was not given rituximab as it was not B-cell type. He was referred to the department of hematology for further management.

In patients presenting with unexplained bilateral nephromegaly with or without acute kidney injury (AKI), lymphomatous infiltration should be a clinical suspicion. Unexplained renal failure or proteinuria, and/or bilateral renomegaly detected on radioimaging should be diagnosed definitively by doing kidney biopsy.[3]

REFERENCES

1. Borowitz MJ, Chan JK. T lymphoblastic leukemia/lymphoma. In: Swerdlow S, Campo E, Lee Harris N, Jaffe ES, Pileri SA, Stein H, et al. (Editors). WHO Classification of Tumours of Haematopoietic and Lymphoid Tissues. Lyon: IARC; 2008. pp. 168-78.
2. Hoelzer D, Gökbuget N. T-cell lymphoblastic lymphoma and T-cell acute lymphoblastic leukemia: A separate entity? Clin Lymphoma Myeloma. 2009;9(Suppl 3):S214-21.
3. Törnroth T, Heiro M, Marcussen N, et al. Lymphomas diagnosed by percutaneous kidney biopsy. Am J Kidney Dis. 2003;42:960-71.
4. Kandel LB, McCullough DL, Harrison LH, et al. Primary renal lymphoma. Does it exist? Cancer. 1987;60:386-91.
5. GellrichJ, Hakenberg OW, Naumann R, et al. Primary renal non-Hodgkin's lymphoma: a difficult differential diagnosis. Onkologie. 2002;25:273-7.
6. Saito S. Primary renal lymphoma: Case report and review of the literature. Uro Int. 1996;56:192-5.
7. Stallone G, Infante B, Manno C, et al. Primary renal lymphoma does exist. J Nephrol. 2000;13:367-72.
8. Tuzel E, Mungan MU, Yorukoglu K, et al. Primary renal lymphoma of mucosa-associated lymphoid tissue. Urology. 2003;61:463-4.
9. Boueva A, Bouvier R. Precursor B-cell lymphoblastic leukemia as a cause of a bilateral nephromegaly. Pediatr Nephrol. 2005;20:679-82.
10. Shi SF, Zhou FD, Zou WZ, et al. Acute kidney injury and bilateral symmetrical enlargement of the kidneys as first presentation of B-cell lymphoblastic lymphoma. Am J Kidney Dis. 2012;60:1044-8.
11. Hartman DS, David CJ Jr, Goldman SM, et al. Renal lymphoma: Radiologic-pathologic correlation of 21 cases. Radiology. 1982;144:759-66.
12. Sheeran SR, Sussman SK. Renal lymphoma: Spectrum of CT findings and potential mimics. Am J Roentgenol. 1998;171:1067-72.
13. Boucheix C, David B, Sebban C, et al. Immunophenotype of adult acute lymphoblastic leukemia, clinical parameters, and outcome: An analysis of a prospective trial including 562 tested patients (LALA87). French group on therapy for adult acute lymphoblastic leukemia. Blood. 1994;84:1603-12.

CASE 90

YOUNG LADY WITH JAUNDICE AND PRURITUS

CASE SUMMARY

A 28-year-old lady presented with fluctuating jaundice and generalized pruritus for the last 6 months without any history of pale stool, nausea, vomiting, hematemesis, melena, abdominal pain, distension or weight loss. She had intermittent, low-grade fever with chills and rigor for same duration and there was history of taking herbal medication 6 months back. There was no history of skin rash, joint pain or sleep disturbance. She was nonsmoker, nonalcoholic and had no family history of similar illness or other familial disease.

On examination, the patient was icteric and skin scratch marks were present in whole body. Other parameters of general examination were normal and vital signs were within normal limit. There were no stigmata of chronic liver disease. On abdominal examination, nontender hepatomegaly was found which was about 2 cm from right costal margin, had regular margin, smooth surface, firm consistency, and upper border of liver dullness was in right fifth intercostal space without any bruit. Nervous system examination showed intact cranial nerves with normal fundoscopic examination. Slit-lamp examination showed no Kayser-Fleischer ring. Other systemic examinations did not reveal any abnormality.

Investigations showed: complete blood count (CBC): hemoglobin (Hb)—10.20 g/dL, white blood cell (WBC)—9,700 µL, platelet—280000 µL, erythrocyte sedimentation rate (ESR)—75 mm in first hour, peripheral blood film (PBF)—normocytic normochromic anemia with fair number of target cells; reticulocyte—1.27%; liver function test—serum bilirubin—total: 11.68 md/dL (direct: 9.12 mg/dL, indirect: 2.56 mg/dL), alanine aminotransferase (ALT)—84 U/L, aspartate aminotransferase (AST)—114 U/L, alkaline phosphatase (ALP)—457 U/L, gamma-glutamyl transferase (GGT)—150 U/L; serum total protein—7.25 g/dL; serum albumin—3.97 g/dL, serum globulin—3.28 g/dL, A:G 1.21, prothrombin time (PT)—12 seconds;

activated partial thromboplastin test (APTT)—30 seconds; ultrasonography (USG)—mild hepatomegaly (13.6 cm), parenchymal echotexture appeared normal, biliary channels were not dilated.

QUESTIONS

1. What differential diagnoses should be considered in this case?
2. What other investigations will you carry out for confirmation?

DISCUSSION

Considering the history, physical examination and investigations, we initially put the following differential diagnoses:
- Chronic hepatitis with cholestasis
- Wilson's disease.

For confirmation of the diagnosis and exclusion of the differentials, we went for further investigations:
- *Serum ceruloplasmin:* 30.2 mg/dL (referral range: 20–60 mg/dL); 24 hours urinary copper: 48.8 µg/day (concentration above 100 µg/24 h confirms Wilson's disease).
- *Viral markers:* Anti-HAV IgM, HBsAg, anti-HBc IgM and total, anti-HCV: Negative.
- *Antinuclear antibodies (ANA):* Negative; antimitochondrial antibody: Negative; anti-smooth muscle antibody: negative; serum *lactate dehydrogenase (LDH):* 449 U/L, Coombs test: direct Anti-HAV IgM, HBsAg, anti-HBc IgM negative and indirect Anti-HAV IgM, HBsAg, anti-HBc IgM positive.
- *Endoscopy of upper gastrointestinal (GIT):* No varix was seen. Features of congestive gastropathy at the body and fundus of stomach.

As we could not come to a conclusion after all of the above investigations, we planned for liver biopsy.
- *Histopathology report of liver biopsy:* Hepatic lobules did not show any significant changes. Portal tract showed fibrosis and mild inflammatory infiltrates, predominantly lymphocytes. Concentric lamellated periductal fibrosis was seen around interlobular bile ducts. No evidence of cirrhosis or malignancy was seen. Comment: Suggestive of sclerosing cholangitis.
- *Magnetic resonance cholangiopancreatography (MRCP):* Multiple skip dilatations were noted at the intrahepatic biliary ducts. Multiple signal void areas were seen in the right lobe of liver segment VII. Common bile duct (CBD) was well-visualized, normal in caliber and homogeneous intraluminal signal intensity. Gallbladder showed normal size. Main pancreatic duct was not dilated. Comment: Suggestive of progressive sclerosing cholangitis.
- *Colonoscopy:* Normal colon and rectum.

Final Diagnosis: Primary Sclerosing Cholangitis

Primary sclerosing cholangitis (PSC) is caused by diffuse inflammation and fibrosis resulting in cholestatic liver disease. The entire biliary tree can be involved and gradually progresses to the obliteration of intrahepatic and extrahepatic bile ducts, biliary cirrhosis, portal hypertension, hepatic failure. PSC is two times more common in men and age of presentation is 25–40 years.[1]

The diagnostic criteria are: Generalized beading and stenosis of the biliary system on cholangiography, absence of choledocholithiasis (or history of bile duct surgery) and exclusion of bile duct cancer by prolonged follow-up. The cause is unknown but it is strongly associated with inflammatory bowel disease, especially ulcerative colitis.[1]

Common symptoms of PSC are fatigue, intermittent jaundice, pruritus, abdominal pain over right upper quadrant, weight loss. Biochemical test presents as cholestatic pattern but ALP and bilirubin levels may vary widely in the patient during the disease course. Antineutrophil cytoplasmic antibody (ANCA), low titers of antinuclear antibody (ANA), anti-smooth muscle antibodies may be found positive; serum antimitochondrial antibody (AMA) is absent. The key investigation of choice is MRCP, revealing multiple irregular stricturing and dilatation, which is considered diagnostic. Endoscopic retrograde cholangiopancreatography (ERCP) is usually reserved for patients who need therapeutic intervention and should follow MRCP. Characteristic features of PSC on liver biopsy are periductal "onion-skin" fibrosis and inflammation, portal edema, bile ductular proliferation. Eventually fibrosis spreads, resulting in biliary cirrhosis; obliterative cholangitis leads to the so-called "vanishing bile duct syndrome."[1]

In our patient, we initially found the typical cholestatic picture characterized by elevated ALP and, later on, typical picture of PSC in liver biopsy and MRCP were also noticed. PSC has close association with ulcerative colitis—which was excluded in our patient by doing colonoscopy.

No curative treatment is available for PSC, but management of cholestasis and its complications are indicated. Ursodeoxycholic acid (UDCA) is mostly used but the evidence supporting this is limited. UDCA has some benefit in reducing colon carcinoma risk. Immunosuppressive agents, including prednisolone, azathioprine, methotrexate and cyclosporine, have been tried; generally, results have been disappointing. ERCP helps to relieve the obstruction in the extrahepatic bile duct by placing a plastic stent or by balloon dilatation.[1]

REFERENCE

1. Ralston SH, Penman ID, Strachan MWJ, et al. Davidson's Principles and Practice of Medicine. 23rd ed. Edinburgh: Churchill Livingstone/Elsevier; 2018. pp. 888-90.

CASE 91

LITTLE GIRL WITH RELAPSED POTT'S DISEASE AND PARAPLEGIA

CASE SUMMARY

A 16-year-old girl, student, immunized as per the standard Expanded Program on Immunization (EPI) schedule presented with the complaints of recurrent weakness of lower limbs, recurrent inability to urinate and defecate, and almost constant pain in her back and neck, which had no aggravating or relieving factor or diurnal variation—for the last 3 years. These were preceded by onset of low-grade fever with evening rise of temperature associated with sweating, but no chills and rigor. After first onset of neck and back pain, her orthopedician advised her to perform some exercises which did not improve her state; rather, one day during exercise, she experienced crucial pain after a clicking sound in her back, followed by weakness in lower limbs and inability to void urine and to defecate. She was diagnosed with *"Pott's disease with dorsal spine compression and vertebral fracture with paravertebral abscess"* and underwent decompressive neurosurgery named "decompression, fusion and stabilization with screw implantation". Category-I anti-tuberculosis (TB) drug was given for 17 months. Patient's paraplegia and bowel-bladder involvement was improved and she was able to walk, but she seldom had back pain after prolonged sitting and was unable to lift weight. After 11 months of completion of anti-TB regimen, her back pain recurred and she eventually developed paraplegia and bowel-bladder incontinence. Then she got admitted to hospital and underwent another neurosurgical procedure named "laminectomy, facetectomy and fixation of D_2, D_3 and D_4 by screw and rods" and started modified Category-II anti-TB drugs with amikacin and levofloxacin, but her symptoms persisted even after a year. So, she got admitted to the Department of Medicine, Dhaka Medical College and Hospital (DMCH).

On general examination, she was ill-looking, mildly anemic and had scar at the back due to previous surgeries. There was no lymphadenopathy. Her vitals were normal. On nervous system examination, higher psychic function including speech and cranial nerve examination including fundoscopy revealed normal findings. Muscle bulk was normal, but tone was increased in lower limbs and muscle power in lower limbs were 1/5 (right) and 3/5 (left). All deep reflexes of all four limbs were exaggerated and plantar response was extensor bilaterally. Ankle clonus was present on both sides. All modalities of sensory perception were diminished below eighth thoracic vertebra. Cerebellar functions were intact and no sign of meningeal irritation was present, but coordination of lower limbs, gait and Rombergism could not be evaluated due to weakness. No abnormality was detected on examination of the rest of the systems.

Complete blood count (CBC) showed hemoglobin (Hb)—13.1 g/dL, white blood cell (WBC)—7,200/mm^3, platelets—272,000/mm^3, erythrocyte sedimentation rate (ESR)—40 mm in first hour. MRI of dorsal spine was done twice—before 1st surgery (Fig. 1) and 2nd surgery (Fig. 2). After first surgery, subsequent histopathological examination of tissue from dorsal spine revealed—histologically consistent with *tuberculosis*. GeneXpert of pus from paravertebral abscess was positive for *MTB* and rifampicin sensitive. Following second surgery, histopathological examination of paravertebral tissue revealed: granulomatous spondylitis, histologically *tubercular spondylitis*. Two more MRIs were done for follow-up (Figs. 3 and 4) while the patient was receiving modified Category-II anti-TB medications.

QUESTIONS

1. What differentials should be considered?
2. How should we manage this difficult case?

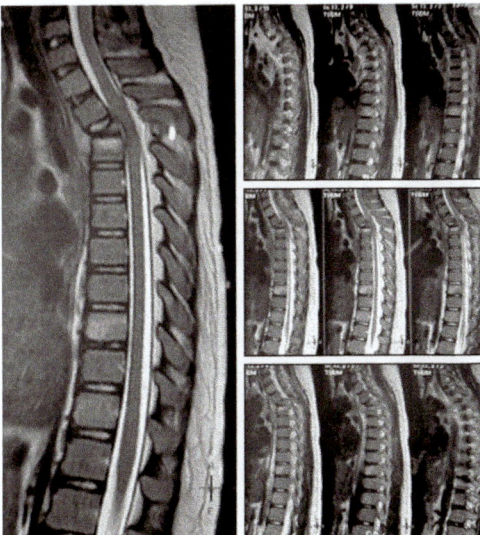

Magnetic resonance imaging done before 1st surgery
Comments: • Tubercular spondylitis (D_3) with pre- and paravertebral abscess along with dorsal spinal cord compression and compressive myelopathy. • Marrow edema at D_4, D_9 and D_{11} bodies. • Disk space between D_8/D_9 is reduced with corresponding end plate irregularities. • Nerve roots at the D_3 level are compressed bilaterally. • Possibility of tubercular spondylodiscitis is also to be considered at D_8/D_9.

Fig. 1: Magnetic resonance imaging of dorsal spine, multiple sagittal cuts, T_2 sequence.

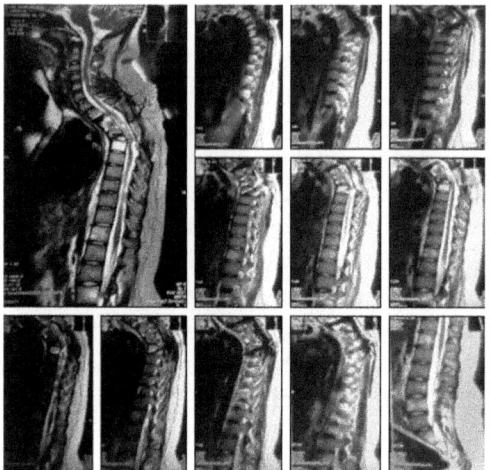

Fig. 2: Magnetic resonance imaging (MRI) of dorsal spine, multiple sagittal cuts, T_2 sequence.

Magnetic resonance imaging done before 2nd surgery

Comments:
- Suggestive of partial collapse of T_3 and T_4 spines with marrow replacement at T_1, T_2, T_3, T_4 and T_{11} spines.
- Paraspinal mass (abscess with granulation tissue) formation at the level of C_7 to T_4 and intracranial extension of the same mass.
- Moderate compression on spinal cord, as well as compression on T_3 and T_4 bilateral exiting nerve roots by the posteriorly protruded collapsed T_3 and T_4 spine along with paravertebral mass (abscess with granulation tissue) possibly tubercular spondylitis.

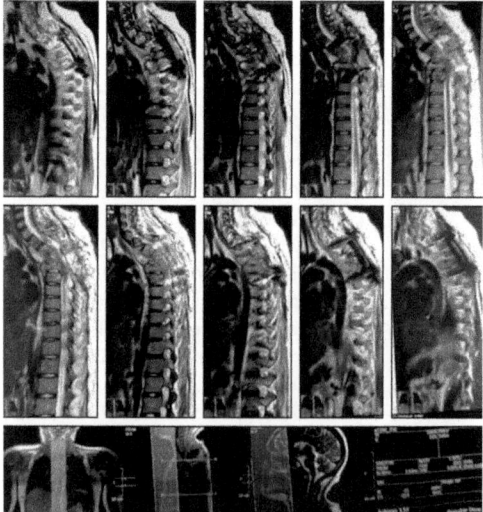

Fig. 3: Magnetic resonance imaging (MRI) of dorsal spine, multiple sagittal planes, T_1 sequence.

Follow-up magnetic resonance imaging (MRI) after 2 months of starting modified Category-II anti-TB medications

Comments:
- Findings suggestive of Pott's disease involving D_1 to D_6 and D_{12} vertebrae with pre- and paravertebral, anterior epidural abscesses and posterior bulging of D_1 to D_6 vertebrae causing thecal sac indentation, significant spinal canal stenosis, cord and corresponding traversing nerve root compression with compressive myelopathy.
- Schmorl's node at lower end-plate of D_9 vertebrae.
- Internal fixation devices, screw and rods at D_1 to D_6 vertebrae levels.

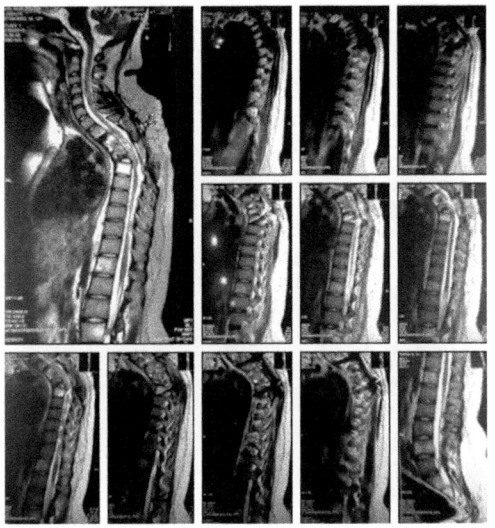

Follow-up MRI done after 9 months of starting Category-II anti-TB medications
Comments: - Pott's disease D_1 to D_5. Severe collapse of D_4 and mild collapse of D_3 bodies. - Transpedicular fixators at D_1 to D_5 levels, right D_1 fixator abut thecal sacs–spinal cord, anterolisthesis of D_3 over D_4 grade I. - Focal myelopathic changes at D_3-D_4 levels. - Hemangioma seen at D_{11} bodies.

Fig. 4: Magnetic resonance imaging (MRI) of dorsal spine, multiple sagittal planes, T_2 sequence.

DISCUSSION

For this young girl with history of low-grade fever and constant neck and back pain with features of cord compression in the form of spastic paraplegia and bowel, bladder involvement, and a definite sensory level—the most likely clinical diagnosis was cord compression due to Pott's disease. This was proved by the investigations and rightly addressed by starting Category-I anti-TB medications and performing surgery. When the girl presented with features of relapse, all the issues were dealt with accordingly by performing a second surgery and starting modified Category-II anti-TB drugs. But unfortunately, her symptoms persisted and she came to us. Our provisional diagnosis was *relapsed Pott's disease with paraplegia* and differentials for the cause of relapsed paraplegia due to dorsal myelopathy were:
- Extensively drug-resistant tuberculosis (XDR-TB)
- Nontuberculous *mycobacterium* (NTM) infection
- Deep fungal infection.

We repeated the relevant investigations which did not reflect any active disease. MRI of spine was repeated (Figs. 5 and 6) and no pre- or paravertebral lesion was detected. Though her symptomatic improvement regarding paraplegia and bowel-bladder incontinence was not tangible, the patient was afebrile and stable. As evident from the history and serial MRI of spine, she had compression-collapse of multiple thoracic vertebrae, and resultant significant spinal canal stenosis. Though the two surgeries performed were attempted at correcting the deformities, the anatomical distortion of the spinal

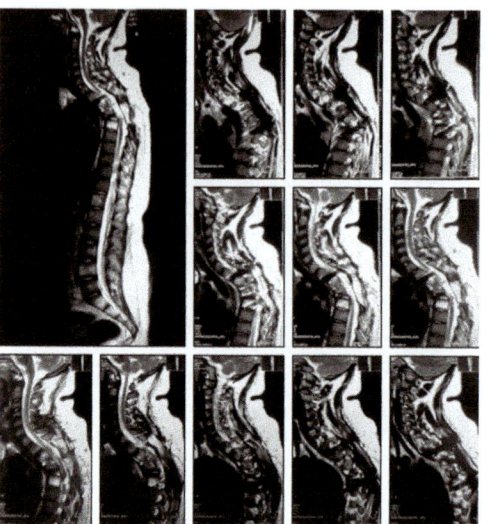

Magnetic resonance imaging done after hospital admission (Figs. 5 and 6)	
Comments: • No pre- and paravertebral lesion detected. • Evidence of laminectomy. • Fusion of D_3–D_4 noted with obliteration of intervening disk space? Inflammatory.	

Fig. 5: Magnetic resonance imaging (MRI) of spine, multiple sagittal planes, T_2 sequence.

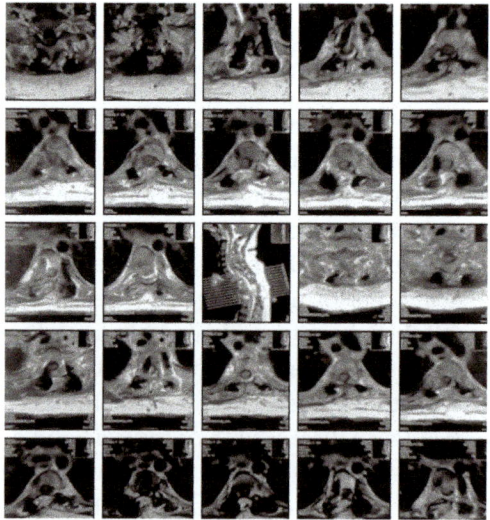

Fig. 6: Magnetic resonance imaging (MRI) of spine, multiple axial cuts, T_1 sequence.

canal and surrounding structures was undeniable. So, after much discussion, we concluded that her persistence of symptoms could be explained by late-onset paraplegia due to mechanical pressure on the cord. Depending on clinical judgement, we avoided further invasive investigations, and continued the Category-II anti-TB drugs for 2 years and ensured physiotherapy.

Final Diagnosis: Relapsed Pott's Disease with Paraplegia due to Mechanical Cord Compression

The patient eventually responded, and after completion of anti-TB therapy, she resumed her normal daily activities with difficulty and residual disability. She is still receiving regular sessions of physiotherapy including electrical stimulation therapy. In her last follow-up, she informed us that she could move her left leg, but her right leg was still very weak. Despite this, she had started going to school again.

In 1779, Percival Pott described the first modern case of spinal tuberculosis (TB); hence, we call it Pott's disease. Of all TB patients, nearly 1–2% have skeletal system involvement, of which spinal TB is the most common form (50% of skeletal TB).[1] Pott's disease can be drastic in presence of neurologic deficit attributable to substantial spinal disfigurement, and neural structures compression. Although any part of the spine can be affected in spinal TB, the thoracolumbar junction is the most common site of involvement.

There are two discrete types of spinal TB: spondylodiscitis (the classic form), and spondylitis without disk involvement (atypical form). The intervertebral disk involvement is secondary to spread from adjacent infected vertebra in adults, while it is largely due to the vascularized nature of the intervertebral disk in children. The basic lesion in Pott's disease is a combination of osteomyelitis and arthritis, usually affecting multiple vertebrae. The anterior aspect of the vertebral body adjacent to the subchondral plate is commonly involved. Spinal TB can cause progressive bone destruction leading to vertebral collapse and kyphosis, cold abscess formation (from infection extension into adjacent ligaments and soft tissues), spinal canal narrowing (abscesses or granulation tissue or direct dural invasion) resulting in spinal cord compression and neurologic deficits.[2]

In the active stage, patients present with typical systemic symptoms. The spine is stiff and movement is restricted due to pain, with gibbus tender on percussion. The typical night cries are due to movement between the inflamed surfaces during sleep, when persistent paraspinal muscle spasm around the involved vertebral bodies relaxes. A cold abscess may be present. Unusually, the patient may initially present with neurological deficit. Abscess or sinus can track along the fascial plains or course of the neurovascular bundles and present far away from the vertebral column. Paraplegia due to spinal TB has been classified into two main groups:[3]

- *Group A:* Early-onset paraplegia—this is the active phase of the vertebral disease, usually within the first 2 years of the onset. The underlying pathology is inflammatory edema, granulation tissue, tuberculous abscess, caseous tissue or, rarely, ischemic lesion of the cord.
- *Group B:* Late-onset paraplegia—appears many years (more than 2 years) after the disease had persisted in the vertebral column. Neurological complication may be due to recurrence of the disease or owing to mechanical pressure on the cord. The most common underlying pathology

is caseous tissue, tuberculous debris, sequestra from vertebral body and disk, internal gibbus, vertebral canal stenosis or severe deformity.

X-ray spine, computed tomography (CT) scans and, mostly, MRI can be very useful for early detection of vertebral involvement.

Pott's disease warrants treatment with multiple anti-TB drugs. Treatment must be continued for at least 6-9 months, and sometimes, up to 9-12 months. Immunodeficient patients may need lifelong drug therapy to prevent recurrence. External bracing is the intervention of choice, allowing rehabilitation and self-care. Surgery (spinal fusion, rod placement) may finally be needed to relieve cord compression, correct abnormal curvature of the spine, or resolve spinal instability secondary to loss of bone mass.

Prognosis is variable. Some individuals recover completely, particularly with prompt and aggressive treatment. Advanced disease may cause long-term disability even after cure of the bacterial infection. Depending on the severity of symptoms, spinal fusion may be effective in relieving discomfort. Owing to different modalities of medical and surgical management, the outcomes of spinal TB are varied.

REFERENCES

1. He M, Xu H, Zhao J, Wang Z. Anterior debridement, decompression, bone grafting, and instrumentation for lower cervical spine tuberculosis. Spine J. 2014;14(4):619-27.
2. Rasouli MR, Mirkoohi M, Vaccaro AR, Yarandi KK, Rahimi-Movaghar V. Spinal tuberculosis: diagnosis and management. Asian Spine J. 2012;6(4):294-308. doi:10.4184/asj.2012.6.4.294
3. Agrawal V, Patgaonkar PR, Nagariya SP. Tuberculosis of spine. J Craniovertebral Junction Spine. 2010;1(2):74-85.

CASE 92

YOUNG MAN WITH HEPATOSPLENOMEGALY AND MONOCLONAL GAMMOPATHY

CASE SUMMARY

A 30-year-old male weaver, resident of Sirajganj (part of north-central Bangladesh) presented with fever for the past 5 months and significant weight loss. Fever was intermittent with chills and rigor, usually subsided with sweating on taking antipyretics but recurred after several hours and highest recorded temperature was 104°F. Weight loss was documented to be 14 kg in the last 5 months. He also complained of anorexia, persistent abdominal discomfort and generalized weakness. He did not give any history of cough, hemoptysis and hematemesis or bleeding from any other site, jaundice, back pain or joint pain. He had no significant travel history, or contact with patient of tuberculosis. He was nonsmoker and nonalcoholic.

On examination, the patient was ill-looking, cachectic and moderately anemic. Pulse was 80 beats/min, BP—120/80 mm Hg, temperature—103°F, and respiratory rate was 16 breaths/min. There was no bleeding spot and no bony tenderness. On abdominal examination, nontender hepatomegaly was found, which was about 5 cm from right costal margin, had regular margin, smooth surface, firm consistency and upper border of liver dullness was in right 5th intercostal space without bruit. Splenomegaly was also present and about 7 cm from left costal margin in the anterior axillary line toward the right iliac fossa. It was firm in consistency, nontender with smooth surface. Examination of other systems revealed normal findings.

On investigation, findings were: *Complete blood count (CBC)*: White blood count (WBC)—2900/µL, hemoglobin (Hb)—9.30 g/dL, platelet—1,60,000/µL, erythrocyte sedimentation rate (ESR)—83 mm in first hour, peripheral blood film (PBF)—normocytic normochromic anemia with bicytopenia. *Liver function test*: serum bilirubin—23 µmol/L, alanine aminotransferase (ALT)—84U/L, prothrombin time (PT)—13 seconds, serum albumin—2.28 g/dL, serum

Fractions	%	Ref.%	g/L	Ref.g/L
Albumin	26.8	55.8-66.1	21.4	40.2-47.6
Alpha1	5.4	2.9-4.9	4.3	2.1-3.5
Alpha 2	7.5	7.1-11.8	6.0	5.1-8.5
Beta 1	3.3	4.7-7.2	2.6	3.4-5.2
Beta 2	3.0	3.2-6.5	2.4	2.3-4.7
Gamma	54.0	11.1-18.8	43.2	8.0-13.5

TP: 80   A:G: 0.37

Figs. 1A and B: Serum protein electrophoresis. (A:G, albumin to globulin; TP, total protein; Ref: Reference)

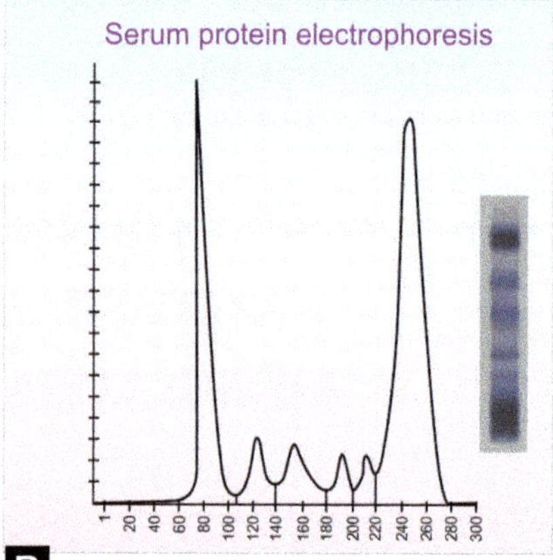

creatinine—0.89 mg/dL, serum urea—15 mg/dL, febrile antigens—negative, C-reactive protein (CRP)—46 ng/mL, blood culture (CS)—no growth. *Urine routine examination (RE)*: protein—++, sugar—nil, pus cell—2-4/HPF, RBC—nil; ultrasonography (USG)—moderate hepatosplenomegaly. *Bone marrow study*: cellularity—hypercellular, myeloid to erythroid (M:E) ratio—normal, erythropoiesis—active and normoblastic, granulopoiesis—active and maturing into segmented form, megakaryocyte—normal in number, lymphoid cell—normal in number, plasma cells—increased in number. About 20-25% of marrow-nucleated cells were plasma cells showing atypical cytology with fair number of plasmablasts. Comment: Features suggestive of reactive marrow. However, possibility of plasma cell dyscrasias should be ruled out by serum protein electrophoresis. *Serum protein electrophoresis*: There was a diffusely increased band in the gamma region (Figs. 1A and B). An underlying monoclonal band could not be excluded. Therefore, immunofixation was recommended.

QUESTIONS

1. What are the differential diagnoses you should consider?
2. What other investigations will you consider for confirmation?

DISCUSSION

Considering the history, physical examination and investigations, we initially put the following differential diagnoses:
- Visceral leishmaniasis (kala-azar)
- Chronic myeloid leukemia
- Multiple myeloma

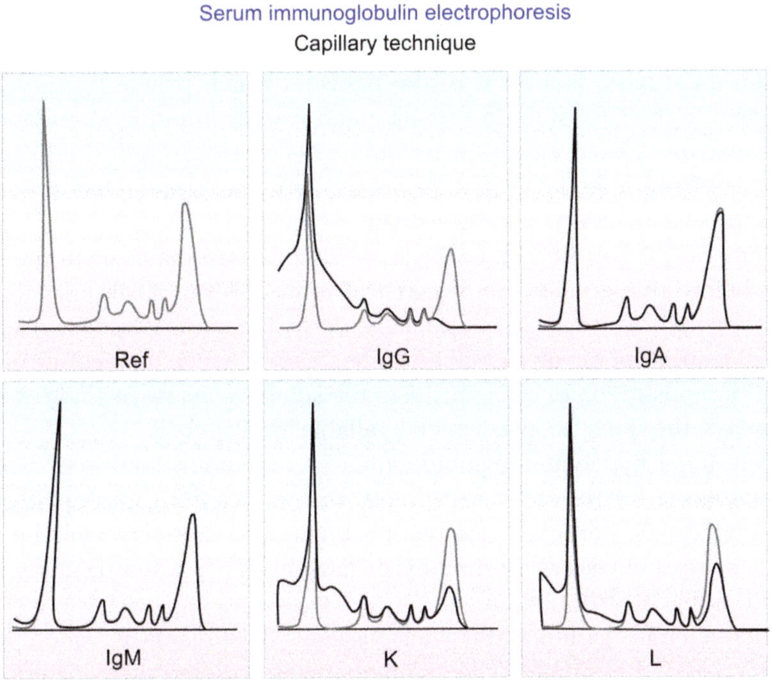

Serum immunoglobulin electrophoresis
Capillary technique

Fig. 2: Serum immunoglobulin electrophoresis.

- Disseminated tuberculosis
- Lymphoma.

For confirmation of the diagnosis and exclusion of the differentials, we went for further investigations:
- *Urine for Bence-Jones protein*: Positive
- Serum calcium (corrected): 8.9 mg/dL (8.8–10)
- *Serum immunoglobulin electrophoresis:* Capillary immunoglobulin electrophoresis showed a moderate immunoglobulin G (IgG) heavy chain band and also a moderate kappa light chain band (Fig. 2).
- *Immunochromatographic test (ICT) for kala-azar (rK39)*: Positive
- *Splenic aspirate study*: Smears showed lymphocytes at various stages and histiocytes. Small numbers of Leishman-Donovan (LD) bodies were seen within and outside the histiocytes. The background showed blood. Suggestive of visceral leishmaniasis.

Final Diagnosis: Visceral Leishmaniasis

Visceral leishmaniasis is a slowly progressive indigenous disease caused by protozoa of *Leishmania* genus. It is transmitted by the bite of an infected female phlebotomus sandfly that inoculates promastigotes into the host skin. The disease presents in four different forms with a wide range of clinical features:

visceral leishmaniasis or kala-azar, cutaneous leishmaniasis, mucocutaneous leishmaniasis, and diffuse cutaneous leishmaniasis.

The amastigote is a form of the parasite, which primarily infects the reticuloendothelial system in kala-azar and usually found in abundance in bone marrow, spleen and liver. Immunity becomes compromised causing persistent fever, anemia, liver and spleen enlargement, and if left untreated, opportunistic infection may cause death.

Sometimes, it is difficult to diagnose visceral leishmaniasis in the early stage before the appearance of classical triad of fever, splenomegaly and pancytopenia that results in considerable delay. Diagnosis is usually made by clinical features of the disease in an endemic area, which then confirmed by either demonstration of the parasite in the splenic aspirate or indirect tests. Nowadays, the rK39 test kit is widely available for diagnosis.

Polyclonal hypergammaglobulinemia is a common feature of visceral leishmaniasis. Kala-azar, as an etiology of monoclonal gammopathy, has been implicated in only few case reports. It may also cause cryoglobulinemia. These features of visceral leishmaniasis have been proposed resulting from chronic antigenic stimulation.[1,2]

Monoclonal gammopathy in visceral leishmaniasis should be differentiated from monoclonal gammopathy of undetermined significance (MGUS). Treatment of visceral leishmaniasis results in disappearance of M spike. However, the recognition of this correlation is important in endemic areas as M spike-positive patients might be harboring leishmaniasis. Though these cases are rare, but are a potentially treatable cause of monoclonal gammopathy; therefore, in endemic areas, visceral leishmaniasis should be considered in the differential diagnosis of monoclonal gammopathy.

REFERENCES

1. Ghosh AK, Dasgupta S, Ghose AC. Immunoglobulin G subclass-specific antileishmanial antibody responses in Indian kala-azar and post-kala-azar dermal leishmaniasis. Clin Diagn Lab Immunol. 1995;2(3):291-6.
2. Garcia-Menendez L, Lopez SC, Eroles FAL, Lahera MM, del-Canto GJ, Sanz AC. Monoclonal component in visceral leishmaniasis: a rare association that can lead to misdiagnosis. Rev Clin Esp. 1998;198:517-20.

CASE 93

YOUNG FEMALE WITH RECURRENT ABDOMINAL PAIN

CASE SUMMARY

A 31-year-old female, diabetic and normotensive presented with abdominal pain for the past 10 years, headache and weight loss for 3 years. The abdominal pain was so severe that, each time the pain occurred, she needed admission in the local hospital, where her pain subsided after conservative management. She also underwent elective cholecystectomy, but her symptom did not improve. During one such episode, she came to a medical university hospital of Bangladesh and was diagnosed as a case of chronic calcific pancreatitis and was treated by removal of pancreatic calculi as well as pancreatic duct with lateral pancreaticojenunostomy and jejunojejunostomy. After the surgery, she was symptom-free for 5 years, after which the pain recurred in the same manner. Then, 3 years back, she started having almost constant generalized headache. She also reported significant unintentional weight loss in the course of the last 3 years.

On examination, her body build was below average. Vital signs were normal. No other abnormality was detected in her general and systemic examinations.

Investigations showed neutrophilic leukocytosis; peripheral blood film—normal; chest X-ray—normal; serum electrolyte—normal; ultrasonography of abdomen—multiple pancreatic stone with bilateral renal stones; serum calcium level—10.5 mg/dL. Serum albumin was low and renal function tests were normal.

QUESTIONS

1. What are the differentials?
2. What should be the next step of investigation?

DISCUSSION

This patient with recurrent abdominal pain had evidence of multiple stones in pancreas and kidney. Hypercalcemia could explain all her symptoms. Though the calcium level was not as high as expected, yet, low serum albumin of this patient could be the cause. The total serum calcium was 11.8 mg/dL. Then we checked phosphate and magnesium and both were low. This made it a case of hypercalcemia with hypophosphatemia. Also there was hypomagnesemia; so, parathyroid hormone test was performed which was 124.5 pg/mL (very high). Parathyroid scan findings were consistent with parathyroid adenoma/hyperplasia (Fig. 1).

Final Diagnosis: Primary Hyperparathyroidism due to Parathyroid Adenoma

Primary hyperparathyroidism is a condition characterized by an inappropriate excess secretion of parathyroid hormone. The elevated hormone levels result in hypercalcemia and hypophosphatemia, which causes serious medical sequel, including renal colic, peptic ulcer disease, pancreatitis, osteoporosis, polyuria and depression.

Primary hyperparathyroidism is caused by a single parathyroid adenoma in 90% of patients.[1] Rarely, patients may develop hyperparathyroidism secondary to a parathyroid carcinoma.

Imaging studies, including parathyroid scintigraphy should be performed only after the diagnosis of primary hyperparathyroidism is established on the basis of biochemical findings. Surgery is usually recommended in age less than 50 years, renal stone, renal impairment, osteoporosis, peptic ulcer disease, significant hypercalcemia more than 11.4 mg/dL.

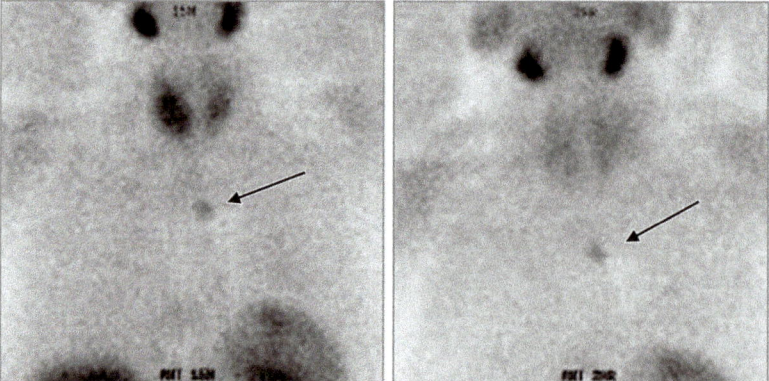

Fig. 1: Parathyroid radioisotope scanning showing adenoma.

This young lady developed bilateral renal stone, so we referred her to surgery department. Cinacalcet, a calcimimetic, is a treatment option for those, who cannot undergo surgery.

Parathyroid adenoma can be present as a part of multiple endocrine neoplasia syndromes (MEN 1 or 2). So we checked the growth hormone and calcitonin and all were normal.

REFERENCE

1. Ralston SH, Penman ID, Strachan MWJ, et al. Davidson's Principles and Practice of Medicine. 23rd ed. Edinburgh: Churchill Livingstone/Elsevier; 2018. pp. 663-4.

CASE 94

MIDDLE-AGED LADY WITH UNEXPLAINED ANEMIA

CASE SUMMARY

A 45-year-old housewife presented with generalized weakness, easy fatigability and gradually progressive exertional dyspnea for the past 4 months. Over the last few months, she was diagnosed as unexplained anemia and got several blood transfusions. Her bowel-bladder habit was normal and so was her menstrual and obstetric history. No significant family history was available.

Her physical examination revealed only moderate anemia, without jaundice. Vital signs were within normal limit, lungs were clear. On abdominal examination, there was no organomegaly or ascites.

Investigations showed that her Hb% was low in consecutive blood reports even after a few blood transfusions. Red cell indices showed microcytic hypochromic anemia. Liver and renal function tests were normal. Abdominal ultrasound showed normal appearance of all intra-abdominal organs. Previous peripheral blood film was insignificant. Bone marrow study showed erythroid hyperplasia. One Hb electrophoresis report was normal. Her iron profile was also within normal limit. But the reticulocyte count was increased with normal Coombs' test. Colonoscopy and endoscopy reports were also normal.

QUESTIONS

1. What are the differential diagnoses?
2. What is the next step of investigation?

DISCUSSION

The clinical presentation and microcytic hypochromic blood picture are suggestive of two most common causes: iron-deficiency anemia (IDA) and hereditary hemolytic anaemia. But previous PBF, bone marrow studies were insignificant. Serum iron profile was normal. However, reticulocytosis was present. So, regardless of the Hb electrophoresis report, we repeated the PBF and it revealed the raised amount of reticulocytes with the "Golf Ball" appearance (Fig. 1). It is the characteristic appearance of hemoglobin H (HbH) subtype of alpha thalassemia. Then, Hb electrophoresis was repeated in capillary gel method and it confirmed HbH disease with raised HbH percentage. Later, we arranged the genetic testing in complex PCR method (Fig. 2) and it also confirmed the HbH disease.

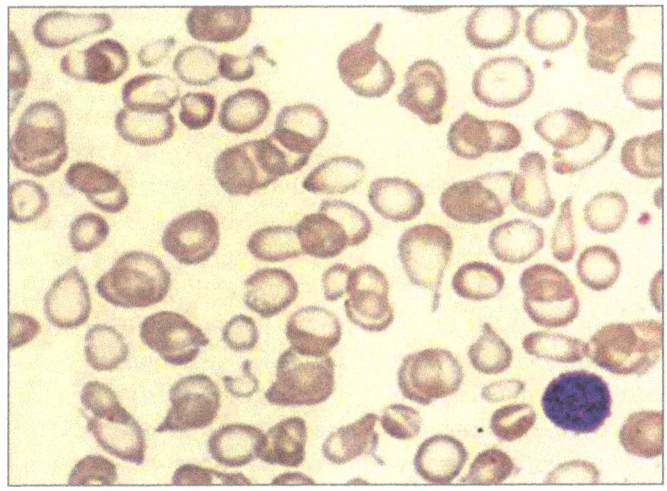

Fig. 1: "Golf ball" appearance of RBC.

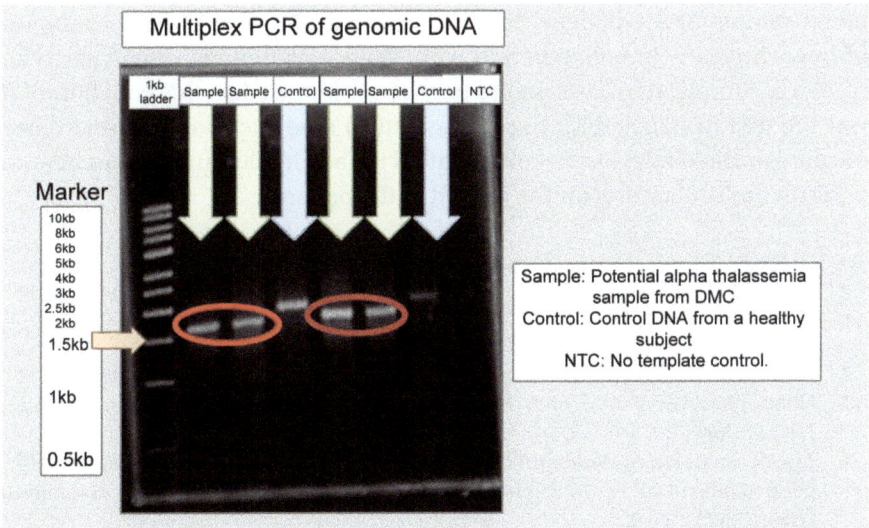

Fig. 2: Multiplex PCR of the patient's genomic DNA using 16 primers specific for the detection of seven most common alpha thalassemia deletions. The gel image shows the presence of α2 3.7 deletion; when compared with the product sizes for the respective primer pairs.

She, along with her family, was counseled regarding the disease and now she is under regular follow-up.

Final Diagnosis: Hemoglobin H (HbH) Disease

Hemoglobin H (HbH) disease is a form of alpha thalassemia which is characterized by one copy of the normal alpha-globin gene and the loss of rest of the three alpha-globin genes, which results in abundant formation of HbH.[1] HbH is characterized by a high ratio of beta-globin to alpha-globin. The epidemiological studies show that the HbH disease is predominantly more common in Southeast Asia, the Middle East and the Mediterranean countries.[2]

HbH disease should always be considered in patients with mild-to-moderate microcytic hypochromic hemolytic anemia and hepatosplenomegaly which is unexplained by other causes. Heinz bodies are detected on blood smears after cresyl blue staining. The "Golf-ball" appearance of the red cells (cells with HbH inclusion bodies) with supravital stain after prolonged incubation is also indicative of HbH disease. Capillary gel electrophoresis of Hb is more diagnostic which may reveal the presence of HbH even up to 30%. Diagnosis is confirmed by genetic testing in PCR method.[3-5]

Although the benefits of molecular diagnosis are immense, it has not been widely used in Bangladesh. However, in recent years, molecular diagnosis has drawn much attention of the clinicians because of their high resolving power in solving complicated cases. In our case, the clinicians teamed up with the Biochemistry and Molecular Biology department of Dhaka University, Bangladesh, to conduct the molecular analysis of the blood sample of the patient. This can be regarded as one of the examples of how clinicians in collaboration with Molecular Biology researchers can resolve a complicated case. To the best of our knowledge, this collaboration was the first in Bangladesh to solve a clinical case successfully, which may encourage the clinicians to collaborate with academics and researchers to perform molecular tests for the benefit of the patients.

REFERENCES

1. Chui DH. Alpha-thalassemia: HbH disease and Hb Bart's hydrops fetalis. Ann NY Acad Sci. 2005;1054:25–32.
2. Harteveld CL, Higgs DR. α-thalassaemia. Orphanet J Rare Dis. 2010;5:13.
3. Chandrashekar V and Soni M. Hemoglobin Disorders in South India. ISRN Hematology, 2011.
4. Liu YT, et al. Rapid detection of alpha-thalassaemia deletions and alpha-globin gene triplication by multiplex polymerase chain reactions. Br J Haematol. 2000;108(2):295–9.
5. de Mare A, Groeneger AH, Schuurman S, et al. A rapid single-tube multiplex polymerase chain reaction assay for the seven most prevalent alpha-thalassemia deletions and alpha alpha alpha (anti 3.7) alpha-globin gene triplication. Hemoglobin. 2010;34(2):184–90.

CASE 95

YOUNG LADY WITH PALPITATION AND HYPOPLASTIC UPPER LIMB

CASE SUMMARY

A 23-year-old young lady presented with palpitation for the last 22 days, after delivering a healthy baby. It was associated with breathlessness which increased with activity and on lying flat. There was no associated leg swelling. She had recurrent episodes of cough and breathlessness on exertion since childhood. She was the second child of non-consanguineous married couple. Her parents and siblings were normal in health. This was the first time she got admitted in hospital for shortness of breath.

Examination revealed slopped right shoulder, rudiment abnormal thumb on left hand (Fig. 1), and right hand deformity (absent thumb and radial deviation of hand) that is radial clubhand (Fig. 2), which was present since birth. Blood pressure was 90/60 mm Hg, pulse was 90 b/min, respiratory rate was 38/min, and oxygen saturation was 86%. Jugular venous pressure (JVP) was not raised. No edema or hepatomegaly was found. No obvious deformities were observed in lower limbs or elsewhere. Cardiovascular examination revealed hyperdynamic precordium, left parasternal systolic

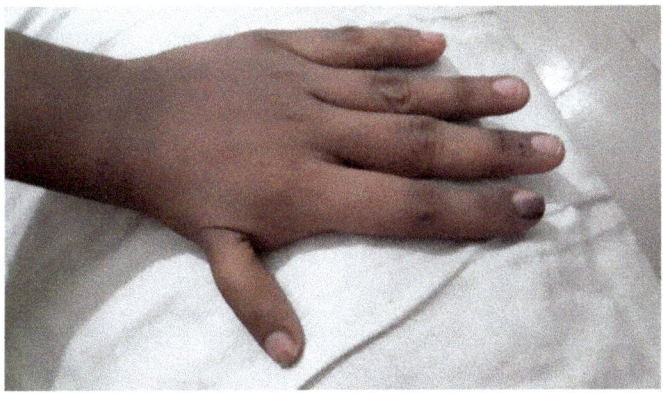

Fig. 1: Left hand—rudimentary thumb.

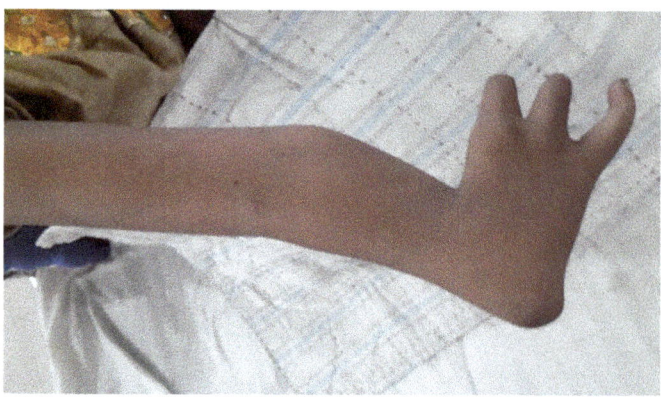

Fig. 2: Right upper limb—absent thumb and index finger with underdeveloped distal phalanges.

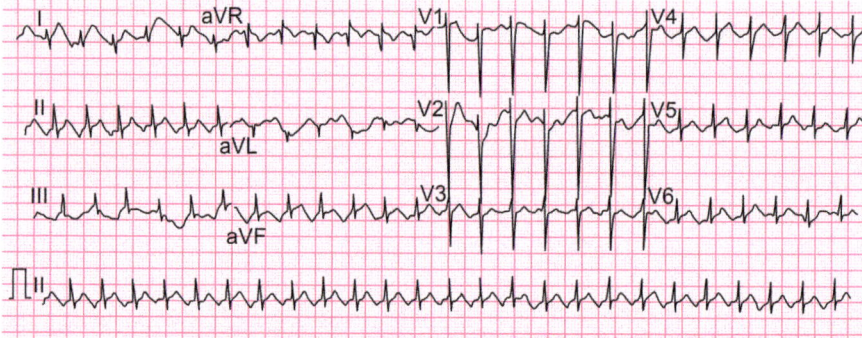

Fig. 3: Supraventricular tachycardia.

lift, palpable P2, and a pansystolic murmur all over the precordium more prominent in left parasternal area with no radiation. Basal crackles were present bilaterally.

Electrocardiography (ECG) showed supraventricular tachycardia (Fig. 3). Chest X-ray showed cardiomegaly with prominent pulmonary vascular markings with scoliosis (Fig. 4). Plain X-ray of right hand showed absence of first and second metacarpal bone and underdeveloped distal phalanges of rest of the finger (Fig. 5). Two-dimensional echocardiography showed ventricular septal defect (VSD) with pulmonary hypertension (HTN) (Figs. 6A and B). Her hemogram was within normal limit. Renal and liver function tests were normal.

QUESTION

1. What is your provisional diagnosis?

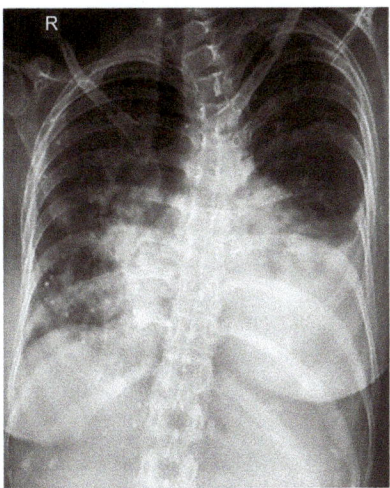

Fig. 4: Cardiomegaly with prominent pulmonary vascular markings with scoliosis.

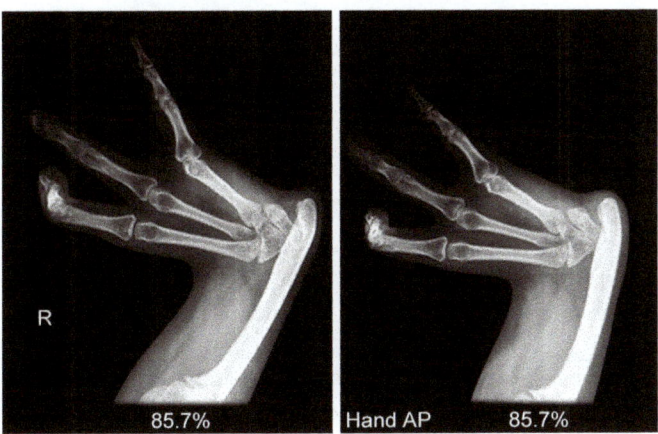

Fig. 5: Absent first and second metacarpal bone with rudimentary distal phalanges.

DISCUSSION

This young lady came to us in her postpartum period with aggravation of palpitation and breathlessness which had been persistently present since childhood, along with her skeletal deformities. All of this indicated a congenital pathology; and after carrying out examinations and targeted investigations, we reached the diagnosis of atriodigital dysplasia syndrome- also called Holt-Oram syndrome (HOS).

Final Diagnosis: Holt-Oram Syndrome

Holt-Oram syndrome is an autosomal dominant disorder. This is caused by mutations on chromosome 12q24.1 which inactivate the gene *TBX5*.

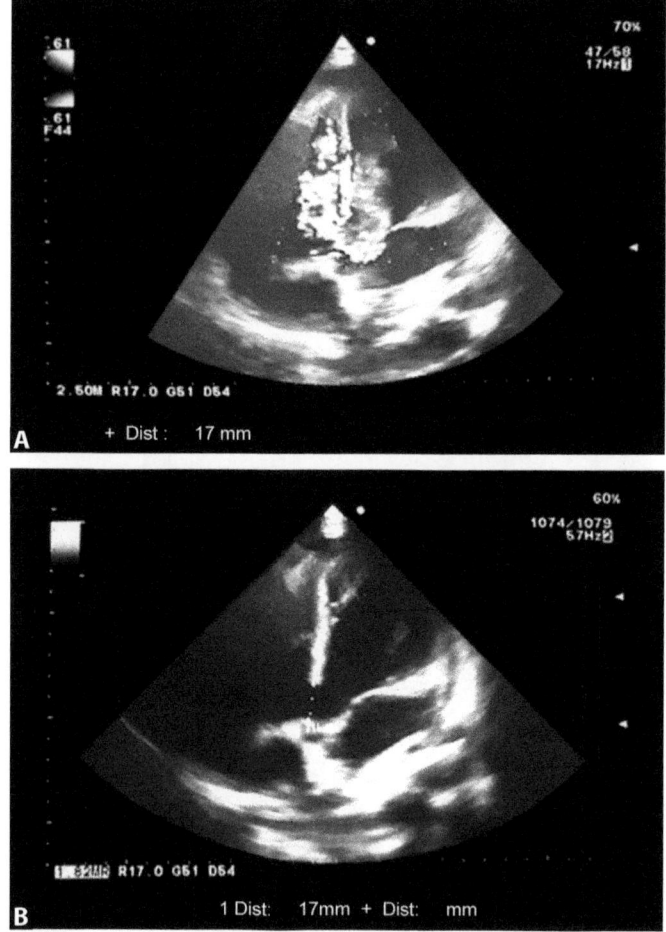

Figs. 6A and B: Echocardiogram showing ventricular septal defect (VSD) with pulmonary hypertension (HTN).

Holt and Oram first elaborated this familial syndrome in a family of nine members spanning four generations. The prevalence of HOS is 1 per 100,000 births.[1-3]

Holt-Oram syndrome usually presents with dysplasia of upper limb ranging from minor radiologic abnormalities to cardiac abnormalities. Deformities which involve skeleton are mainly triphalangeal thumbs, shortness of ulna, shortening of the humerus, radial aplasia, dysmorphism of carpal bones and phocomelia. Most commonly affected structure is thumb. This can be hypoplastic, triphalangeal or absent. Radial hypoplasia, shoulder hypoplasia, clavicle and humerus hypoplasia had also been reported. Skeletal abnormalities rarely involve the lower limbs. This is because the mutant gene interferes with the embryonic differentiation during the 4th and 5th weeks of pregnancy, when the lower limbs are not differentiated. Several clinical and genetic studies noted that almost all cases of HOS had upper extremity involvement; the females had more severe anomalies.[4,5] This feature matches with our case.

Cardiac defects include ventricular septal defect or atrial defect. Other cardiac anomalies can be mitral valve prolapse, mitral stenosis, arrhythmias in the form of atrioventricular blocks. Tetralogy of Fallot and endocardial cushion defects are also noted in subjects with this syndrome. The associated congenital heart defects are determining factors in mortality and morbidity of these patients.[5,6]

Holt–Oram syndrome presented with an associated ventricular septal defect and upper limb musculoskeletal deformity with heart failure, which is a very rare clinical entity. Clinicians should always have a very high index of suspicion in any patient having cardiovascular defect with musculoskeletal defect from birth.

REFERENCES

1. Nourzad G, Baghershiroodi M. A case report on Holt-Oram syndrome (heart-hand). ARYA Atherosclerosis. 2011;7(2):87–92.
2. Basson CT, Bachinsky DR, Lin RC, et al. Mutations in humans cause limb and cardiac malformations in Holt-Oram syndrome. Nature Genetics. 1997;15:30–5.
3. Holt M, Oram S. Familial heart disease with skeletal malformations. Br Heart J. 1960;22:236–42.
4. Oður G, Gül D, Lenk MK, Imirzalioðlu N, Alpay F, Oður E. Variable clinical expression of Holt-Oram syndrome in three generations. Turk J Pediatr. 1998;40:613–8.
5. Araújo Filho R, Alves PM, Carakushansky G, et al. Síndrome de Holt-Oram com persistência de canal AV comum, forma total. Relato de um caso. Arquivos Brasileiros de Cardiologia. 1983;40:397–402.
6. Sletten LJ, Pierpont ME. Variation in severity of cardiac disease in Holt-Oram syndrome. Am J Med Genet. 1996;65:128–32.

CASE 96

YOUNG LADY WITH DISORIENTATION AND BLURRING OF VISION

CASE SUMMARY

A 21-year-old female presented with the complaints of fever for the past 1 month; headache for 10 days and abnormal behavior, disorientation, and double vision for 5 days. Fever was low-grade, continued in nature. Headache was stabbing in nature, involving whole head not associated with vomiting but later associated with double vision and confusion. She did not have any history of pulmonary symptoms, exertional chest pain or previous history of contact with tuberculosis patient. She had no recent history of travel. She was not immunized as per the Expanded Programme on immunization (EPI) schedule. Before admission in hospital, she received treatment with ceftriaxone and amikacin.

The young lady was conscious but confused and disoriented. GCS score was 13/15. General examination findings were normal except she was mildly anemic. Nervous system examination revealed right-sided 6th nerve palsy. Fundoscopic examination revealed bilateral papilledema. There was no other neurological deficit or signs of meningeal irritation. Other systemic examinations revealed nothing abnormal.

Investigations showed complete blood count (CBC): Hb—10.5 g/dL, total WBC—10,200/mm^3 (N—35%, L—55%), platelets—400,000/mm^3; serum creatinine—0.7 mg/dL. Urine routine microscopic examination was normal. Mantoux test (MT)—24 mm (positive). CSF study revealed increased protein and slightly decreased glucose with elevated WBC count, predominantly lymphocytes (protein—80 mg/dL; glucose—30 mg/dL; leukocyte—100, L 95%, PMN 5%). Adenosine deaminase (ADA) was 7.6 IU/L. GeneXpert of CSF for *Mycobacterium tuberculosis* was negative.

QUESTIONS

1. What next investigation should be done?
2. What might be the diagnosis?

DISCUSSION

Patient presented with prolonged low-grade fever and headache associated with disorientation and blurry vision. Examination revealed papilledema and 6th nerve palsy. Clinical features and CSF findings (predominantly lymphocytic infiltration with elevated protein, decreased glucose) were suggestive of tubercular infection. Though GeneXpert was negative, yet other features were highly consistent with tubercular meningitis. So our next investigation of choice was MRI of brain with contrast which revealed enhancement of the basal meninges and hydrocephalus—suggestive of tubercular basal meningitis (TBM).

Final Diagnosis: Basal Meningitis due to Tuberculosis

Anti-tuberculosis drugs with steroid were started. The patient responded quickly and became well-oriented within a week of starting anti-TB regimen.

The incidence of CNS tuberculosis is dependent on the prevalence of tuberculosis in the general population.[1] Various manifestations and complications of TBM such as convulsion, cranial nerve palsy, stroke, low Glasgow Coma Scale score, vision loss, and hydrocephalus have been reported.[2] Headaches in these patients is due to involvement of the meninges and other inflammatory changes that produces hydrocephalus and stroke.[3]

Characteristic of TB is the involvement of basal meninges. The basal enhancement, hydrocephalus, tuberculomas, and infarcts are more common in tubercular meningitis than in pyogenic meningitis.[4]

Though the MRI finding of basal enhancement is not pathognomonic for TBM, specially when present in isolation, yet it should be correlated with other associated imaging features and clinical presentation like hydrocephalus.[5-7] So imaging like MRI along with CSF findings has an important role in establishing the diagnosis.

REFERENCES

1. Garg RK. Tuberculosis of the central nervous system. Postgrad Med J. 1999;75:133–40.
2. Kumar S, Verma R, Garg RK, Malhotra HS, Sharma PK. Prevalence and outcome of headache in tuberculous meningitis. Neurosciences. (Riyadh, Saudi Arabia). 2012;21(2):138–44. doi:10.17712/nsj.2016.2.2015678.
3. Raut T, Garg RK, Jain A, Verma R, Singh MK, Malhotra HS, et al. Hydrocephalus in tuberculous meningitis: Incidence, its predictive factors and impact on the prognosis. J Infect. 2013;66(4):330–7.
4. Chowdhury V, Gulati P, Sachdev A, Mittal SK. Sonography in pyogenic and tubercular meningitis: A comparative study. Indian J Radiol Imag. 1991;1:7–10.
5. Theron S, Andronikou S, Grobbelaar, Steyn F, Mapukata A, Du Plessis J. Localized basal meningeal enhancement in tuberculous meningitis. Pediatr Radiol. 2006;36(11):1182–5.
6. Andronikou, Savvas and Wieselthaler, Nicky. Modern imaging of tuberculosis in children: Thoracic, central nervous system and abdominal tuberculosis. Pediatr Radiol, 2004;34:861–75. DOI: 10.1007/s00247-004-1236-2.
7. Andres MM, Austine JU, Paguia MPR. Tuberculous meningitis basal cistern enhancement pattern on CT imaging. TB Corner. 2016;2(5):1–9.

CASE 97

MIDDLE-AGED MAN WITH PROLONGED FEVER, ANOREXIA AND WEIGHT LOSS

CASE SUMMARY

A 65-year-old businessman presented with 3.5 months' fever, anorexia and weight loss. The fever was low-grade with evening rise of temperature associated with night sweats without chills and rigor, subsided by taking antipyretic. Highest recorded temperature was 101°F. He experienced anorexia which was not associated with dysphagia, nausea, vomiting, abdominal fullness or alteration of bowel habit; and lost about 10 kg weight in the last 3 months. One and half years earlier, the patient underwent transurethral resection of bladder tumor (TURBT) due to transitional cell carcinoma of urinary bladder followed by intravesical chemotherapy (six doses of mitomycin C). Follow-up urethrocystoscopy revealed presence of residual tumor, for which second TURBT was done and chemotherapy was repeated. Both postoperative periods were uneventful. He denied having cough, hemoptysis, chest pain, respiratory distress, hematemesis, melena, loin pain, hematuria, unconsciousness, headache, convulsion, joint pain or skin rash. He had no contact with bird or bat-droppings, and did not meet any known tuberculosis (TB) patient and gave no significant travel history.

He was ill-looking with below average body build, mildly anemic, without any lymphadenopathy, clubbing, jaundice or abnormal pigmentation. His vitals were normal with no postural drop. All systemic examination findings were normal.

Investigations showed, his hemoglobin (Hb) level was 11 g/dL, mean corpuscular hemoglobin (MCH)—26.3 pg, mean corpuscular hemoglobin concentration (MCHC)—33.1 g/dL. Erythrocyte sedimentation rate (ESR) was 30 mm in first hour. Electrocardiogram (ECG) and chest skiagram revealed no abnormality. Urinalysis showed trace proteinuria with 2–3 pus cells/high power field of microscope (HPF) but no red blood cells (RBCs). Creatinine and serum electrolytes were normal. Bilirubin was 0.4 mg/dL, alanine

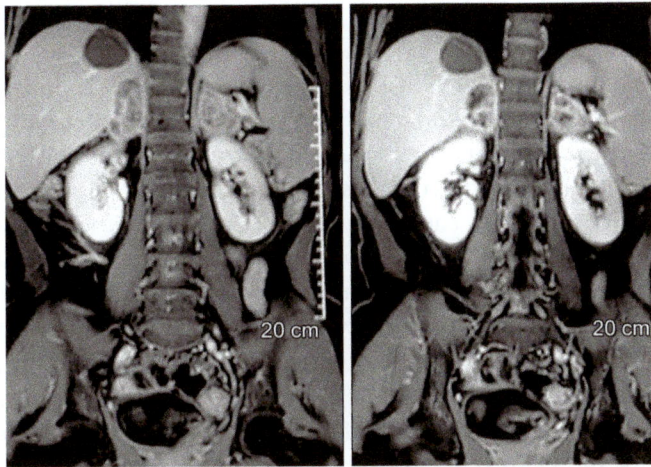

Fig. 1: Magnetic resonance imaging (MRI) of abdomen with contrast, multiple coronal planes showing bilateral adrenal masses and hepatic cyst.

transaminase (ALT) 31 U, alkaline phosphatase (ALP) 290 U. Abdominal ultrasonography revealed *space - occupying lesions (SOL) in right lobe of liver* (focal fat infiltration or hemangioma or resolving abscess) and cystitis. Computed tomography (CT) scan of the whole abdomen with intravenous and oral contrast gave the impression of *bilateral adrenal masses (most probably adrenal metastasis) and simple cyst in right lobe of the liver.* Magnetic resonance imaging (MRI) of abdomen also commented *bilateral adrenal masses [right: (4.3 × 2.2) cm, left: (4.5 × 3) cm]—possible metastasis, hepatic cyst in right lobe of liver (4 × 3.2) cm*, mild thickening of left lateral wall of urinary bladder without invasion of muscularis propria (Fig. 1). Regarding the cyst in the right lobe of liver, we reviewed the previous investigation reports and found that in an ultrasonogram of abdomen done 4 years back—the cyst was of the same size, which conferred that it was a simple hepatic cyst.

QUESTIONS

1. What are the differential diagnoses?
2. What further investigations should be carried out to reach the final diagnosis?

DISCUSSION

For this patient, apart from diabetes mellitus and hypertension with status post-transurethral resection of bladder tumor (TURBT), our differential diagnoses were:
- Tuberculosis of adrenal glands

- Deep fungal infection of adrenal glands
- Recurrence of malignancy with adrenal metastases.

As warranted by the differentials, CT-guided fine needle aspiration cytology (FNAC) was done from masses of both adrenal glands, and the cytopathology report revealed: "Smear shows adequate cellular material containing plenty of degenerating polymorphs, lymphocytes and histiocytes on the background of extensive caseation necrosis. A few epithelioid cells seen in the background. Diagnosis: *granulomatous inflammation, possibility:* tuberculosis. Histoplasmosis cannot be ruled out. Advice: please correlate clinically." Clinically, the patient was neither toxic, nor markedly febrile which made the diagnosis of tuberculosis doubtful. So, we sent the slides for review to another laboratory and the report said, "Smear shows *Histoplasma capsulatum* on the background of epithelioid histiocytes, lymphocytes, polymorphs and cellular debris." Then we went for fungal staining which showed presence of numerous fungi of species *Histoplasma capsulatum* on the background of epithelioid histiocytes, lymphocytes, polymorphs and cellular debris. Diagnosis: **Histoplasmosis**.

Final Diagnosis: Disseminated Histoplasmosis with Bilateral Adrenal Involvement with Diabetes Mellitus, Hypertension and Status Post-TURBT

Histoplasma capsulatum, a dimorphic fungus, found in the environment, particularly in soil containing large quantities of bat or bird droppings—is the culprit behind histoplasmosis. There are no defined zones of distribution of histoplasmosis in Bangladesh. The fungus is endemic in Ohio and Mississippi river valleys, but also lives in parts of Central and South America, Africa, Asia and Australia.[1] People in endemic areas, mostly those with exposure to contaminated soil, acquire the disease by inhaling fungal microconidia.

Histoplasmosis may present in three ways: pulmonary, progressive disseminated and primary cutaneous histoplasmosis. Symptomatic infections typically present as an influenza-like illness (fever, chills, headache, malaise, myalgia and cough and chest pain) 3–17 days after exposure. Acute pulmonary histoplasmosis is often self-limiting. Sequelae include chronic pulmonary histoplasmosis, broncholithiasis, pulmonary nodules, pericarditis, mediastinal granuloma or fibrosis. Rarely, progressive disseminated form of the disease affects the immunocompromised patients and inhabitants of endemic areas at extremes of age. It manifests as acute progressive disease in immunocompromised hosts or chronic disease in immunocompetent individuals.[2]

Adrenal involvement is typically seen with disseminated chronic histoplasmosis which has a predilection for immunocompromised individuals. In case of our patient, he was diabetic for the last 7 years and received chemotherapy twice for bladder tumor, putting him at risk, though, he did not have prior respiratory complaints and his chest skiagram was normal. As in this case, histoplasmosis often presents with similar constellation of clinical features as tuberculosis and is often missed. Furthermore, it shares pathological characteristics of necrotizing granulomas and caseous necrosis with tuberculosis, explaining the first FNAC report of our patient.

Histoplasma antigen detection in urine and/or serum is the most widely used and most sensitive method for diagnosing acute histoplasmosis. Other methods include antibody tests, culture and microscopy. In disseminated histoplasmosis, abdominal imaging findings of mild to moderate hepatomegaly with or without splenomegaly is usual, along with lymphadenopathy and splenic focal hypodense lesions.[3] In adrenal histoplasmosis patients, bilateral adrenal masses are generally found, with varied imaging features. Ultrasonography may reveal uniformly hypoechoic to heterogeneous echotexture. CT findings of bilateral symmetrical adrenomegaly with preservation of the contour of the gland, central hypodensity with peripheral enhancement and presence of calcification has also been described.[4] The differential diagnoses of bilateral adrenomegaly include metastasis, lymphoma, adrenal hemorrhage, sarcoidosis and infections (histoplasmosis, tuberculosis, cryptococcosis, coccidioidomycosis and blastomycosis). Presence of central hypodensity and peripheral rim enhancement of the adrenals narrow down the differentials to tuberculosis and histoplasmosis. Frequently, the only demonstrable site of active disease is the adrenal gland. Hence, adrenal FNAC can suggest the diagnosis which can be further consolidated by urine antigen, culture and polymerase chain reaction.[4,5]

Management of disseminated histoplasmosis includes treatment with amphotericin B followed by itraconazole and replacement of glucocorticoid and mineralocorticoid if there is evidence of adrenal insufficiency. Duration of the antifungal treatment may be 3–12 months, according to disease severity and immunological status of the patient.

In our TB-burdened country, though the diagnosis of adrenal histoplasmosis seems a little far-fetched, yet, it should definitely be considered in patients presenting with constitutional symptoms and unilateral or bilateral adrenal masses with or without adrenal insufficiency. When suspected, image-guided FNAC should be performed straight away, as if untreated—a significant number of patients with adrenal histoplasmosis may progress to life-threatening adrenal insufficiency.

REFERENCES

1. Bahr NC, Antinori S, Wheat LJ, et al. Histoplasmosis infections worldwide: thinking outside of the Ohio river valley. Curr Trop Med Rep. 2015;2(2):70–80. doi:10.1007/s40475-015-0044-0

2. Vyas S, Kalra N, Das PJ, et al. Adrenal histoplasmosis: An unusual cause of adrenomegaly. Indian J Nephrol. 2011;21(4):283-5. doi:10.4103/0971-4065.78071.
3. Radin DR. Disseminated histoplasmosis: abdominal CT findings in 16 patients. Am J Roentgenol. 1991;157(5):955-8.
4. Rozenblit AM, Kim A, Tuvia J, et al. Adrenal histoplasmosis manifested as Addison's disease: unusual CT features with magnetic resonance imaging correlation. Clin Radiol. 2001;56(8):682-4.
5. Schonfeld AD, Jackson JA, Smith DJ, et al. Disseminated histoplasmosis with bilateral adrenal enlargement: diagnosis by computed tomography-directed needle biopsy. Tex Med. 1991;87(4):88-90.

CASE 98

YOUNG BOY'S LONG JOURNEY WITH UNRESOLVED ABDOMINAL PAIN

CASE SUMMARY

An 18-year-old boy, non-smoker, non-alcoholic presented with intermittent pain in the upper abdomen for the last 6 years. Pain was moderate in intensity, burning in nature with radiation to the back, aggravated by taking meal, not relieved by medication and usually persisted for 15–20 minutes. Pain was associated with severe anorexia and occasionally with vomiting. Vomitus was moderate in amount, contained undigested food particles, not mixed with blood, not bile-stained, non-projectile and usually occurred following meal. Along with these complaints, he visited several physicians, also got admitted in different hospitals and received varied modalities of treatment with partial immediate symptomatic improvement but nothing resolved his condition completely. He gave history of recurrent painful oral ulcer. Later, he also developed peri-orbital swelling. Systemic enquiry revealed no history of fever, cough, chest pain, night sweat, joint pain, diarrhea, scanty micturition, hematuria, easy bruising, rash, headache, visual disturbance, hearing problem, heat/cold intolerance. He denied history of taking nonsteroidal anti-inflammatory drugs (NSAIDs). Before admission, about 8 months back, he received anti-tubercular drugs empirically for 6 months, without any improvement. His birth history was uneventful with good cry and respiration. Feeding pattern and appetite was normal in early childhood with normal growth and development up to the age of 12 years. Since his symptoms started, his mother noticed stunted growth and poor weight gain. All his family members were apparently healthy.

On examination, the patient was ill-looking, undernourished and face was puffy (Fig. 1). He was moderately anemic. Vital signs were within normal limit. Leukonychia was present. His pubic and axillary hair were absent. Bipedal leg edema was present. Oral cavity was normal. Abdominal examination was unremarkable, except epigastric tenderness. His higher psychic function was

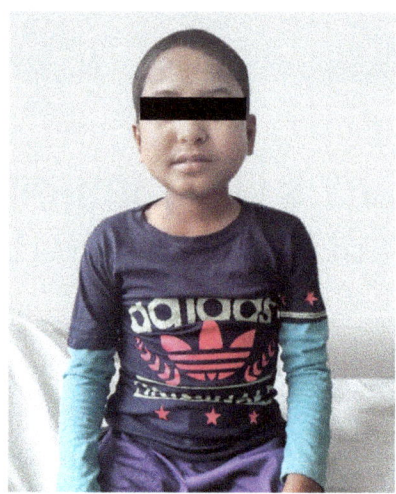

Fig. 1: Young boy with stunted growth and puffy face.

intact with normal intelligence. Other systemic examination revealed no abnormality.

Investigations showed: hemoglobin was 9 g/dL. MCV, MCH, MCHC were normal. ESR was 24 mm in first hour. CRP was 45 mg/L. Peripheral blood film revealed normocytic normochromic anemia. Serum amylase and lipase were normal. Serum albumin level was 17 g/dL (35-50 g/dL) but other liver function and renal function tests were normal. USG of the whole abdomen revealed no abnormality. CT abdomen revealed only mild ascites. Iron profile, vitamin B12 assay and folic acid level were normal. Endoscopy of upper GIT showed multiple big ulcers at body, antrum and pre-pyloric mucosa of stomach (Fig. 2). Histopathology report showed "inflamed and ulcerated gastric mucosa. Ulcer base revealed edema and infiltration by many acute and chronic inflammatory cells. The gastric pits were scanty. These were irregular and showed invasion by polymorphs." Barium follow through revealed normal caliber and mucosal pattern throughout the whole length of small intestine. Fasting gastrin level was 15 pg/mL (13-115 pg/mL). Hormone analysis revealed GH level—7 ng/mL (0.06-5.0 ng/mL), FSH—0.48 mIU/mL (0.7-11.1 mIU/mL), LH—0.53 mIU/mL (0.8-7.6 mIU/mL), testosterone level was 2.15 ng/mL. Serum TSH, ACTH, prolactin, parathyroid hormone (PTH) levels were normal. Anti-*Helicobacter pylori* IgG was negative. Stool routine examination was normal, and stool culture and sensitivity revealed no growth of pathogens.

QUESTIONS

1. What investigations should be done next?
2. What management is appropriate for this patient?

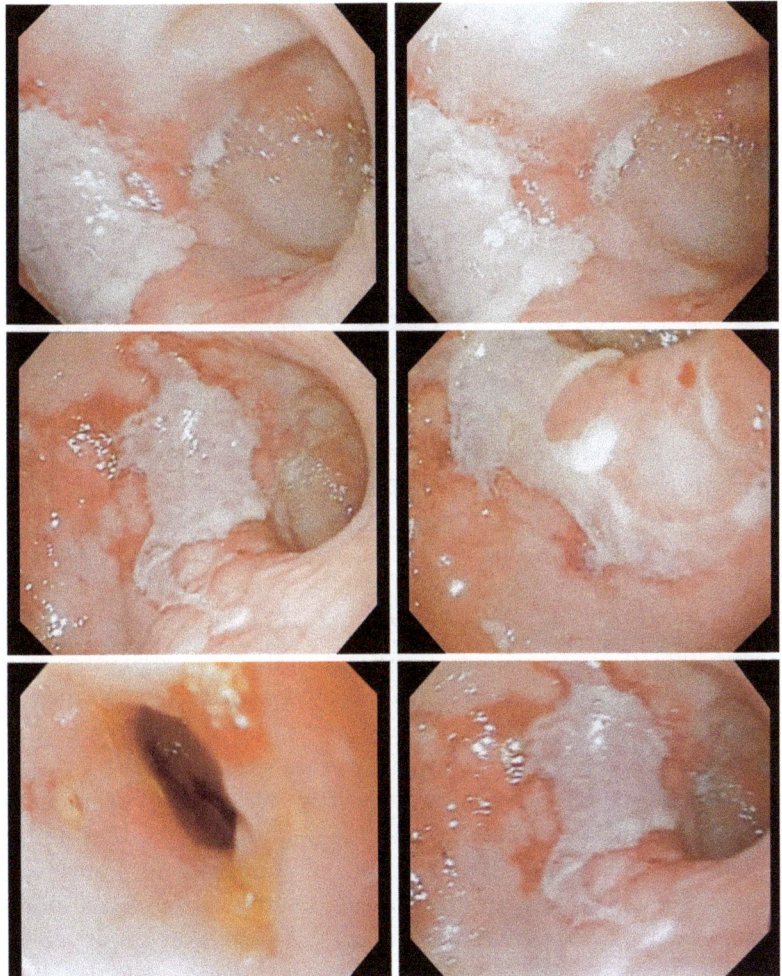

Fig. 2: Upper GI endoscopy showing multiple big ulcers at body, antrum and prepyloric mucosa of stomach.

DISCUSSION

Patient presented with intermittent upper abdominal pain for prolonged period. Chronic pancreatitis was excluded by negative blood investigations but endoscopy of upper GIT revealed multiple discontinued big ulcers which were non-healing with conventional treatment that the patient received during these 6 years of illness.

Causes of recurrent peptic ulcer such as Zollinger-Ellison syndrome, *Helicobacter pylori* infection were excluded. But several clues like recurrent oral aphthous ulcer, multiple non-healing skipped gastric ulcers, stunted growth, poor weight gain, delayed puberty were indicating chronic

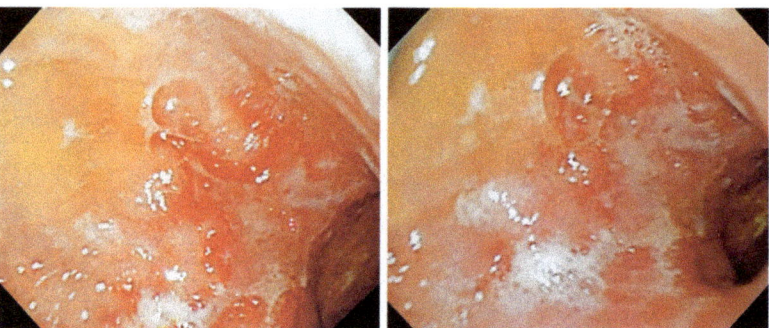

Fig. 3: Follow-up endoscopy showing reduction in ulcer size and improvement of inflammation.

inflammatory lesion involving gastrointestinal tract. His anemia and features of hypoalbuminemia can also be explained by his poor appetite, less food intake and probable underlying inflammatory condition. Our strong suspicion was Crohn's disease.

We did the following investigations:
- *Colonoscopy:* Seen up to 10 cm of terminal ileum. A small (5 cm) subpedunculated polyp was seen at 8 cm from anal verge. The mucosa, vascular pattern and lumen of whole colon, rectum and terminal ileum appeared normal.
- *Fecal calprotectin:* 379 µg/g (reference value—<50 µg/g).

As patient's condition was deteriorating, we started treatment with prednisolone, mesalazine and azathioprine. Within 3 weeks of commencing treatment, patient's condition improved, abdominal pain subsided and he gained about 4 kg weight after starting treatment. We did a follow-up endoscopy, which revealed reduction in ulcer size and improvement of inflammation (Fig. 3).

Final Diagnosis: Crohn's Disease (Isolated Gastric Involvement)

Crohn's disease can involve any part of the gastrointestinal tract from mouth to anus. It most commonly involves terminal ileum and cecum, and less commonly can cause isolated colon involvement.[1]

Crohn's disease of stomach is not common and usually occurs with other lesion anywhere in the gastrointestinal tract.[2] Isolated gastric involvement in Crohn's disease is very rare (less than 0.07%).[3] Only few case reports are documented.[2-4]

Case studies show that usually gastric Crohn's disease presents with epigastric pain, nausea, vomiting and weight loss. These are not pathognomonic of Crohn's disease.[2,3] These symptoms are due to peptic ulcer or obstruction of stomach outlet.[5] Crohn's disease may also manifest with some uncommon presentations, such as impairment of growth, delayed puberty, mouth ulcers, clubbing, chronic iron-deficiency anemia or extra-intestinal manifestations preceding the gastrointestinal symptoms, mainly arthritis or arthralgia, primary sclerosing cholangitis, pyoderma gangrenosum and rarely osteoporosis.[3]

Clinical suspicion and diagnosis of isolated gastric Crohn's disease is difficult and challenging. Upper gastrointestinal endoscopy may reveal combinations of edema, erythema, ulcers, nodularity and cobblestone appearance. The antrum involvement is more than other parts of stomach. Gastric biopsy findings are often nonspecific.[3] Other causes should be systematically excluded to establish the diagnosis. These conditions may include *Helicobacter pylori* infection, tuberculosis, non-steroidal anti-inflammatory drug-induced gastritis, gastrinoma and gastric lymphoma.[3] Inflammatory markers such as fecal calprotectin is also helpful to support the diagnosis.

No studies on the treatment of gastroduodenal Crohn's disease have been reported. Target of the treatment is to relieve the symptoms and to achieve remission. Proton pump inhibitors with steroids are the recommended treatment. Azathioprine and 6-mercaptopurine are effective to maintain corticosteroid-induced remission. Biological agents such as anti-TNF therapy with infliximab have become an effective therapeutic option in steroid-refractory Crohn's disease.[1,6,7]

REFERENCES

1. Zhi XT, Hong JG, Li T, et al. Gastric Crohn's disease: a rare cause of intermittent abdominal pain and vomiting. Am J Med. 2017;130:e181–e185. doi: https://doi.org/10.1016/j.amjmed.2016.12.040.
2. Cary ER, Tremaine WJ, Banks PM, et al. Isolated Crohn's disease of the stomach. Mayo Clin Proc. 1989;64:776–9.
3. Ingle SB, Hinge CR, Dakhure S, et al. Isolated gastric Crohn's disease. World J Clin Cases. 2013;1(2):71–3. doi:10.12998/wjcc.v1.i2.71.
4. Talseth T. Isolated gastric involvement in Crohn's disease: report of a case simulating scirrhus carcinoma. Acta Chir Scand. 1976;42:611–3.
5. Banerjee S, Peppercorn MA. Inflammatory bowel disease. Medical therapy of specific clinical presentations. Gastroenterol Clin North Am. 2002;31:185–202.
6. Shimoyama Y, Kusano M, Hirano Y, et al. Onset of gastric Crohn's disease observed endoscopically. Gastrointest Endosc. 2010;72:1060–1.
7. Kefalas CH. Gastroduodenal Crohn's disease. BUMC Proc. 2003;16:147–51.

CASE 99

YOUNG LADY WITH ABDOMINAL PAIN AND RESPIRATORY DISTRESS

CASE SUMMARY

A 28-year-old housewife presented with recurrent abdominal pain for the past 20 days with respiratory distress and blackening of the tip of the right index finger for 18 days. She developed severe abdominal pain first in epigastric region later spreading to the whole abdomen without any vomiting, or diarrhea. With these complaints, she consulted with a physician and was admitted in a nearby hospital. During her hospital stay, she suddenly developed severe respiratory distress with mild nonproductive cough, chest and back pain without any postural variation, and was refractory to oxygen therapy. As her condition was worsening rapidly, she was referred to intensive care unit (ICU) and kept for 10 days. After improvement, she was discharged from the hospital, but after 2 days she got readmitted in hospital with mild respiratory distress again. On query, she complained of multiple joints pain for the last 2 months. At first, it affected the knees, then both elbows and ankle joints and lastly, small joints of hands; and was associated with mild swelling occasionally. She also had bluish discoloration of fingers of both hands on exposure to cold, which turned reddish on rewarming. During this course of illness, she had no skin rash, oral ulceration, skin tightening, difficulty in deglutition, hemoptysis/hematemesis/hematuria or spontaneous abortion. For joint pain, she took nonsteroidal anti-inflammatory drug (NSAID) (naproxen) and antiulcerant.

General examination of the patient was unremarkable except there was facial flushing and blackening of the tip of the right index finger. On abdomen examination, abdomen was moderately distended, soft and nontender without organomegaly. Percussion note was tympanic all over the abdomen without any shifting dullness. Musculoskeletal system examination revealed no signs of inflammation. Cardiorespiratory and other system examination findings were unremarkable.

Complete blood count (CBC): hemoglobin (Hb)—12.9 g/dL, erythrocyte sedimentation rate (ESR)—20 mm in first hour, white blood cell (WBC)—19,500/cumm and platelets—235,000/cumm. Serum electrolytes: Na—126.9 mmol/L, K—3.44 mmol/L, Cl—94 mmol/L, serum creatinine: 1.41 mg/dL, anti-dengue antibody: negative, C-reactive protein (CRP)—6.74 mg/dL, thyroid-stimulating hormone (TSH)—normal, serum lipase and amylase—normal. Urine routine examination (RE)—pus cell—3-4/hpf, red blood cell (RBC)—nil. Fibrin degradation product (FDP)—17.46 µg/mL, D-dimer—5278 ng/mL, rheumatoid factor (RF)—11.1 IU/mL (negative) and anti-cyclic citrullinated peptide (CCP) antibody—negative. Chest X-ray revealed bilateral patchy opacities in middle and lower zone of lungs. Computed tomography (CT) scan of chest showed diffuse bilateral nonhomogeneous patchy opacities in both middle and lower zone consistent with acute respiratory distress syndrome (ARDS). Ultrasonography (USG) of whole abdomen revealed no abnormality. Endoscopy of upper GIT was normal. Tracheal aspirate for Gram staining and acid-fast bacillus (AFB)—negative.

QUESTIONS

1. What should be the next investigations to reach a diagnosis?
2. What would be the final diagnosis?

DISCUSSION

Several important clues like history of multiple joints pain with Raynaud's phenomenon and blackening of tip of finger pointed towards the diagnosis of connective tissue disorder like systemic sclerosis (SS), systemic lupus erythematosus (SLE) and overlap syndrome.

We did the following investigations to reach the confirmatory diagnosis. After re-admission of this patient, chest X-ray revealed bilateral pleural effusion in both mid and lower zone. Autoantibody profile showed:
- Antinuclear antibody (ANA): strongly positive
- Anti-double stranded deoxyribonucleic acid (anti-dsDNA): positive
- Antiphospholipid antibody: negative
- ENA profile: negative
- Anti-neutrophil cytoplasmic antibodies: negative.

Raynaud's phenomenon is commonly associated with SS and SLE and digital gangrene is more common in SS. But there was no history of skin tightening and also other autoantibodies in extractable nuclear antigen were negative.

So, features and investigations were most consistent with SLE. Our patient presented uniquely with abdominal pain and respiratory distress, which are not very common presentations of SLE. Lupus-induced vasculitis was the possible explanation for her abdominal pain (lupus mesenteric vascultitis) and it also can explain the blackening of the finger.

Acute respiratory distress syndrome (ARDS) due to acute lupus pneumonitis can be the underlying cause of respiratory distress leading to respiratory failure.

The latter presentation with bilateral pleural effusion was due to serositis.

Final Diagnosis: Systemic Lupus Erythematosus with Vasculitis

The classic presentation of SLE is the triad of fever, joint pain and rash in young women. Arthritis or arthralgia is the most common presentation initially, although there may be other constitutional, musculoskeletal, dermatologic, renal, neuropsychiatric, pulmonary, gastrointestinal, cardiac and hematological manifestations as well.[1,2]

REFERENCES

1. Dubois El, Tuffanelli Dl. Clinical manifestations of systemic lupus erythematosus. Computer analysis of 520 cases. JAMA. 1964;190:104–11.
2. Dall'Era M, Wofsy D. Clinical manifestations of systemic lupus erythematosus. Firestein GS, Budd RC, Gabriel SE, MacInnes IB, O'Dell JR, eds. Kelley and Firestein's Textbook of Rheumatology. 10th ed. Philadelphia, Pa: Elsevier Saunders; 2017. pp. 1345–67.

CASE 100

YOUNG MAN WITH PROLONGED FEVER AND RASH

CASE SUMMARY

A 38-year-old gentleman, occasional betel-leaf chewer was admitted with the complaints of fever, reddish facial rash, generalized weakness and weight loss for the last 1 year. His fever was high grade (highest 106°F), started at late night, lasted for 3 to 4 hours, was associated with chills and rigor, and subsided with medications, without sweating. In addition to this, he developed an ulcerative lesion in right side of upper lip, which was initially itchy, bled on scratching, and later became non-itchy, gradually increased in size and persisted for 6 months despite various treatments. Simultaneously, he noticed reddish, painless, non-itchy rash over both malar regions, sparing the nasolabial folds, which seemed more prominent during his febrile episodes, and did not aggravate on sun exposure. Patient also complained of generalized weakness, but could perform his daily activities with difficulty. He had documented unintended loss of 6 kg weight over last 1 year. He did not have cough, chest pain, respiratory distress, or joint pain. With these complaints, he consulted a physician, and biopsy was taken from lip lesion, suggesting the diagnosis of *lymphoma,* based on histopathology; which required confirmation by immunohistochemistry. But, he denied further work-up or treatment, and decided to go abroad to perform further investigations, and to seek a second opinion. There, biopsy was retaken and subsequent histopathological impression was that of a *"benign epithelial hyperplasia"* for which topical medication was prescribed. Then he returned to Bangladesh. The ulcer gradually became smaller and started healing very slowly (Fig. 1), but fever persisted; and with time, his condition deteriorated with new onset of copious hematemesis, scanty epistaxis, and severe low back pain. With this long list of complaints, patient got admitted in Dhaka Medical College and Hospital (DMCH). He did not have headache, dizziness, visual disturbance, or altered bowel-bladder habit. He had no history of contact with pulmonary tuberculosis patient, intravenous drug abuse or unsafe sexual exposure. He

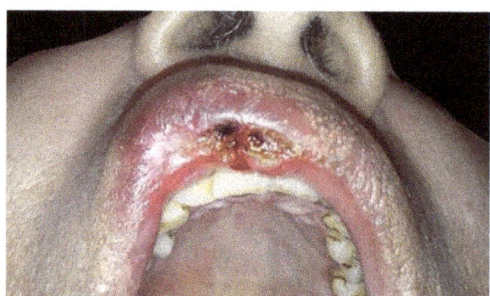

Fig. 1: Partially healed ulcer involving middle and right side of the upper lip.

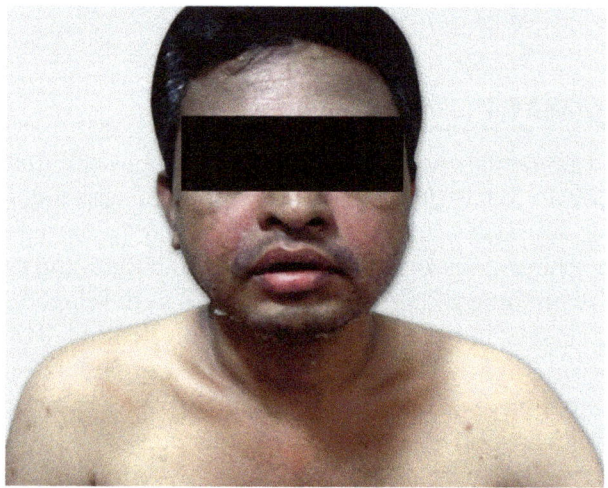

Fig. 2: Photograph of the patient showing malar rash, desquamation, and rash on the upper chest.

was normotensive, nondiabetic, and nonasthmatic. His parents' marriage was not consanguineous, and none of his family members suffered from similar or any other significant familial illness. Over the course of illness, he received several antibiotics (ceftriaxone, cefixime, rifampicin, and doxycycline).

On examination, the patient was ill-looking, moderately anemic, and had a slightly coarse and thick upper lip. Temperature—103°F; pulse—90/min, regular; BP—100/60 mm Hg, without postural drop; R/R—16breaths/min. Erythematous rashes were present on both malar regions sparing the nasolabial folds, and also over the upper chest, with desquamation of skin. Some vesicular lesions with erythematous base were present over the trunk (Fig. 2). A single non-tender lymph node was palpable in left posterior cervical chain, which was about 1 cm × 1 cm in diameter, firm, mobile, free from underlying structure and overlying skin, with no discharging sinus. Bedside urine examination was negative for protein. Liver was palpable about 3 cm from right costal margin, surface—smooth, margin—sharp, non-tender, firm, upper border of liver dullness: in right 6th intercostal space, without hepatic bruit. Spleen was just palpable. GALS screening revealed normal findings, and other systemic findings were unremarkable.

Our investigations revealed, hemoglobin—7.6 g/dL, WBC count—450/mm^3, neutrophil—57%, lymphocyte 51%, platelet count—7,000/mm^3, absolute neutrophil count 290 (normal: 2000-7000), immature granulocytes—6.7%, and corresponding PBF commented pancytopenia. CRP—96 mg/L (normal: <6 mg/L). Urine RME, serum creatinine, serum electrolytes, RBS, stool RME, X-ray chest and ECG were normal. Triple antigen test, HBsAg, anti-HCV, HIV I and II, and ICT for malaria were negative, MT was 3 mm (negative), and blood and urine cultures yielded no growth. Echocardiography revealed normal findings, without any vegetation or thrombus. Ultrasonography of the whole abdomen—mild splenomegaly and moderate amount of gallbladder sludge. CT scan of abdomen—mild hepatosplenomegaly (liver: 15.3 cm in long axis, spleen: 15.1 cm) with mildly dilated portal veins and left renal cortical cyst (Bosniak Type 1) (Fig. 3). Liver function tests showed, serum bilirubin: 1.4 mg/dL, ALT—111 U/L, ALP—72 U/L, serum total protein—7.8 g/dL,

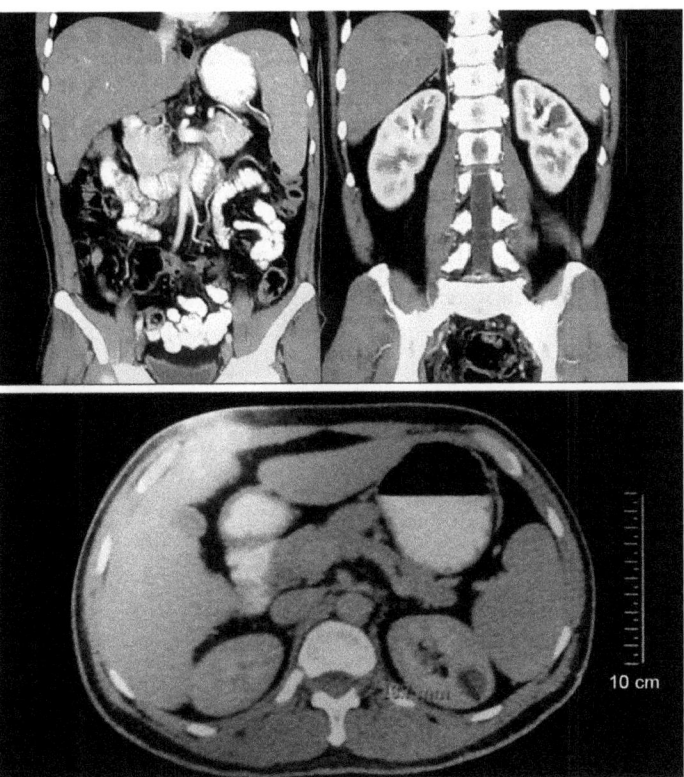

Fig. 3: CT scan of abdomen showing mild hepatosplenomegaly and left renal cortical cyst (Bosniak Type 1).

albumin—4.2 g/dL. *Serum LDH was persistently raised, highest being 2,329 U/L.* ANA, anti-dsDNA, ENA profile, MPO-ANCA and PR3-ANCA were negative. Serum calcium—9.3 mg/dL, inorganic phosphate—3 mg/dL, vitamin D—14.43 ng/mL (deficient). Uric acid—5.5 mg/dL. *Serum ferritin—9,780 ng/mL* (reference value in male: 30–300 ng/mL).

QUESTIONS

1. What are your differential diagnoses?
2. What further investigations are needed to reach the final diagnosis?

DISCUSSION

For this gentleman presenting with prolonged pyrexia, poorly healing lip-ulcer, skin rashes, hemoptysis and epistaxis, low back pain, with mild hepatosplenomegaly, we thought of lymphoma (probably non-Hodgkin lymphoma), hemophagocytic lymphohistiocytosis (HLH), leukemia, and adult-onset Still's disease. Extensive investigations performed over a year could not establish a diagnosis, so we did the following investigations:
- Repeat serum ferritin: >33,511.20 ng/mL (reference value in male: 30–300 ng/mL)
- Fasting lipid profile: normal, except triglyceride—426 mg/dL (increased).
- Serum pro-calcitonin: 1.29 ng/mL (increased)
- Serum fibrinogen: 94 mg/dL (low, reference value: 200-400 ng/mL)
- Bone marrow study: suggestive of acute myeloid leukemia (AML).

At this point, bone marrow was sent for immunophenotyping for full leukemia panel, while the patient was being treated with injectable meropenem, piperacillin and tazobactam combination, along with hydrocortisone, filgrastim, and eltrombopag; but his condition deteriorated quickly, and despite transfer to the intensive care unit (ICU), sadly, he succumbed to death, precluding all our efforts. The bone marrow report is given below:
- Bone marrow immunophenotypic profile for acute leukemia: showed a predominant cell cluster in the lymphocytes region along with very reduced number of granulocytes and monocytes. About 20% of these cells expressed T-cell markers (sCD3, cyCD3, CD4, CD5, CD7, TdT and negative for CD8). Remaining *80% cells were positive for CD56 (40%), CD13, CD38, CD45, HLA-DR* and negative for CD34, CD3, CD5, CD7, CD8, CD10, CD19, CD79a, CD13, CD33, CD117, MPO, CD41a, CD235a, CD71 and CD138. Impression: considering the cell size, percentage (>60% of lymphoid) and immunophenotype findings of critical cells, whole picture was compatible with aggressive NK-cell leukemia (ANKL) with aberrant expression of CD13.

Final Diagnosis: Hemophagocytic Lymphohistiocytosis due to Aggressive NK-cell Leukemia

Hemophagocytic lymphohistiocytosis is a rare and life-threatening primary or secondary condition in which the immune system goes into overdrive, activating too many macrophages and lymphocytes which then phagocytose RBCs, WBCs, and platelets, resulting in self-destruction of tissues and organs, including the bone marrow, liver, and brain. Familial/primary HLH (familial erythrophagocytic lymphohistiocytosis [FEL]) is an autosomal recessive disease, whereas secondary/acquired HLH may be caused by: immunosuppressive drugs, autoimmune diseases, immunodeficiencies, infection, certain types of cancer and/or metabolic diseases. HLH-induced by Epstein-Barr virus or other viral illness, may be due to another genetic condition named X-linked lymphoproliferative disease (XLP).[1-3]

It initially presents with fever, hepatosplenomegaly, pancytopenia, lymphadenopathy, and rash. Cutaneous lesions herald the presence of underlying malignancy, and can aid in early diagnosis.

HLH can be established if (a) and/or (b) below is fulfilled:[1,4]

a. Genetic test: Identifying a mutation in one of the genes responsible for HLH.
b. At least 5 signs or symptoms out of the following eight:
   i. Pyrexia
   ii. Splenomegaly
   iii. Pancytopenia
   iv. Elevated triglycerides levels, or low fibrinogen levels
   v. High ferritin levels
   vi. Hemophagocytosis (the destruction of certain types of blood cells by histiocytes) on bone marrow, spleen or lymph node biopsy
   vii. Reduced/absent NK cell activity
   viii. Elevated blood levels of CD25 (indicating prolonged immune cell activation).

Our patient met majority of the criteria- which were enough to diagnose HLH, and all of his features including generalized weakness, rash, and elevated liver enzymes- could be explained by this.

For primary HLH, allogeneic bone marrow transplantation is one cure. The Food and Drug Association (FDA) has approved an orphan drug— human monoclonal antibody *emapalumab* for primary HLH. Secondary HLH needs treatment according to cause. Prognosis is worst for HLH due to tumors (especially T-cell lymphoma).

The ANKL is a rare neoplasm of mature NK-cells described in the World Health Organization classification.[5] It sporadically affects Asian (mostly China and Japan) and Central and South American populations, and only around 200 cases have been reported in the literature. ANKL frequently complicates fulminant HLH, and usually originates from a single EBV-infected NK cell, hence EBV DNA levels could have been done as diagnostic and prognostic markers. The diagnosis depends on the identification of morphologically and immunophenotypically aberrant leukemia cells. DeVIC chemotherapy (dexamethasone, VP16, ifosfamide, carboplatin) cycles every 3 weeks, followed by allogeneic bone marrow transplantation can be a management option. With or without treatment, ANKL poses a rapidly fatal clinical course with a median survival of around 2 months.[6,7]

Fulminant clinical course, leukemic presentation, and high EBV DNA levels, often with associated hemophagocytosis, should alarm presence of an NK/T-cell neoplasm like ANKL.[7]

REFERENCES

1. Zhang K, Filipovich AH, Johnson J, et al. Hemophagocytic lymphohistiocytosis, familial. GeneReviews. January 17, 2013; http://www.ncbi.nlm.nih.gov/books/NBK1444/.
2. George MR. Hemophagocytic lymphohistiocytosis: review of etiologies and management. J Blood Med. 2014;5:69-86. https://www.ncbi.nlm.nih.gov/pmc/articles/PMC4062561/.
3. Zhang K, Wakefield E, Marsh R. Lymphoproliferative disease, X-Linked. GeneReviews. June 30, 2016; https://www.ncbi.nlm.nih.gov/books/NBK1406/.
4. Zhang L, Zhou J, Sokol L. Hereditary and acquired hemophagocytic lymphohistiocytosis. Cancer Control. 2014;21(4):301-12.
5. Swerdlow SH, Campo E, Pileri SA, et al. The 2016 revision of the World Health Organization classification of lymphoid neoplasms. Blood. 2016;127(20):2375-90. doi:10.1182/blood-2016-01-643569
6. Tang YT, Wang D, Luo H, et al. Aggressive NK-cell leukemia: clinical subtypes, molecular features, and treatment outcomes. Blood Cancer J. 2017;7:660.
7. Nazarullah A, Don M, Linhares Y, et al. Aggressive NK-cell leukemia: a rare entity with diagnostic and therapeutic challenge. Human Pathology: Case Reports. 2016;4:32-7. https://doi.org/10.1016/j.ehpc.2015.08.001.

CASE 101

YOUNG DIABETIC MALE WITH PERSISTENT PYURIA AND DRASTIC WEIGHT LOSS

CASE SUMMARY

A 40-year-old male, resident of Chattogram (in the southeastern part of Bangladesh), presented with the complaints of high-grade continued fever with chills and rigor with evening rise of temperature for the past 2.5 months; with severe anorexia and 18 kg weight loss in this period. His bowel-bladder habits were normal. When his fever continued despite a proper course of antibiotics, he got admitted in a local hospital and underwent open cholecystectomy for cholelithiasis with uncontrolled diabetes mellitus. Even after the operation and completion of another course of antibiotic, his fever persisted—compelling him to seek further evaluation. He neither had dysuria, cough, breathlessness or hemoptysis; nor had history of jaundice, unsafe sexual exposure, contact with smear-positive pulmonary tuberculosis patient, or of drinking raw cow-milk.

The patient was ill-looking with below-average body build and had a cholecystectomy scar at the right subcostal region. He was mildly anemic, dehydrated with a coated tongue, pyrexic, tachycardic and had clubbing. He had no rash or abnormal pigmentation. Abdominal examination revealed non-tender hepatosplenomegaly (liver: 3 cm, spleen: 3 cm). Cardiovascular and other systemic findings were unremarkable.

Investigations showed CBC: mild anemia (Hb—10.4 g/dL, MCV—71.1 fL), PBF—microcytic hypochromic anemia. ESR was persistently elevated, highest being 56 mm in first hour. Fasting plasma glucose was 3.1 mg/dL, 2 hours after breakfast plasma glucose was 6.8 mg/dL. Serum creatinine was normal, ALP was 429.9 U/L. Repeated urinalysis over 3 months showed persistent pyuria (albumin: +, pus cells: plenty), but none of the corresponding urine cultures yielded growth. Chest skiagram was normal. Ultrasonogram of whole abdomen commented mild hepatosplenomegaly, mild pelvicalyceal system dilatation with bilateral small renal calculi with cystitis, mildly enlarged prostate. Blood culture in FAN method yielded no growth of bacteria.

QUESTIONS

1. What are the differential diagnoses?
2. What investigations are necessary to pinpoint the diagnosis?

DISCUSSION

Initially, our provisional diagnosis was recurrent UTI as repeated urinalysis revealed plenty of pus cells every time. But our patient was nonresponsive to antibiotics. So, for this patient with prolonged fever coming from a malaria endemic zone presenting with hepatosplenomegaly and sterile pyuria, we considered following differentials:
- Disseminated tuberculosis
- Chronic malaria
- Chronic kala-azar.

Repeat ultrasonogram showed *mild hepatosplenomegaly* with early stage benign enlargement of prostate (BEP). ICT for malaria and kala-azar were negative and malarial parasite was not found in thick and thin blood films. We repeated the blood and urine cultures and this time, urine culture yielded growth of *Enterococcus* species (colony count: 4×10^3/mL). Despite treatment with sensitive antibiotic, patient remained febrile and pyuria persisted. Meanwhile, we sent his urine for Gene Xpert for *Mycobacterium tuberculosis* (MTB) test and report revealed *urine GeneXpert: positive for MTB, rifampicin resistance: not detected.* For further evaluation, hepatic and splenic biopsy could have been done to detect tuberculous involvement.

Final Diagnosis: Renal Tuberculosis (Disseminated TB)

Tuberculosis (TB) is a contagious infection that can present with a variable clinical picture, making the diagnosis difficult. Renal TB may be part of a disseminated infection or a localized genitourinary disease. Tuberculosis of the kidney and urinary tract is most commonly caused by the human tubercle bacillus, *Mycobacterium tuberculosis*, but the bovine tubercle bacillus, *Mycobacterium bovis*, occasionally can be responsible. Patients of tuberculosis of the urinary tract present with lower urinary symptoms, and suspicions of tuberculosis are aroused only when there is no response to the usual antibacterial agents or when urine examination reveals pyuria in the absence of a positive culture on routine media. Other symptoms that sometimes occur include back, flank and suprapubic pain; hematuria; frequency; and nocturia—which overlap with conventional bacterial UTI. Renal colic is uncommon, occurring in fewer than 10% of patients, and constitutional symptoms such as fever, weight loss and night sweats are also unusual. Only one-third of patients have an abnormal chest skiagram.[1]

This patient was diabetic for the last 7 years and mostly had poor glycemic control, putting him at risk of disseminated tuberculosis. He had prolonged fever, significant weight loss, hepatosplenomegaly, but his chest skiagram was normal. So, repeated investigations, several unresponsive antibiotic therapies, and a cholecystectomy later—we finally reached the diagnosis of disseminated tuberculosis on the basis of positive urinary GeneXpert and started standard anti-TB medication to which the patient responded well.

Despite presence of confounding clinical informations, going back to the basic lesson of early suspicion of renal tuberculosis in patients with persistent culture-negative pyuria would be of great benefit to both the patients and the physicians.

REFERENCE

1. Eastwood JB, Corbishley CM, Grange JM. Tuberculosis and the kidney. J Am Soc Nephrol. 2001;12(6):1307-14.

Index

Page numbers followed by *f* refer to figure and *t* refer to table.

A

Abdomen 158
  acute 290
  computed tomography scan of 109*f*, 180*f*, 285*f*, 307*f*, 353*f*
  distended 108, 169
  lower 63
  lump in 270
  magnetic resonance imaging of 339*f*
  ultrasound of 155
  X-ray of 289*f*
Abdominal mass, asymptomatic 56
Abscess
  Collar stud' 219
  hepatic 47
  intra-abdominal 63, 64
  paravertebral 314
  splenic tubercular 158
  tubercular splenic 158
Accidental tongue 12
Acid-fast bacilli 31, 45, 142, 288
  stain 187
Acidosis 140
Acquired granulomatous inflammatory disease 175
Acquired immunodeficiency syndrome 142
Actinomyces
  genus 46
  israelii 46
Actinomycosis 46, 173
  disseminated 46
Activated partial thromboplastin time 6, 7, 113, 218, 249
Activated prothrombin complex concentrate 8
Acute respiratory distress syndrome 279, 280, 349, 350
Acute rheumatic fever 38, 39
  diagnosis of 39*t*
Adalimumab 146
Addison's disease 155
Adenocarcinoma 98, 202
  colonic 98

Adenosine
  deaminase 142, 169, 291
  diphosphate 268
Adrenal insufficiency, life-threatening 341
Adrenal mass, bilateral 154, 339, 339*f*
Adriamycin 85
Adult T-cell lymphoblastic
  leukemia 308
  lymphoma 308
Adult-onset Still's disease 144, 354
Aedes mosquitoes 187
Agglutination test 261
Alanine aminotransferase 6, 30, 74, 123, 147, 215, 217, 229
Alanine transaminase 194
Albendazole 181, 209
  plus praziquantel 273
Albumin 18, 245
Alkaline phosphatase 10, 96, 109, 230, 311
Allopurinol 148
Alpha-fetoprotein 201
Amastigotes 131
Amenorrhea 124
  primary 122
American College of Rheumatology 164
Amikacin 336
Amnesia 122
Amphotericin B 216, 303
Anakinra 36, 146
Anasarca 113
Anemia 124, 139, 145, 215, 224, 328
  mild 172, 206
  moderate 217
  severe 6, 140, 150
Angioedema 40
Angioid streaks 265, 265*f*, 266
Angiotensin-converting enzyme 199, 212, 250
  inhibitors 40
Anisochromia 109
Anisocytosis 109
Aniso-poikilocytosis 51
Ankle joints 230

Anorexia 62, 78, 100, 141, 177, 248, 262, 338
  severe 343
Antecubital fossa 264*f*
Antibiotics 100, 260
  therapies, unresponsive 359
Antibody
  antimitochondrial 194
  antiphospholipid 218, 349
  profile 71
Anti-cyclic citrullinated peptide 13, 252, 349
Anti-cytomegalovirus 10
Anti-double stranded deoxyribonucleic acid 164, 349
Anti-Echinococcus antibody 271
Antigen antibody 289
Anti-hepatitis
  A virus 9
  B core 74
  C virus 9, 74, 93, 120, 261
  E virus 190
Antihistamines 11
Anti-human immunodeficiency virus 91, 142
Antileukemic drugs 198
Antineutrophil cytoplasmic antibody 313
Antinuclear antibody 6, 13, 59, 71, 74, 93, 123, 153, 164, 183, 194, 195, 204, 206, 218, 234, 275, 289, 299, 312, 313, 349
  positive 35
Antiphospholipid syndrome 153
  treatment of 153
Antiplatelet drug 268
Antiretroviral therapy 132
Anti-ribonucleoprotein 184
Anti-Sjögren's syndrome 35, 134, 289
Anti-smooth muscle antibodies 74, 194
Antistreptolysin O 38, 134
Antithyroglobulin antibody 179
Antithyroid peroxidase 59
Antithyroperoxidase 79
Anti-tissue transglutaminase 83, 161
Anti-tuberculosis
  drugs 163
  medication 190
Anti-voltage-gated calcium channel 296
Appetite 86

Arsenicosis
  chronic 32
  management of 33
Artemisinin combination therapy 139
Arteria dorsalis pedis arteries 70
Arthralgia 18, 34, 51, 66, 70, 73, 153, 224, 262, 297
Arthritis 86, 156
Ascites 63, 290
Aspartate aminotransferase 30, 87, 190
Aspiration, ultrasound-guided 64
Ataxia 127
Atriodigital dysplasia syndrome, diagnosis of 333
Atrium, right 249
Atrophic thyroiditis, autoimmune 179, 180
Aura 304
Autoantibody profile 145
Autoimmune disease 153
Autosomal recessive disease 355
Avascular necrosis, steroid induced 27
Azathioprine 21, 144-146, 254
Azithromycin 228

B

Back pain 66, 96, 149, 169, 233, 348
  history of 86
Balloon dilatation 313
Bartter's syndrome 23
Basal ganglia 59*f*, 60
Basal meningitis 337
Bee stings, multiple 278, 279
Behçet's disease 142
Bell's palsy 42
Bence-Jones protein 323
Beta-glucocerebrosidase enzyme 124
Bezafibrate 195
Bicytopenia 229, 307
Bilateral medial medullary syndrome 16
  causes of 17
Biliary cirrhosis 313
Bilirubin 134
  normal 123
Biosynthetic human growth hormone 125
Bladder
  disturbance 25
  dysfunction 1
  tumor, resection of 338, 339

Blastomyces dermatitidis 302
Blastomycosis 302, 341
Bleeding
    diathesis 7, 267
    episodes 5
    gastrointestinal 265
Blisters, multiple 34
Blood
    glucose, capillary 138
    lipoprotein profile 125
    pressure 18, 22, 141, 157, 182, 206, 236, 279
    reports, routine 291
    sugar, random 267, 304
    transfusion 6, 34, 281, 328
        history of 260
    urea 246
Bone 175, 239
    malignancies, primary 92
    marrow 234, 242, 302
        examinations 75, 194
        smear 197*f*
        study 110, 308
        suppression 146
    mineral density 97, 230, 242
    pain 133, 193, 197
    scan 98*f*
Bony metastasis 98
Bortezomib 14
Bowel habit, alteration of 338
Bowel wall edema 290
Brain 175
    diffusion-weight image MRI of 16*f*
    magnetic resonance imaging of 50*f*, 79*f*, 105*f*, 106*f*, 128*f*, 200*f*, 237*f*, 305*f*
    metastasis 239
    olivopontocerebellar degeneration, latest magnetic resonance imaging of 128*f*
Brainstem 16, 107
    dysfunction, signs of 16
    encephalitis 16
Breast postmastectomy, carcinoma of 175
Breath, shortness of 122, 288, 331
Breathlessness 333
Brittle nail 159*f*
Bronchiectasis 179
Bronchioloalveolar cell carcinoma 98
Bronchoalveolar lavage fluid 18
Broncholithiasis 156
Brucella 262
    abortus 261
    melitensis 261
Brucellosis 261, 286
    symptoms of 262
Bruch's membrane 265
B-type natriuretic peptide 249
Buccal mucosa, hyperpigmentation of 30*f*
Budd-Chiari syndrome 282
Bulla-spread sign 34
Bullous pemphigoid 35
Bullous systemic lupus erythematosus 35
Burkholderia 89
    pseudomallei 88
        growth of 88*f*
Burr hole, multiple 95
Butterfly rash 133

C

Calcium 100, 134
    channel blocker 40
    pyrophosphate dihydrate 23
Campylobacter jejuni 85
    infection 84
Carbohydrate antigen 203
Carbon monoxide 72
Carboplatin 356
Carcinoembryonic antigen 203, 288
Carcinoma stomach 238
Carcinomatosis cerebri 238
Cardiac cirrhosis 250
    treatment of 250
Cardiac defects 335
Cardiac failure 250
Cardiovascular disease 231
Cardiovascular system 265
Cardioverter defibrillator, implantable 248
Carotid artery, internal 94
Carpal bones 334
Castleman disease 235
Cefadroxil 44
Cefixime 34, 352
Ceftazidime 89
Ceftriaxone 336, 352
Celiac disease 222

Cell
   count 142, 152
   malignant 68, 175
Cellular debris 340
Cellular fibroblastic proliferation 64*f*
Central nervous system 120, 187, 192, 302
   disease 231
   tuberculosis 192
Cephalosporin 228
Cerebellar degeneration 201
Cerebellar function 58, 315
Cerebellar signs 128
Cerebellar system 294
Cerebellum 60*f*, 129
Cerebral infarct, acute 49
Cerebral involvement, nature of 239
Cerebral malaria 139
Cerebral sinus venous thrombosis 282
Cerebral venous sinus thrombosis 305
Cerebrospinal fluid 16, 127, 160, 167, 187, 190, 234
   analysis 212
Cerebrovascular accident 107
Cervical lymph node 302
Chemotherapy 175, 338
Chest
   computed tomography scan of 19*f*, 63*f*, 246
   high-resolution computed tomography of 179*f*, 276*f*
   inspection of 45*f*
   pain 25, 70, 73, 93, 133, 199, 206, 221, 263, 274, 343, 348
      exertional 336
   percussion 180
   radiography of 242
   right upper 217
   wall pain 149
   X-ray 157, 261
Chikungunya 187
   encephalitis 187
      diagnosis of 188
   virus 187
Chlamydia 228
   trachomatis 228
Cholecystectomy 325
Cholelithiasis 53
Cholesteryl ester storage disease 124, 125

Cholestyramine 11
Chronic arsenic exposure, signs of 32
Chronic inflammatory
   cell 75, 175*f*
   demyelinating polyneuropathy 235
Chronic liver disease 31, 76, 122, 124, 193, 194, 236, 239
   diagnosis of 74, 238
Chronic sinusitis 206
   history of 179
Churg-Strauss syndrome 20
Chylous ascites 291, 292
Cicatrization 263
Ciliary function test 179
Ciprofloxacin 175
Circumoral paresthesia, history of 1
Cirrhosis 195
Clindamycin 34
Clofazimine 135, 148
Clopidogrel 267
Coccidioidomycosis 341
Coeliac disease 102, 161
Cold abscess 219
   formation 319
Cold intolerance 177
Colitis, chronic nonspecific 194
Colonoscopic biopsy 102
Colonoscopy 158, 312, 346
Common bile duct 312
Complete blood count 6, 9, 90, 127, 141, 147, 152, 155, 157, 173, 183, 186, 196, 199, 229, 260, 267, 274, 301, 304, 311, 315, 321, 336, 349
Confusion 336
Conjunctival mucosa 34
Conn's syndrome 23
Connective tissue disease 145, 184
Consciousness 245
Constipation 211
Contraceptives, injectable 108
Convulsion 1, 93
Coombs' test 35, 109, 183, 194, 225, 298, 328
Coronary artery bypass surgery 250
Corticosteroid 135
   intravenous 50
Cotrimoxazole 175
Cough 25, 70, 133, 199, 203, 221, 274, 343

chronic nonproductive 277
history of 66
mild nonproductive 348
persistent 294
Cranial nerves 107, 200
Cranial neuropathy 201, 201
Craniotabes 1
C-reactive protein 13, 18, 39, 63, 87, 113, 134, 141, 147, 172, 199, 206, 252
Creatine kinase 234
Creatine phosphokinase 252, 275, 279
Creatinine kinase level 254
Crohn's disease 346, 347
Crow-Fukase syndrome 234
Cryptococcosis 341
Cryptococcus 176
Cyclophosphamide 85, 121, 146, 151, 207, 254, 293, 310
Cyclosporine 254
Cyst, simple 339
Cystitis 339
Cytopenia 197
Cytoplasmic antineutrophil cytoplasmic antibodies 59, 120, 207, 212

D

Dapsone 135, 148
Darier-Roussy syndrome 148
Dark-field microscopy 107
Deep fungal infection 317
Degenerative disk disease 97
Deglutition 348
Dengue
  antibody, positive 113
  syndrome 113
Denovo mutation 129
Dental hypoplasia 1
Dentate nucleus 59
Deoxyribonucleic acid 164, 183, 218, 222, 252, 289
Dercum's disease 148
Dermatan sulfate 231
Dermatofibroma 148
Dermatomyositis 175
  amyopathic 253
Dexamethasone 151, 356
Dextrocardia 178f, 179f
Diabetes mellitus 175, 340, 357
Diarrhea 100, 159, 211, 280, 343, 348
  bloody 297
  chronic 81, 221

Diastolic dysfunction 249
Diffuse large cell non-Hodgkin lymphoma 308
Digital subtraction angiogram 94
Disease-modifying antirheumatic drugs 306
Disseminated histoplasmosis 155, 340
  management of 341
  progressive 155
Disseminated tuberculosis 68, 173, 192, 358
  diagnosis of 359
Distal convoluted tubule 23
Diurnal variation 314
Dizziness 108, 118, 224, 245, 278, 351
Domperidone 86
Dorsal spine
  compression 314
  magnetic resonance imaging of 91f, 106f, 315f, 316f
Dorso-lumbar spine 97
Doxorubicin 121, 137, 293, 310
Doxycycline 228, 352
Drastic weight loss 357
Dress syndrome 115, 116
  diagnostic criteria of 116t
Drug abuse 130
  intravenous 260, 281
Drug reaction 115
Duodenal ulcer 27
Duodenitis
  chronic nonspecific 83
  erosive 289
Duodenum 160
Dysarthria 127
Dysautonomia 201
Dysphagia 1, 12, 15, 16, 34, 70, 71, 153, 224
  management of 71
Dyspigmentation 147
Dyspnea 277
  exertional 12, 274
  recurrent 40
Dystonia 4
Dystrophic calcification 175, 264

E

Ear
  nose and throat 171
  pain 212

Echinococcus granulosus 180, 272, 272*f*
Echocardiography 169, 304
Edema 224
  bipedal 161
Ejection fraction 225
Elbow joints 306
Electrolytes 223
Electrophoresis 52
Elevated protein 337
Emapalumab 355
Encephaloduroarteriosynangiosis 95
Encephalomalacia 40-42
Encephalomyelitis 201
Encephalomyosynangiosis 95
Encephalopathy 188
  hepatic 122, 236, 239
Endocardial cushion defects 335
Endocrinopathy 234
Endoscopic retrograde
    cholangiopancreatography
    203
Enterobacter 45
Enterococcus 176
  faecalis 91
  species 358
Enzyme-linked immunosorbent assay
    35, 164
Eosinophilia 101, 115, 194, 229
Epidermis, atrophy of 254
Epididymal mass 68*f*
Epididymo-orchitis, right-sided 192
Epigastrium 301
Epilepsy, secondary 41, 42
Episodes, recurrent 209
Epistaxis 34, 118, 233, 267
Epithelial cell 275
Epithelioid cells 285
Epithelioid histiocytes 340
Epstein-Barr virus 355
Erosions 34
Erythema 147
  nodosum 134, 156
    leprosum 135
Erythrocyte sedimentation rate 18, 37,
    39, 51, 70, 73, 96, 113, 119, 134,
    139, 141, 147, 155, 163, 199,
    206, 210, 212, 215, 217, 227,
    260, 284, 288, 298
Escherichia coli 176, 190, 218
Esophageal stenting 71
Esophageal varices 123
Etanercept 146
Evans syndrome
  etiology of 299
  primary 299
Ewing's sarcoma 120, 121
Excision biopsy 308
Exercise test 296
Extensive parenchymal lung disease 19*f*
Extensively drug-resistant tuberculosis
    317
Extractable nuclear antigen 7, 35, 71,
    134, 153, 184, 234, 275
  profile 252
Extracutaneous systemic disease 148
Extrahepatic bile ducts 11
Extrahepatic portal vein obstruction 282
Eye 199
  movement, rapid 56
  pain 159, 212
  red 221

F

Facial hyperpigmented lesions 67*f*
Facial nerve palsy 212
Facial numbness 199
Fahr's disease 60, 61
  diagnosis of 60
Fahr's syndrome 61
Familial erythrophagocytic
    lymphohistiocytosis 355
Fasting lipid profile 354
Fatal respiratory failure 16
Fatigue 262
Fecal calprotectin 346
Fever 25, 34, 37, 66, 86, 113, 115, 144,
    149, 186, 189, 203, 215, 227,
    301, 338, 351
  and jaundice, prolonged 215
  fluctuating 260
  history of 96, 152, 169, 294, 343
  intermittent 163
  low-grade 297
  occasional low-grade 100
  prolonged 157
  recurrent 251
Fiber electromyography, single 295
Fibrin degradation product 227
Fibrinogen degradation product 113
Fibronectin 268

Fibro-osseous lesions, benign 64
Fibrosing mediastinitis 156
Fibrosis 195
Fibrotic ring 45
Fibrous dysplasia 64, 65
Fine needle aspiration cytology 56, 68, 82, 158, 200, 285, 291, 295, 302, 340
Fissure, interhemispheric 237, 237f
Fitz-Hugh-Curtis syndrome 228
Flaccid paraparesis 29
Fludarabine 7
Fluid-attenuated inversion recovery 49
Fluorescent treponemal antibody absorption 107
Flupentixol 7
Folate levels 105
Folic acid supplements 100
Follicle-stimulating hormone 78
Follicular lymphoma 293
    low-grade 292
Foot, inversion of 229
Fractures, recurrent 241
Fresh frozen plasma 218
Fundoscopy 127, 229
Fungal infection 155
    disseminated 302

G

Gait, hemiplegic 41
Gallbladder 312
Gammaglobulins, elevated titers of 204
Gamma-glutamyl transferase 9
Gastric adenocarcinoma 99, 239
Gastric biopsy 238
Gastric cancer 239
Gastric lymphoma 347
Gastric outlet obstruction 27
    history of 27
Gastric ulcer 27
    histopathology of 28f
Gastrinoma 347
Gastritis
    diffused hemorrhagic 289f
    hemorrhagic 289
Gastrointestinal manifestation 102
Gastrointestinal symptoms 154, 280
Gastrointestinal system examination 172

Gastrointestinal tract 123, 175, 203
Gaucher's disease 110, 124
Genetic disorders 305
Genital mucosa 34
Genitourinary tract 175
Genu valgum 229
Giant cell
    lesions 64
    tumor 64, 65
        recurrent 63
Giardiasis 102
Gitelman's syndrome 23
    acquired 24
    diagnosis of 24
Glanzmann's thrombasthenia 268, 269
Glasgow coma
    scale 73, 78, 93, 139, 186, 217
    score 191
Glomerulonephritis 20, 110
Glucocorticoid 72, 207
Glycosaminoglycans 230, 231
Gold standard test 289
Gomori methenamine-silver nitrate 302
Goodpasture's syndrome 20
Gottron's papule 252, 254
Gram negative coccobacilli 87
Gram staining 349
Granulocyte predominance 146
Granuloma 68, 89, 291
Granulomatosis 20, 207
Gronblad-Strandberg syndrome 265
Gum bleeding 193

H

Hand
    deformity, right 331
    radial deviation of 331
Hansen's bacilli 134
Hard palate 154
Head injury 25
Head, computed tomography scan of 298f
Headache 5, 34, 66, 108, 118, 122, 152, 189, 211, 212, 233, 278, 304, 338, 343, 351
    frontal 159
Hearing
    difficulties 15
    impairment 231

Heart
　defects, congenital 335
　disease 185
　　ischemic 12
　sign 16
Helicobacter pylori infection 239, 345, 347
Heliotrope rash 252
Helminthiasis 102
Hemangioma 339
Hemarthrosis, history of 267
Hematemesis 5, 73, 122, 221, 236, 267, 281, 311, 338, 348
　episodes of 240
　history of 25
Hematocrit 6, 172
Hematologic tests 223
Hematopoietic stem cell
　therapy 72
　transplantation 151
Hematuria 5, 224, 267, 297, 308, 338, 343, 348
Hemiparesis 199, 217, 219
Hemoglobin 18, 52, 67, 87, 108, 134, 160, 172, 183, 186, 194, 196, 203, 217, 227, 233, 241, 251, 274, 288, 291, 301, 344
　disease 329
　electrophoresis 52
　H disease 329, 330
　normal 152
Hemoglobinopathies 54
Hemoglobinuria 140
Hemolysis 36, 216
Hemolytic anemia
　autoimmune 216, 299
　hereditary 328
Hemophilia
　acquired 8
　　idiopathic 7
Hemoptysis 66, 73, 199, 206, 267, 348
　history of 274
Hemorrhage 138, 305
　intracerebral 93, 297
Hemorrhagic disease, life-threatening 269
Heparin sulfate 231
Hepatic cyst 272*f*, 339, 339*f*
　multiple 271
　simple 339

Hepatic failure 250, 313
　acute 113
Hepatic fibrosis, congenital 282
Hepatic involvement, acute 228
Hepatitis 115, 192
　B 93, 222
　B virus 7, 222, 237, 249
　　infection 154, 222
　C virus 7, 249
　drug-induced 190
　moderate chronic 123
　nonspecific reactive 112
Hepatotoxicity 36
High protein, causes of 170
High-frequency repetitive nerve stimulation test 295
Hilar lymphadenopathy, bilateral 148
Hip
　joint 26*f*, 62
　pain 62, 63
Histiocytosis 97
Histoplasma
　antigen 341
　capsulatum 155, 340
Histoplasmosis 340, 341
　acute pulmonary 155
　chronic cavitary pulmonary 155
Hodgkin's disease 286
Hodgkin's lymphoma 92
Hoffman's sign 294
Holt-Oram syndrome 333, 335
Homer-Wright pseudorosettes 57
Hormone, antidiuretic 170
Horner's syndrome 56
Human immunodeficiency virus 93, 113, 120, 160, 222
　disease, stage of 142
　infection 131
Human leukocyte antigen 37, 97, 269
Hurler syndrome 230
Hybrid lesions 65
Hydatid cyst
　hepatic 179, 270, 271
　recurrent 271
Hydatid disease 272
Hydrocephalus 191
Hydroxychloroquine 146, 148, 184, 185, 290
Hypercalciuria 23
Hypercholesterolemia 125

Hyperkeratosis 263
Hyperparathyroidism 242, 326
Hyperpigmentation 30f, 154, 154f
Hyperplasia
   benign epithelial 351
   nodular regenerative 112
Hypersensitivity syndrome, drug-
      induced 115
Hypertension 110, 118, 340
Hypertriglyceridemia 125
Hyperviscosity syndrome, causes of 117
Hypocalciuria 23
Hypochloremia 245
Hypochondriac region, right 284
Hypochondrium 109
   right 301
Hypochromasia 51
Hypoechoic lesion 286
Hypoechoic parenchyma 9
Hypogammaglobulinemia 272
Hypogastric region 190
Hypoglossal palsy 16
Hypoglycemia 140
Hypokalemia 23, 24
Hyponatremia
   mild 245
   severe 80
   symptoms of 246
Hypopituitarism, partial 80
Hypoplastic upper limb 331
Hypothyroidism 60, 110, 179
   primary 80, 170, 179

I

Ifosfamide 121, 356
Iliac bones 64
Iliac fossa, right 86
Imipenem 89
Immotile ciliary syndrome 179
Immunoblot assay 35
Immunochromatographic test 131, 137, 323
Immunoglobulin
   G4 113, 204
   intravenous 254, 300
Immunohistochemistry 308
Immunosuppressive drugs 69
Indigestion, chronic 211
Infarction
   bilateral 16
   hepatic 112

Infections 176
Inflammation, granulomatous 285, 340
Inflammatory bowel disease 83, 161, 222, 286
Inflammatory cell, acute 175
Inflammatory syndrome 156
Infliximab 36, 146
Injection benzathine penicillin 107
Insulin sensitizing agents 195
Interstitial pneumonia 277
   nonspecific 277
Intestinal lymphangiectasia, primary 161
Intestinal taeniasis 210
Intracellular pathogens 130
Intracerebral hemorrhage, acute 219, 298f
Intracranial space-occupying lesions 106
Intracytoplasmic sperm injection 180
Intrahepatic bile ducts 11
Intrahepatic cholestasis, benign
      recurrent 10
Intrauterine death 153
Iron
   deficiency anemia 328
   profile 52
Isoprinosine 167
Itching 9, 25, 100
Itraconazole 156, 303
Ivermectin 103

J

Jaundice 1, 9, 25, 44, 113, 140, 169, 203, 215, 267, 281, 284, 301, 311
   fluctuating 311
   history of 221, 297
   intermittent 313
   recurrent 9
Jejunum 83
Jerky movements, recurrent 166
Joint 175
   fixed deformity of multiple 2f
   interphalangeal 183
   multiple small 37
   pain 144, 169, 186, 221, 241, 263, 338, 343
      asymmetric 51
      multiple 152
   swelling, history of 152

Jugular venous pressure 331
Juvenile idiopathic arthritis 3

K

Kala-azar 52, 75, 76, 109, 131, 216, 322, 323, 358
   chronic 358
Kartagener syndrome 179-181
Kayser-Fleischer ring 2, 123, 166, 191, 229, 311
Keratan sulfate 231
Kidney 89
   disease 229
   enlarged 307
   injury 310
      acute 140, 279, 280
   left 91
Knee
   arthritis 86
   joint 144, 230, 306
      pain, severe right 22
   left 37
Knocked knees, bilateral 229
Knodell score 75
Knuckle rash 252, 253*f*
Koilonychia 90, 159
Kupffer cells 75
Kyphosis 319

L

Lactate dehydrogenase 113, 225, 312
Lambert-Eaton myasthenic syndrome 201, 295
Lamina propria 84*f*
Lamivudine 131
Langerhans cell histiocytosis 176
Lax skin 263
Leg
   and abdomen, swelling of 248
   edema 34
   swelling, bilateral 233
   ulcer 182
Leishmania 76
   donovani 131
      bodies 216
Lenalidomide 14, 151
Lepromatous leprosy 176
Leprosy 42, 135
Leptospirosis 115, 299

Lesions, occupying 339
Leukemia 115, 118, 198, 308, 309, 354
   acute 299
      lymphoblastic 197, 308
   chronic myeloid 322
Leukocytosis 96, 146
Leukoerythroblastic blood picture 298
Leukonychia 90, 221
Leukopenia 134, 145, 215
Liddle's syndrome 23
Light-headedness 224
Limb weakness 58, 294
Limbic encephalitis 201
Lip swelling 41*f*
   after treatment, significant improvement of 43*f*
Lipid profile 304
Lipogranuloma 175
Lipoprotein, high-density 125, 249
Liposomal amphotericin B, doses of 76
Liver 89, 239, 285*f*
   biochemistry of 76
   biopsy 10, 75, 77, 110, 123, 124
      basis of 122
      histopathology report of 312
   disease 124
   dullness, upper border of 55
   enhancement of 227
   enzyme 47, 155
      abnormalities 250
   fibroscan of 10, 110
   function test 157, 169, 204, 237, 261, 291, 301, 304, 321, 332, 353
      abnormal 146
   involvement 32
   mass 56
   parenchyma 237
   right lobe of 339
   stiffness 74
   upper border of 236
Loin pain 338
Loose skin over axilla, folds of 264*f*
Low back pain 90, 149, 196
Lower limb 100, 294
   edema, acute 44
   left 70
   right 91
Lower lip, predominantly 40
Lumbar disc herniation 92
Lumbar region, left 63

Lumps 90, 147
  and bumps, multiple 147
Lung 175, 239
  cancer, small cell 201, 295
  involvement 32
  nodules 156
Lupus enteritis 164, 290
  underlies 290
Lupus vulgaris 68, 175
Luteinizing hormone 123
Lymph node 175, 239, 293, 297, 308
  axillary 297
  biopsy 302
  histopathology of 308
  metastatic 201
  para-aortic 292
Lymphadenitis 219
  granulomatous 301
Lymphadenopathy 115, 146, 149, 307
  abdominal 83
  intra-abdominal 31f
  para-aortic 291
  unmasking of cause of 163
Lymph nodes 40
Lymphoblastic lymphoma 308
Lymphocyte 186, 285, 340
  count 160
  intraepithelial 161
Lymphocytic infiltration, predominantly 337
Lymphohistiocytosis, hemophagocytic 354, 355
Lymphoid cells, dense infiltration of 84f
Lymphoid follicles 83
Lymphoid hyperplasia 292
Lymphoid tissue 85
Lymphoma 91, 115, 120, 158, 175, 176, 308, 309, 354
  diagnosis of 351
  low-grade 173
Lymphomatous infiltration 309, 310
Lymphopenia 147
Lymphoplasmacytic infiltrate 204
Lymphoproliferative disorder 83, 84f
Lysosomal storage disease 124

M

Macrophages 175
Maculopapular rash, desquamated 114f
Magnesium 22
  supplements 24
Magnetic resonance cholangiopancreatography 271, 312
Malabsorption 71, 161
  syndrome 84, 102, 222
    strongyloidiasis leading to 102
Malaise 34, 115, 262
Malakoplakia 172, 173, 175, 176
Malar rash 352f
Malaria 109, 137
  chronic 358
  diagnostic test for 138
  multidrug resistance 140
  severe 139
Mantoux test 83, 134, 147, 155, 157, 225
Mass lesion 173
Massive hepatomegaly 108
Massive lymphadenopathy 172
Mean corpuscular hemoglobin 338
  concentration 338
Mean corpuscular volume 215
Measles infection 167
Mebendazole 209
Mediastinal granuloma 156
Mediastinal lymphadenitis 155
Mediastinal lymphadenopathy 173, 174f, 204
Medulloblastoma 120
Melena 5, 73, 236, 267, 311, 338
  episodes of 240
Melioidosis 88
  disseminated septicemic 88
Melkersson-Rosenthal syndrome 42
Melphalan 151
Menstrual regulation, history of 228
Mental development 196
Meropenem 89
  injection 88
Mesenchymal tumor 265
Mesenteric abnormalities 290
Mesenteric vein thrombosis 282
Metabolic bone disease 230
Metabolic diseases 355
Metacarpophalangeal joints 37
Metastasis 339
  hepatic 56
Methotrexate 21, 146, 148, 184, 207, 254
Methylprednisolone 156

Michaelis-Gutmann bodies 173, 175, 175f
Microcytic hypochromic
  anemia 44, 141
  blood 328
Micturition, frequency of 48
Mid-abdominal pain 100
Mitomycin C, doses of 338
Mitral regurgitation, mild 249
Mixing study 7t
Monoclonal gammopathy 234, 321, 324
Monoclonal paraprotein 150
Monocytes 175
Mononuclear cell 87
Mononucleosis, infectious 286
Montoux test 172
Morning stiffness 241
Morning vomiting 25
Motor function 138, 196
Moyamoya disease 95
  appearance of 94
  causes of 95
  familial 95
  typical angiographic appearance of 94f
Mucopolysaccharidosis 230
  diagnosis of 230
Mucosa, scalloping of 84f
Mucosal edema 289
Multifocal encephalitis 237
Multi-organ involvement 207
Muscle
  biopsy 252
  bulk 2
  hematoma 267
  weakness 152
Musculoskeletal
  disease 231
  examination 251
  manifestations 3, 71
  sequelae 146
  system 6, 306, 348
Myalgia 260
Myasthenia gravis 201, 295
Mycobacteria 142
Mycobacterium
  avium 176
  bovis 358
  leprae 135
  tuberculosis 31, 69, 176, 190, 219, 336, 358
Mycophenolate mofetil 21
Myelodysplastic syndrome 175
Myeloid cells 118
Myeloma 118
  multiple 150, 242, 322
Myelopathy 107, 201
Myeloproliferative
  disease 118
  neoplasms 118
Myocarditis 115
Myoclonic jerk 56
  movement 167
Myxedema 170

N

Naproxen 348
Nasal intonation 199
Nasal regurgitation 294
Nausea 62, 159, 211, 248, 278, 280
Neck
  side of 263
  swelling 217
  veins, engorged 248
Necrotic neoplasms 46
Needle aspiration cytology 62
Neisseria gonorrhoeae 228
Neoplastic bone lesion 62, 63f
Nephritis, interstitial 115
Nephrotic-range proteinuria 18
Nephrotoxicity 36
Nerve stimulation test, repetitive 296
Nervous system 123
  examination 58, 96, 100, 152, 311
Neural leprosy, pure 135
Neuroblastoma 56, 120
  adrenal 56
  pseudorosettes pattern of 57f
Neuroectodermal origin 120
Neuroleptics 4
Neurologic examination 212
Neurologic manifestation 103
Neurological symptoms 117
Neuromyotonia 201
Neuropsychiatric
  abnormality 104
  disorders 107
Neurosyphilis 106, 107

Neutropenia 299
Neutrophil 46, 186
Neutrophilic leukocytosis 6, 82, 91, 245, 325
Nevirapine 131
Niclosamide 211
Night sweat 25, 66, 343
Nitrofurantoin 86
NK-cell leukemia 354
   aggressive 355
Nodular hepatic tuberculosis 286
Nodular swellings, multiple 90
Nonalcoholic farmer 144
Nonalcoholic fatty liver disease 194
Nonalcoholic steatohepatitis 195
Non-Hodgkin lymphoma 92, 292, 354
Non-sanguineous fluid 44
Nonsmoker and betel-leaf chewer 171
Nonsteroidal anti-inflammatory drug 5, 24, 96, 113, 182, 185, 236, 266, 267, 284, 288, 306, 343, 348
Nontender hepatomegaly 51
Nontender hepatosplenomegaly 229
Nontuberculous mycobacterium infection 317
Normal pressure hydrocephalus 127
Normocalciuria 23
Normocytic anemia 6, 96, 119, 134
Normocytic normochromic anemia 101, 157, 163, 241, 311
Nuclear ribonucleoprotein, small 35

O

Occult blood test 160
Octreotide 162
Odynophagia 171
Offensive dark-colored stool 193
Oligomenorrhea 78
Oliguria 224, 248
Open lung biopsy 246
Ophthalmologic disease 231
Opsoclonus-myoclonus 201
Oral
   doxycycline, course of 44
   glucose tolerance test 30
   moniliasis 68
   prednisolone 144
   quinine sulfate 137
   steroids 116
   tolerance tests 223
   ulcer 70, 221
   ulceration, history of 133
Organomegaly 234
Organs, intra-abdominal 328
Orofacial granulomatosis 42
Orogenital ulcerations 141
Orthopnea 177
Osteoarthritis 13, 236
Osteoarticular manifestations 198
Osteolytic lesions, multiple 150
Osteomalacia 242, 243
Osteomyelitis 89
Osteopenia 3f, 196
   severe 198
Osteoporosis 97, 97f, 242, 326
Osteosclerotic myeloma 234
Otitis media, chronic 180
Outpatient department 147, 233
Overlap syndrome 184, 349

P

Pacemaker implantation, permanent 249
Pain, abdominal 25, 44, 51, 62, 117, 189, 190, 193, 203, 211, 221, 227, 263, 284, 288, 311, 313, 325, 326, 348
Pale stool 9
   history of 311
Palmar erythema 74f, 117, 248
Palpitation 25, 93, 224, 297, 331
Pancreas 175
Pancreatic ascites 170
Pancreatic calculi, removal of 325
Pancreatitis
   autoimmune 204
   chronic calcific 325
   IgG4-related autoimmune 204
Pancytopenia 281, 355
Papilledema 160
   bilateral 217
   causes of 161
Paracetamol 186
Paralysis 56
Paraneoplastic cranial neuropathy 201
Paraneoplastic syndrome 16, 201, 202
Paraplegia 314, 317, 318
Paraspinal sympathetic ganglia 56

Parathyroid
  adenoma 326, 327
  hormone 59, 61, 196, 229, 230, 344
Paratracheal lymphadenopathy 92
Paraventricular white matter 59f
Parenchyma, hepatic 281, 284
Parenchymal lung disease, diffuse 253, 275, 276f
Parent's screening 52
Paresthesia 29, 224
Parietal lobe, left posterior 105
Parkinson's plus syndrome 60
Parkinsonism 4
Parotid gland, bilateral 68
Parvovirus B19 53
Patent foramen ovale 95
Pelvic
  collection, moderate 227
  infection symptoms 228
  inflammatory disease 228
Penicillamine 146
Penicillin 7
Peptic ulcer
  causes of recurrent 345
  disease 27, 326
Periadenitis 219
Pericarditis 156
  suggestive of 228
Perinuclear antineutrophil cytoplasmic antibodies 120, 207, 212
Periodic acid-Schiff 156
Peripheral blood 328
  film 13, 53f, 82, 87, 96, 119, 123, 160, 183, 217, 222, 227, 237, 260, 267
Peripheral hypereosinophilia 116
Peripheral nerve
  damage 21
  thickened 133
Peripheral nervous system 129
Peripheral neuropathy 201
Peripheral primitive neuroectodermal tumors 120
Periportal fibrosis 75
Pes cavus 229
Pharyngeal muscle 254
Phenytoin 7
Phocomelia 334
Phonophobia 189, 304
Photophobia 189, 304
Photosensitivity 34

Pigmentation, abnormal 193
Pitting leg edema, bilateral 12
Pituitary autoimmunity 80
Plasma cell dyscrasia 234
Plasmodium falciparum 139
Platelet 51, 169
  aggregation
    test 268
    lack of 269
  alloimmunization 269
  functional disorder 268
  persistently low 87
Pleomorphic purpura 217
Plethora 118
Pleural effusion, right-sided 114
Pleuritic chest pain, recurrent 277
Pneumococcal vaccine 180
Pneumonia 89
Pneumonitis 115
POEMS syndrome 32, 234
  diagnostic for 235t
Polyangiitis 20, 207
  microscopic 20
Polyarthralgia 66
Polyarthritis 37, 306
  progressive 1
Polyclonal hypergammaglobulinemia 324
Polycystic kidney and liver 307
Polycythemia 118
  rubra vera 118
Polymerase chain reaction 131, 187
Polymorphonuclear neutrophils 45
Polymyositis 185
Polyneuropathy 234
Portal hypertension 313
Portal vein 291
  thrombosis 281, 282
Postcholecystectomy state 91
Post-head injury 40-42
Postictal confusion 122
Postradiotherapy 175
Postural drainage 181
Postural variation 348
Potassium 22
Pott's disease 314, 317, 319
  relapsed 318
Praziquantel 211
Prednisolone 85, 151
Prednisone 293, 310

Pregnancy 305
   loss 153
Primary care hospital 278
Primigravida 37
Primitive neuroectodermal tumor 120
Probably adrenal metastasis 339
Progressive nodular swellings, history of 44
Prominent spleen 237
Prostate 89
   benign enlargement of 358
   enlargement of 149
   specific antigen 201
Protein
   C deficiency 282
      symptomatic 282
   S deficiency 282, 305
      symptomatic 282
   S, reduced 305
Proteus 176
Prothrombin time 6
Proton pump inhibitor 193
Proximal interphalangeal joints 251, 5, 306
Pruritus 118, 313
   young lady with 311
Pseudomonas aeruginosa 176
Pseudoxanthoma 264
   elasticum 265
Psychiatric manifestations 167
Psychiatric symptoms 4
Psychosis, young lady with 182
Pubic hair 124
Puerperium 305
Pulmonary disease 231
   severe 156
Pulmonary disorders 246
Pulmonary edema 279f
Pulmonary fibrosis 71
Pulmonary function tests 277
Pulmonary hypertension 71, 72, 185, 332, 334f
   risk for 185
Pulmonary manifestation 102
Pulmonary regurgitation, moderate 249
Pulmonary tuberculosis 127, 246, 247, 285
Pulmonary venous congestion 45
Pulmonary-renal syndrome, middle-aged lady with 18

Punctum 147
Pupillary light reflexes 104
Purpura 297
Purpuric rash 133
Pus cells 357
Pyelonephritis with hypertension, recurrent 150
Pyogenic peritonitis 170
Pyrexia 355
Pyuria, persistent 357

Q

Quadriparesis 22
Quadriplegia 15
Quinolones 176

R

Ramsay-Hunt syndrome 213
Rapid diagnostic tests 140
Rash 113, 251, 343, 351
   on back 253f
Raynaud's phenomenon 5, 18, 66, 71, 122, 153, 184, 224, 274
Real-time reverse transcriptase 188
Recurrent crying bouts 1
Red blood cell 18, 45, 53, 58, 96, 163, 183, 187
Red granulation tissue 172
Reddish skin nodules, painful 133
Redness 306
Renal and bone marrow 116
Renal dysfunction 308
Renal function 155
   test 243, 304, 325, 332
Renal impairment 326
Renal inflammation 21
Renal insufficiency 150
Renal involvement 307
Renal lymphoma 309
Renal stone 326
Renal tuberculosis 358
Renomegaly 306
Residual tumor 338
Resistance 310
Respiratory distress 73, 140, 152, 338, 348
Respiratory rate 18, 236, 331
Respiratory system examination 18, 55, 251

Respiratory tract infection, repeated 230
Retina, Bruch's membrane of 265
Retinal hemorrhage 266
Retroperitoneal fibrosis 204
Retroperitoneum 175
Reynauds's phenomenon, signs of 71
Rhabdomyolysis 279, 280
Rheumatic disease 184
    inflammatory 184
Rheumatic heart disease 38
Rheumatoid arthritis 175, 182
Rheumatoid factor test 13, 252
Rhodococcus equi 176
Rib
    fractures, multiple 3*f*
    right-sided 64
Ribonucleic acid 167
Rickets 3, 230
    with hydrocele 230
Rifampicin 11, 135, 352
Right knee 37
    arthralgia 86
    arthritis 23
Rinne and Weber test 212
Rituximab 21, 36, 146, 293
Roglobulin antibody 79
Rosacea 42
Round cell tumors 120
Rudimentary distal phalanges 333*f*

S

Sacroiliac joint infiltration 98*f*
Sarcoidosis 120, 135
Scanty lymphocyte 148
Scanty micturition 343
Scarring 263
Sclerosing cholangitis 204
    primary 313
Sclerosing panencephalitis, subacute 167
Sclerosing sialadenitis 204
Sclerosis
    aortic 249
    multiple 16, 49, 60
Sclerotic bone lesions 235
Scoliosis 333*f*
Scrotal edema 291
Scrotum, USG of 68*f*
Sebelipase alfa 125
Secondary healthcare center 189

Seizure 107
Sensory
    disturbance 93
    modalities 41, 58
Sepsis 145, 299
    overwhelming 75
Septic arthritis 89, 145
Septicemia
    with 89
    without 89
Serositis 226
Serum 202
    albumin 30, 141, 160, 196, 212, 229, 325
    level 291
    alpha-fetoprotein 109
    amylase 203
    antinuclear antibodies 10, 261
    bilirubin 190, 237, 321
    calcium 147, 212, 242, 323
    ceruloplasmin 10, 312
    copper 105
    level 166
    cortisol 82
    creatinine 18, 63, 134, 147, 157, 163, 190, 206, 241, 246, 270, 298
    electrolyte 30, 147, 163, 190, 212, 246*t*
    ferritin, repeat 354
    fibrinogen 354
    globulin 30
    immunoglobulin electrophoresis 323, 323*f*
    lactate dehydrogenase 298
    lipase 203
    pro-calcitonin 354
    protein electrophoresis 97, 322, 322*f*
    sodium 78
    uric acid 267
    vitamin B12 234
Sexual exposure, unprotected 130, 281
Sharp's syndrome 184
Shawl sign 252
Sheehan's syndrome 80
Shifting dullness 227
Shigella 176
Shock 140
Short stature 122, 230
Shoulder
    dislocation, bilateral 3*f*
    joint, right 1

Sickle cell 53
   anemia 53
   disease 53, 118
Sickle syndromes 53
Sickling test 52
Sinus 219
Situs inversus 180*f*
Skeletal deformity 229, 230
Skin 278
   biopsy 153, 252
   changes 66, 234
   changes syndrome 234
   involvement 116
   lesion 21, 107, 154
      hyperpigmented 66, 67
   manifestations 71
   overlying 5
   pustule, biopsy of 46
   rash 70, 115, 152, 224, 338
   thickened 177
   with hypertension, malakoplakia of 175
Sleep pattern, abnormal 224
Slit lamp examination 166
Slurring of speech, middle-aged male with progressive 58
Small intestinal disease, immunoproliferative 83, 84
Smoke, puff of 95
Soft stool, frequent passage of 209
Soft tissue 294, 309
   density mass 155
   mass, removal of 171
Solar keratosis 29
Somatropin 125
Sore throat 141, 146, 297
Speech disturbance 15
Spinal cord 16
Spinal metastasis 92
Spinal tuberculosis 319
   types of 319
Spine
   generalized osteopenia of 197*f*
   magnetic resonance imaging of 97*f*, 318*f*
Spinocerebellar ataxia 128, 129
Spleen 89
Splenectomy scar 74
Splenic aspirate study 323
Splenic lesion 158

Splenomegaly 86
Spontaneous abortion 348
Spontaneous gum bleeding 117, 267
Staphylococcus aureus 176, 183
Status post-splenectomy 75
Steroid therapy 204, 205
Stiff's person syndrome 201
Still's disease, relapsed 146
Stomach
   adenocarcinoma of 98
   cancer of 99
   infiltrating adenocarcinoma of 239
   prepyloric mucosa of 345*f*
Stool
   examination 210, 223
   incontinence 93
   occult blood test 225
Storage disease 110
Straight leg raise test 90
Streptomycin 190
Stroke 93
   recurrent 106
Strongyloides stercoralis 27, 102
   infection 27
Strongyloidiasis, treatment for 103
Subcutaneous adipose tissue 134
Subcutaneous nodules, multiple 119
Subcutaneous sarcoidosis 148
Subfertility 179
Submammary folds 119
Submandibular lymph node 163
Submandibular lymphadenopathy 171
Submandibular region 90, 172
Sulfonamide 7
Supraclavicular node, right 219
Supraclavicular regions, right 172
Suprahepatic vein 282
Suprarenal gland, right 56
Supraventricular tachycardia 332*f*
Swallowing difficulty 58
Sweats 262
Swelling 177, 193, 241, 306
   generalized 159
   nodular subcutaneous 147
Symmetrical sensory motor polyneuropathy 29
Syndrome of inappropriate antidiuretic hormone secretion 246, 247
Synovitis, chronic 87

Systemic amyloidosis
  primary 14
  treatment for 14
Systemic corticosteroids 175
Systemic lupus erythematosus 6, 20, 68, 110, 164, 184, 218, 225, 254, 275, 290, 300, 307, 349
  diagnosis of 111*t*, 275
  manifestation of 275
Systemic lupus international collaborating clinics 164
Systemic sclerosis 71, 153, 185, 349
Systolic dysfunction 225
Systolic functions 242

T

Tacrolimus 254
Taenia 210
  saginata 210, 211
  asiatica 210
  rhynchus 210
  solium 210
Taeniasis 211
Takatsuki disease 234
Target cells 51
Target sign 289, 290
T-cell lymphoblastic
  leukemia 308
  lymphoma 309
Testicular atrophy 248
Testosterone 344
Tetralogy of Fallot 335
Thalidomide 148, 151
Thighs, part of 263
Thoracic surgery, past history of 62
Thrombocytopenia 149, 150, 163, 183, 194, 215, 299
  autoimmune 300
  immune 299
Thrombocytosis 101, 118
Thrombophilia 282
Thrombotic thrombocytopenic purpura 218
Thyroid 40, 109
  function test 13, 82, 160
  gland 108, 175
  stimulating hormone 123, 134, 203
Thyroiditis, autoimmune 181

Thyroxine 108
  total 123
Tinnitus 25, 212
Tissue biopsy 121
  histopathology of 84*f*
Tongue
  amyloidosis 14
  dorsal surface of 13*f*
  fissure in 41*f*
  middle-aged gentleman with enlargement of 12
  nodules over posterior part of 172*f*
  posterior part of 172
  smooth 100
  with hypertension, malakoplakia of 175
Transient ischemic attacks 95
Transjugular intrahepatic portosystemic shunt 250
Trauma, history of 93, 203
Traumatic brain injury 40
Treponema pallidum 106, 107
  antibody 107
  hemagglutination assay 228
Tricuspid valve 250
Triiodothyronine 123
Trimethoprim-sulfamethoxazole 176
Tropical sprue 102
Trunk, skin of 34
Tubercle bacilli 286
Tubercular basal meningitis 337
Tubercular epididymo-orchitis 68
Tubercular lymphadenitis, stages of 219
Tubercular peritonitis 170
Tubercular spondylitis 315
Tuberculosis 130, 143, 157, 192, 218, 247, 263, 315, 337, 338, 341, 347
  abdominal 192
  arthralgia 68
  extrapulmonary 247
  intestinal 102, 192, 221
  isolated hepatic 285
  lymphadenitis 68
  treatment-completed 20
Tuberculous granulomata 286
Tuberculous lymphadenitis 219
Tumor
  cells 293
  markers 109
  of bone, secondary 242

U

Ulceration 147
Ulcerative colitis 204, 313
Ulcers, multiple 171
Unconsciousness 199, 338
    sudden 78
Upper abdomen 51, 270
Upper abdominal
    discomfort 108
    pain 55, 157
Upper eyelid 251, 294
    swelling 252, 253f
Upper gastrointestinal tract 98, 169, 190, 222, 238
    endoscopy of 45, 74, 82, 109, 114, 194, 225, 238f, 289f, 302
Upper limb 294
Upper respiratory infection 18
Urinalysis 227
Urinary copper 166
Urinary GeneXpert, positive 359
Urinary incontinence 93, 122, 127
Urinary total protein 275
Urinary tract infection 86, 92, 218
Urine
    metanephrine in 56
    protein test 18
    red-colored 297
    retention of 96
    routine examination 13, 157, 275, 322
        microscopic 6
    stream 206
Urosepsis 219
Ursodeoxycholic acid 11, 313
Uterus 124

V

Vaccination 15
Valvular disorders 94
Variceal bleeding 236
Variceal ligation, endoscopic 281
Varicella zoster virus 213
Vascular endothelial growth factor 235
Vascular involvement 32
Vasculitis 218
    systemic lupus erythematosus with 350
Venereal disease research laboratory test 93
Ventricular septal defect 332, 334f

Vertebral compressions, multiple 197f
Vertebral fracture 314
Vertigo 25, 212
    episodes of 117
    history of 93
Vietnamese tuberculosis 88
Vincristine 85, 121, 293, 310
Viral encephalitis 238
Viral illness 355
Viral markers 312
Visceral leishmaniasis 75, 76, 131, 216, 323, 322, 324
    diagnosis of 131
Vision
    blurring of 93, 159, 233, 304, 336
    dimness of 199
    double 199, 336
Visual acuity, impairment of 199
Visual disturbance 5, 15, 171, 263, 343, 351
Visual impairment 58
Visual problems 66
Vital signs 119, 212
Vitamin
    A 81
    B12 101, 105, 127
    C 44
    D 59, 81, 229, 230, 244
        deficiency 243
        resistance 243
Vitiligo 12
Vitronectin 268
Voice, hoarseness of 58
Vomiting 25, 62, 73, 159, 189, 278, 280, 304, 348
    and weight loss, middle-aged man with 25
von Willebrand disease 6
von Willebrand factor 268

W

Waldenström macroglobulinemia 117
Waldmann's disease 161
Warfarin 267, 283
Weakness 278
Wegener's granulomatosis 20
Weight gain and breathlessness 177
Weight loss 34, 154, 157, 169, 199, 206, 211, 233, 262, 338
Whipple's disease 176

White blood
  cell 44, 58, 82, 87, 160, 163, 169, 186, 189, 267, 270, 298
  count 119
Whitish segments, per anal discharge of 210*f*
Whitmore's disease 88
Whole blood transfusions, multiple units of 221
Willebrand factor 6
Wilson's disease 3, 124, 191, 230, 312
  diagnosis of 4
  hepatic 4
Woven bone, curvilinear trabeculae of 64*f*
Wrist joint 306
  X-ray of 2

X

Xanthoma 176

Z

Zidovudine 131
Ziehl-Neelsen stain 134
Zollinger-Ellison syndrome 345

EU GSPR Authorised Reprsentative
Logos Europe, 9 rue Nicolas Poussin
1700, La Rochelle, France
Phone: +33 (0) 6 67 93 73 78
E-mail: contact@logoseurope.eu

www.ingramcontent.com/pod-product-compliance
Ingram Content Group UK Ltd.
Pitfield, Milton Keynes, MK11 3LW, UK
UKHW050427150426
5217IPUK00019B/1282